A NURSE'S
SURVIVAL GUIDE TO

LEADERSHIP AND MANAGEMENT ON THE WARD

Titles in this series:

A Nurse's Survival Guide to the Ward 2E
A Nurse's Survival Guide to Leadership and Management
   on the Ward
A Nurse's Survival Guide to Drugs in Practice
A Nurse's Survival Guide to Critical Care

Survival Guide to Midwifery

For Elsevier:

Commissioning Editor: Susan Young
Development Editor: Catherine Jackson
Project Manager: Gail Wright
Senior Designer: Sarah Russell

A NURSE'S SURVIVAL GUIDE

LEADERSHIP AND MANAGEMENT ON THE WARD

Jenny Thomas RN BSc(Hons) CMS PGCHE

Consultant in Health Care Management

Senior Lecturer, London South Bank University, London, UK

CHURCHILL
LIVINGSTONE

ELSEVIER

EDINBURGH   LONDON   NEW YORK   OXFORD   PHILADELPHIA   ST LOUIS   SYDNEY   TORONTO   2006

CHURCHILL
LIVINGSTONE
ELSEVIER

First Published as *'Survival Guide for Ward Managers, Sisters and Charge Nurses'* 2006
Reprinted as *'A Nurse's Survival Guide to Leadership and Management on the Ward.'* 2009

ISBN: 978-1-4377-1747-1
Formerly: 978-0-4431-0324-7

British Library Cataloguing in Publication Data
A catalogue record for this book is available from the British Library

Library of Congress Cataloging in Publication Data
A catalog record for this book is available from the Library of Congress

Note
Knowledge and best practice in this field are constantly changing. As new research and experience broaden our knowledge, changes in practice, treatment and drug therapy may become necessary or appropriate. Readers are advised to check the most current information provided (i) on procedures featured or (ii) by the manufacturer of each product to be administered, to verify the recommended dose or formula, the method and duration of administration, and contraindications. It is the responsibility of the practitioner, relying on their own experience and knowledge of the patient, to make diagnoses, to determine dosages and the best treatment for each individual patient, and to take all appropriate safety precautions. To the fullest extent of the law, neither the Publisher nor the Author assumes any liability for any injury and/or damage to persons or property arising out of or related to any use of the material contained in this book.

The Publisher

Working together to grow
libraries in developing countries

www.elsevier.com | www.bookaid.org | www.sabre.org

ELSEVIER   BOOK AID International   Sabre Foundation

ELSEVIER   your source for books, journals and multimedia in the health sciences

www.elsevierhealth.com

The publisher's policy is to use **paper manufactured from sustainable forests**

Printed in China

Contents

Preface   xi
Acknowledgements   xiii
Abbreviations   xv

Chapter 1
Be clear about your role and responsibilities   1
Be clear about what 24-hour responsibility means   2
Be clear about what makes a good leader   4
Make sure your decisions are informed ones   6
Clarify your objectives   8
Understand your legal responsibilities   9
Be clear about your line manager's role   11
Remember you are the patients' overall advocate   13
Don't take on other people's pressures   14
Balance your clinical work with administrative duties   16
Be aware of the impact of your role on others   17

Chapter 2
Define and prioritise your workload   25
Define your workload   26
Organise your office   28
Control your diary   30
Keep up with your emails   32
Cut interruptions   33
Don't waste time with unnecessary reading   34
Reduce your meetings and get the best out of those you do choose to attend 36
Chair meetings effectively   38
Learn to let go through delegation   39
Be proactive   41

Chapter 3
Create a positive working environment   45
Have a plan   46
Set meaningful objectives with your team   48
Be a good listener   49
Feedback with sincerity   51
Know your staff well   52
Never talk disapprovingly of others   54

Get your staff to take more responsibility   55
Have a system for dealing with patients' visitors   56
Deal with conflict   58
Implement clinical supervision   59

Chapter 4
Manage and treat your staff well   63

Get to know your HR advisor   64
Write everything down   66
Make appraisals work   67
Know how to handle unacceptable behaviour   69
Deal with poor performance   71
Know when and how to discipline   72
Actively manage sick leave   73
Ensure all staff have appropriate training, development and support   76
Inform and involve your team   78
Implement self-rostering   80

Chapter 5
Make sure care is patient-centred   83

Maintain your clinical skills   84
Ensure that all patients have a full assessment and care plan   86
Be clear about what health care assistants can and cannot do   88
Eliminate long handovers   89
Use task-orientated care only when appropriate   91
Work towards primary nursing   92
Make sure patients are informed   93
Improve care through audit and benchmarking   96
Don't accept poor standards of care when short-staffed   98
Take the lead on ward rounds   99

Chapter 6
Get your budget right   105

Know what your budget is   106
Prioritise PAY   107
Go through your budget statement each month   110
Manage annual leave   112
Manage your allowance for unplanned absence   113
Plan your study leave allowance   115
Get your staff involved in NON PAY   116
Be more active in the business planning process   118
Don't do anything without identified funding   119
Meet regularly with your finance advisor   121

Chapter 7
Respond well to complaints 125
Work on the content, not number of complaints 126
Take appropriate steps before you investigate 128
Investigate sensitively 129
Know when to stop the complaint investigation 132
Consider holding a meeting with the complainant 134
Follow six key steps during the meeting 135
Write a good final response letter 137
Follow up the complaint with action 142

Chapter 8
Instigate a rolling recruitment programme 147
Review the post with the person who is leaving 148
Write good adverts and application packages 150
Shortlist and arrange interviews properly 151
Get the best out of the interview process 153
Follow up all candidates personally 155
Arrange a good induction programme 157
Continually explore all other avenues to get staff 158
Don't discriminate 160
Succession plan 162
Fully involve your team in all aspects of recruitment 163

Chapter 9
Be politically aware 167
Understand how health care is managed nationally 168
Know your board of directors and their priorities 171
Choose your meetings carefully 173
Network – get to know the right people 174
Be diplomatic 176
Work with your director of nursing 178
Get recognition for your work 180
Choose your mentor and mentees with care 181
Plan ahead for your own needs 182

Chapter 10
Look after yourself 187
Recognise symptoms of stress 188
Recognise and deal with any staff stress 190
Get yourself a mentor 192
Set up a peer support group or action learning set 194

Train up your deputy ward manager   196
Get a union representative or steward on your team   198
Choose carefully whom you talk to and what you say   199
Get over mistakes and move on   201
Drink plenty of water and eat regularly   202
Remember it's only a job   204

Chapter 11
Be a good role model   209
Be smart   210
Make a good first impression   211
Always smile and be positive   213
Speak clearly   214
Be relaxed and in control   216
Make your writing distinguishable   218
Be aware of how others see you   220
Set an example with your choice of language   222
Never moan or gossip about others   223
Don't stagnate   224

Chapter 12
Manage your manager   227
Clarify expectations   228
Work with, not against, your manager   230
Act, if an important decision has been made without your consultation   231
Act, if a change in another department has a knock-on effect in yours   233
Don't be pressurised into taking on extra work without funding   235
If you are doing extra work without funding, take action   237
Keep the communication channels open   238
Write good and timely reports   239
Actively manage incidents, mistakes and accidents   241
Know how to conduct a good investigation   243

Chapter 13
Manage difficult people and difficult situations   247
Manage a difficult manager   248
Deal with that problematic colleague   250
Manage any allegations of bullying or harassment   251
Manage staff complaints   253
Make sure staff are not being used or abused by others   254
Don't tolerate any form of racism or other discrimination   256
Take action when staffing levels are dangerously low   258
Break up any cliques   259

Be specific about expanding nursing roles 261
Be proactive with enforced moves or mergers of services 264

Chapter 14
Manage difficult staff
267
Staff who refuse to look professional or wear proper uniform 268
Staff who refuse to accept change 270
Staff who can't seem to prioritise their work 271
Staff who are lazy 273
Staff who have alcohol problems 274
Members of staff who don't get on 276
Staff who are careless and sloppy 277
Staff who manipulate situations for their own gain 278
Staff who moan and whinge 280
Staff who are continually late for duty 282

Chapter 15
Get the best advice
287
Know where to go for legal advice 288
Know where to go for professional advice 289
Utilise the wide range of services from the chaplaincy department 290
Use but don't abuse the nurse specialists 291
Help patients and relatives access the right advice 293
Keep up-to-date with risk management issues 295
Consult policies, procedures and guidelines 296
Maximise computer access 297
Utilise the knowledge and skills of your nursing colleagues 299
Utilise the practice development team 300

Chapter 16
Question external directives
305
Is another link nurse role really needed? 306
Has the bed manager considered all other options? 308
Was that audit really necessary? 309
Has your line manager questioned the decision? 310
Are performance targets worth lowering the quality of care for? 311
Are senior managers aware of the implications of their decision? 312
Are consultant/specialist decisions always right? 313
Ask your union steward for assistance 315
Don't hesitate in contacting the chief executive 316
Rely on your own common sense 317

Index 319

Preface

The role of ward manager is so important yet so overlooked in today's health care system. Where has the ward manager's 'voice' gone? Unfortunately, the role has become so huge that some are struggling to keep up with the day-to-day demands of running shifts and completing all the paperwork, that they do not have the time or energy left to lead nursing. There are few specific training programmes, which means that learning often takes place through trial and error. This is not the most effective way to build up the skills and confidence required to lead. In addition, it is a rather isolated role at a time when support is probably most needed in your career.

I spent many years as a ward manager, yet it was not until I reached senior manager/deputy director level that I finally found out the things I should have known back then. Nobody told me how to run a budget; I just started receiving budget statements each month. Nobody told me how to write a complaint response letter; I just guessed. In fact, I still didn't know until I spent a year afterwards working in a complaints department!

I attended numerous management courses and learned about various management theories and models, but few gave specific information on how to do things. I still picked up most of my job through experience. Nobody showed me how to compile an 'off-duty' in order to remain within budget, and I have yet to meet a ward manager who has been shown.

I now provide teaching programmes, facilitate workshops and support groups for ward managers and matrons, and have been asked many times which book I got my information from. But there was no book. Not until now! Most of the content in this book is taken from more than 20 years of personal experience and observations. I gained a lot of this information from all the jobs I have had in health care since being a ward manager.

This is basically a 'how-to' book. When you need to look up how to do something, the last thing you need to do is wade through lots of theory and background reading.

You will find this book helpful whether you are planning to be a ward manager, have recently taken on the role or even if you have many years of experience in the role. Matrons will also find it a useful guide for teaching and developing their teams. Although the book is aimed specifically at ward managers, it can be applied to clinical managers of any setting including A&E, ICU and outpatients.

The first eight chapters concentrate on the basic skills required for the ward manager's role. The next few chapters (9–12) give information on how to be more effective in your role. And finally, Chapters 13–16 discuss common problems for ward managers, suggested solutions and where to go for the most appropriate advice.

This book can be easily read through from cover to cover. It contains useful action points at the end of each chapter, which you may wish to use to inform your personal development plan. It can also be used as a handy reference book in times of need. You can look up quickly how to write up a serious incident investigation, for example, or how to calculate your ward's study leave allowance.

Although the content of the book is mainly based in the context of the NHS, it is also relevant for those working in private health care. Most private health care companies base their policies and procedures on at least those required within the NHS sector.

I hope you enjoy reading this book and that it provides you with the support and practical information you need to do the job effectively, and to keep yourself sane in what must be one of the most difficult and demanding jobs within health care management.

I have purposefully not included separate sections on leadership and management, clinical governance or quality. I didn't feel you would be inclined to read whole chapters on these subjects. In fact, these themes are included but run generally throughout the book. I may have missed something out which you feel is vital to the role. Any feedback would be gratefully received. You can email me at jenny.thomas1@ntlworld.com. I will be happy to read your comments and consider suggestions for future editions.

London 2006

Jenny Thomas

Acknowledgements

A big thank you to my colleague Louise Terry (senior lecturer in law and ethics) for her valuable contributions to Chapter 1. Thanks also to Paul Deemer (NHS Employers) who contributed the benefit of his wide experience in human resources and helped to shape Chapters 4, 8, 13 and 14.

Abbreviations

AOB	any other business
BNF	British National Formulary
CNO	Chief Nursing Officer
CNST	Clinical Negligence Scheme for Trusts
CPR	cardiopulmonary resuscitation
CRB	Criminal Records Bureau
DHSSPS	Department of Health, Social Services and Public Safety
ECDL	European Computer Driving Licence
ECG	electrocardiogram
FAQs	frequently asked questions
HCA	health care assistant
HDU	high dependency unit
HIW	Healthcare Inspectorate Wales
HR	human resources
HSS	health and social services
ITU	intensive treatment unit
JCNC	Joint Consultative and Negotiating Committee
JSSC	Joint Staff Side Committee
KSF	knowledge and skills framework
LHB	local health board
MRSA	methicillin-resistant *Staphylococcus aureus*
NIO	Northern Ireland Office
NMC	Nursing and Midwifery Council
NSF	national service framework
OH	occupational health
PALS	patient advice and liaison service
PCT	primary care trust
PRHO	pre-registration house officer
RCA	root cause analysis
RCN	Royal College of Nursing
SAFF	service and financial framework
SHA	strategic health authority
SLA	service level agreement
WTE	whole time equivalent

CHAPTER 1

BE CLEAR ABOUT YOUR ROLE AND RESPONSIBILITIES

Be clear about what 24-hour responsibility means 2

Being called at home is unacceptable 2

Your role is to minimise risk 3

Professional accountability as a nurse manager 3

Being held legally accountable for the actions of others 4

Be clear about what makes a good leader 4

Manager or leader? 4

Skills of a good ward leader 5

Make sure your decisions are informed ones 6

Advice from your line manager 6

Advice from your mentor 6

Advice from your clinical supervisor 6

Advice from your HR department 7

Advice from your finance department 7

Advice from other ward managers 7

Clarify your objectives 8

Review your objectives regularly 8

Other sources of knowledge 8

360-degree feedback 9

Understand your legal responsibilities 9

Tensions between roles of nurse and manager 9

Staffing shortages 10

Sending staff to other wards 10

Vicarious liability 11

Expanded roles 11

Duty to report concerns 11

Be clear about your line manager's role 11

Shadow your manager 12

'Act up' in your manager's absence 12

Build up a good working relationship 12

Remember you are the patients' overall advocate 13

Patients feel vulnerable 13

Patients need strong leadership at ward level 13

Don't take on other people's pressures 14

Be wary of nonclinical managers 15

Don't allow other people's emergencies to become yours 15

Balance your clinical work with administrative duties 16

Reduce your patient caseload 16

Be aware of the impact of your role on others 17

Doctors and other health care professionals 17

Student nurses 18

Patients and relatives 18

Hospital management 18

Beyond your control? 19

When you become a nurse manager your responsibilities change. Most of your education and experience to date will have been focused on clinical practice, but the manager's role requires a very different set of skills. You now manage a team of staff with a set budget and are responsible for maintaining an environment in which people can work well.

Being a good nurse does not necessarily mean that you are naturally a good nurse manager. The two roles are very distinct. As a nurse, you are responsible for providing patients with a high standard of care. As a nurse manager you are responsible for ensuring that patients get a high standard of care through others. It takes time and experience to learn the art of being a good manager. Clarifying exactly what is expected of you in your role is the first major step.

BE CLEAR ABOUT WHAT 24-HOUR RESPONSIBILITY MEANS

Ward managers carry 24-hour responsibility for the ward. This means you are required to ensure that systems and processes are in place for patients to receive a high standard of care from your team, day and night, irrespective of whether you are there or not. It also means that you could be liable for poor patient care when you are not there if it is evident that you did not do everything to ensure that those systems and processes were in place. This includes:

● the appropriate development and support of your staff
● appropriate policies, guidelines and standards
● adequate 'off-duty' rotas
● appropriate risk management activities.

The individual nurses in your team are registered professionals and therefore responsible and accountable for their own actions or inactions, under the terms of their registration. However, as the nurses' manager, you may be liable if you do not provide the right working conditions for your team to provide good care.

BEING CALLED AT HOME IS UNACCEPTABLE

The term '24-hour responsibility' does not mean that you should be accessible out-of-hours. It is a common misconception that the ward manager should be available at all times. There have been instances when on-call or site managers have called ward managers at home or on their mobiles to sort out issues. You do not receive any payment for this, so it's unwise to encourage it. Home distractions or tiredness could impair your response.

It is different if you have not done your job properly. For example, if some staff do not turn up for work on your ward one day and it is not clear on the 'off-duty' who should be working that shift, then that is your responsibility. You have not ensured adequate cover in your absence, and you need to be contacted to clarify matters. However, if members of your staff go off sick when you are not there, leaving shifts uncovered, it is the responsibility of the manager on site to deal with the problem.

It is also not appropriate for members of your own team to be calling you at home. Your role is to empower them to make their own decisions and not to have to call you out-of-hours for advice. When you are not there, it is the responsibility of your organisation and you to ensure that other senior managers are there to turn to for advice and support in emergencies. This is usually your line manager during office hours and some sort of on-call or site manager out-of-hours. If there is no such system properly in place, you could be liable for failing to address this omission.

YOUR ROLE IS TO MINIMISE RISK

The 24-hour responsibility aspect entails minimising the risk of anything untoward happening by ensuring:

- the appropriate health & safety procedures are in place
- the appropriate resources are available, including staff
- all members of your team have full access and have been made aware of all the appropriate policies and guidelines to inform them of the standards expected
- all members of your team have had appropriate induction and ongoing development to ensure they are competent in their role.

PROFESSIONAL ACCOUNTABILITY AS A NURSE MANAGER

The Nursing and Midwifery Council (NMC) does not offer any specific guidance on the accountability of nurse managers other than Clause 8.4 in the Code of Professional Conduct, which states that: 'When working as a manager, you have a duty towards patients and clients, colleagues, the wider community and the organisation in which you and your colleagues work. When facing professional dilemmas, your first consideration in all activities must be the interests and safety of patients and clients.' (NMC 2004).

In 2002, one of the reasons for removing a matron from the register was cited as placing 'unreasonable demands on staff'. A unit manager was also removed for 'failing to take appropriate action when a patient was assaulted by a member of staff' (NMC 2002). In other words, as a manager who is also an NMC registrant, you are failing to uphold the Code of Professional Conduct if you do not put the interests of the patients first in any managerial decisions that you make.

If you are working under extreme pressure or there are staffing shortages out of your control, you must report it to the appropriate senior manager and be able to demonstrate that you have made every effort to remedy the situation. This is made clear in Clause 8.3 of the Code of Professional Conduct: 'Where you cannot remedy circumstances in the environment of care that could jeopardise standards of practice, you must report them to a senior person with sufficient authority to manage them . . . This must be supported by a written record.' (NMC 2004).

BEING HELD LEGALLY ACCOUNTABLE FOR THE ACTIONS OF OTHERS

Your legal accountability is a grey area but there have been cases where a person has been liable personally for someone else's incompetence. This is illustrated clearly in the case of Trustees of London Clinic v Michael Alan Edgar (2001) where a surgeon was held liable for the inactions of nursing staff. After an operation for scoliosis a 12-year-old girl was left paralysed when nursing staff failed to inform the surgeon she could no longer move her toes. The nurse assigned to the patient was described as 'inexperienced'. The conduct of the nursing team was described as 'unforeseeably irrational' and 'negligent', with a charge nurse who at one point saw the wrong forms being used, so transcribed the records saying she could not move her toes but did not query it. The hospital settled out of court but then recovered £30,000 from the surgeon because his handover was held to have been 'so routine as to be automatic' despite the fact that the original operation was successful and he had remained on site overnight in order to address any postoperative complications.

BE CLEAR ABOUT WHAT MAKES A GOOD LEADER

MANAGER OR LEADER?

OK, so your job title is a 'manager'. This does not automatically make you a good leader. Your job is to manage staff and resources to ensure that patients on your ward receive a good standard of care. If you lead well, your job as a manager will be made far easier. The job of a manager is to ensure people get things done, whereas a leader guides and inspires people and asks them how we can get things done. A good leader also enables their team to question whether the things need doing in the first place.

Nowadays, leadership is divided into two distinct styles: transactional and transformational. Transactional leadership seems to be the term that applies to the older managerial style, i.e. the setting of tasks and giving rewards to those who achieve them. Transformational leadership is more about influencing others to do things. The transformational leader is more charismatic and inspirational. They are more considerate towards individuals. They stimulate people to be more creative and to challenge the system.

Transformational leadership

Transformational leadership is currently recommended as the model of leadership within the health care setting. That is, it is being taught on all the clinical leadership courses. It is debatable as to whether transformational leadership is the model that is actually being used throughout practice at the moment. The current emphasis on meeting targets can be viewed as transactional. However, a transformational leader will not only ask their team how targets can be met, they will also question the targets and look at alternative solutions if they are detrimental to the overall patient care. So even in a transactional organisation, you can be transformational in your approach.

To become more transformational in your style, it would be worth considering the five practices of good leadership that were revealed following an analysis of leadership research by Kouzes & Posner (2002). These are to:

- inspire a shared vision
- model the way
- challenge the process
- encourage the heart
- enable others to act.

Inspire a shared vision. Get the team together and ask them about where they all want to be in the future, or more realistically in a year's time. Facilitate them to set specific objectives together that they are all willing to work towards.

Model the way. Set an example about the standards you want your team to achieve and give them regular individual feedback about their progress. Show them how to cut through the bureaucracy.

Challenge the process. Continually question and look for ways of improving care in your ward. Encourage your staff to question decisions made by others (including other health professionals), by having the appropriate knowledge, confidence and support in order to do so.

Encourage the heart. Maintain morale by being continually optimistic and encouraging your staff in their work. Praise them when they do things well.

Enable others to act. Empower your staff by investing in their development and support and help them to make important decisions and take risks.

SKILLS OF A GOOD WARD LEADER

Research by the Royal College of Nursing (RCN) into the specific roles of a ward leader identified five major requirements. These were used as the basis of a ward leadership development programme (Cunningham & Kitson 2000). They are:

- management of self
- building and maintaining effective relationships with other staff
- focusing on the patient
- internal and external networking
- increasing political awareness.

Much of the current NHS agenda is geared towards leadership development at all levels within the organisation. Various development programmes are available for ward managers (e.g. Kings Fund 2005, NLIAH 2005, RCN 2005). It's worthwhile accessing one of these types of programmes which are focused on clinical leadership rather than general management.

MAKE SURE YOUR DECISIONS ARE INFORMED ONES

ADVICE FROM YOUR LINE MANAGER

Try not to rely on your line manager as your only source of advice. They are not necessarily the best people to guide you in your work. Not all line managers have been ward managers and know what the role entails. And of those who have had experience, how can you be sure that their experience is any better than yours and that they are giving you the right advice?

Sometimes nurses rely too heavily on the next person up within the hierarchical system. Nowadays, being more senior does not necessarily mean that you have the most relevant experience. That's not to say you should ignore the advice and guidance of your line manager. Indeed there are some very good and experienced matrons and service managers. However, it is always advisable to seek guidance from a variety of sources so that you can make an informed choice.

ADVICE FROM YOUR MENTOR

At this level, you should get yourself a mentor; preferably someone several ranks higher than you. If possible, try and get one of the board directors to be your mentor. Most board directors are keen to mentor someone from the clinical setting within their own organisation. A senior manager from another hospital or even a non-health care setting would be advantageous, particularly in helping you with human resource (HR) issues (see Ch. 10 for further information on mentorship in management).

ADVICE FROM YOUR CLINICAL SUPERVISOR

It would also be wise to have a clinical supervisor. You need to have someone who is more expert than you in your specialist area to help you reflect and learn from your clinical practice. This could be a nurse specialist, consultant doctor or nurse or another more experienced ward manager.

Build up a good relationship with your mentor and/or clinical supervisor so that you can contact them in times of need, rather than just meet them at set times.

ADVICE FROM YOUR HR DEPARTMENT

Do not rely on your line manager or colleagues for advice regarding personnel issues. You may be able to benefit from their experience with similar issues but make sure you also consult with HR before making any decisions. If you have problems with your staff such as inappropriate behaviour, sickness/absence problems or incompetence, your HR department will be able to provide the most up-to-date and appropriate information.

Make sure you build up the appropriate networks before any problem arises. You should be meeting with your HR advisor on a monthly basis to build up a good working relationship. This will help enormously in times of crisis.

ADVICE FROM YOUR FINANCE DEPARTMENT

If you are going to make any changes at all which may involve extra staff or resources, always consult with your finance advisor first. It is their job to calculate the cost of any changes and to advise you what the best course of action is in terms of resources.

Build up links with your finance advisor. They can help you become involved in the business planning process for your directorate and you will become far more knowledgeable and effective in accessing appropriate resources.

ADVICE FROM OTHER WARD MANAGERS

Another incredibly valuable resource often ignored by many ward managers is that of other more experienced ward managers. Why do so many ward managers work alone without searching out the support from their more experienced peers? If you don't have some sort of group where ward managers get together to share experiences, guide and support each other, it would be a good idea to develop one yourself (see p. 194).

Remember that if you make decisions that affect your staff or patients based on the advice of one person alone, you cannot blame them if your decision was the wrong one. If there is a serious incident, for example, and you take a course of action that your manager advised, you may remain fully responsible for the outcome of that decision. So get advice from others as well before you make that decision. Make sure all your decisions are informed ones.

CLARIFY YOUR OBJECTIVES

Within three months of starting your job you must have a formal performance review with your manager to clarify your objectives. If your manager does not arrange this automatically, take the lead and make it happen. You should have three months first to settle in and identify what needs doing and any further skills that you require to meet those needs.

Your manager will also have specific objectives that you are required to fulfil. These may relate to government targets such as the number of complaints, MRSA rates or financial targets. You may have targets such as implementing team nursing, self-rostering or increasing staffing levels. The aim of the performance review is to clarify your objectives together. At your first meeting, you should:

● review where you are now
● agree your objectives and how these will be achieved
● identify the skills you require to achieve the objectives.

A performance review at this stage will ensure that you both agree what your priorities are. There will always be more demands than you can meet. You have to agree with your manager which tasks are more important. You may see that all the patient information leaflets need updating, for example, but if you do not have enough staff to fulfil your minimum staffing requirements, your priority will be to recruit more staff over the next six months. Having this set out formally will stop you taking on lots of extra tasks.

It will stop you going off in a different direction to that of your manager. You should also discuss and understand your line manager's own objectives. Part of your role is to assist your manager in achieving their organisational objectives. You should be working together towards the same goals. The performance review process helps to ensure this happens.

REVIEW YOUR OBJECTIVES REGULARLY

Every time you find that there are more things that need to be changed or improved, do not go ahead and attempt to add it to your workload. Concentrate on your objectives. If you feel that your long-term priorities need to change, arrange a meeting with your manager to discuss and, if necessary, change your agreed objectives.

Review your progress towards your objectives with your manager regularly. Priorities change frequently and your objectives should reflect these changes. In addition, frequent reviews help you and your manager understand and appreciate your role and responsibilities.

OTHER SOURCES OF KNOWLEDGE

One problem with being a ward manager is how do you know what you need to know? How do you know that you are doing the job right? This is especially poignant if your manager has never been a ward manager, has only a few years experience or their experience in the role is limited to one ward only.

Having a wider network is key to ensuring you have access to a wider source of knowledge. Take time to set up good links with other ward managers and departments such as HR, finance and facilities. Assess where you are now. You can use your job description to guide you or the knowledge and skills framework (KSF) and build on that assessment. Alternatively, assess yourself using the questionnaire provided in Appendix 1.1. This may help you to identify areas for improvement.

360-DEGREE FEEDBACK

Another way of assessing where you are now is to undertake a 360-degree review. This is becoming an increasingly popular method of gaining feedback from others. It involves filling in a questionnaire assessing yourself against certain criteria and asking your managers, your team and your peers to also fill in the same questionnaire about you and your performance.

You can develop your own questionnaire. Alternatively, there are numerous types of set questionnaires that you can use to assess specific or general aspects of your work such as communication skills or specific leadership skills.

If you do decide to undertake a 360-degree review, it would be wise to do it in conjunction with someone who has good feedback skills. Enlist the help of someone such as your mentor or line manager to help you:

● deal with any negative feedback in a constructive manner
● focus on your strengths and identify any areas for improvement.

UNDERSTAND YOUR LEGAL RESPONSIBILITIES

Addressing adverse incidents and accusations of negligence costs the NHS a lot of time and money and causes managers and staff immense anxiety. Legal actions can take years to resolve, meaning years of stress. You may have to defend your actions or inactions in court.

Most nurses are aware of their legal and professional liability for their individual practice. Patients are owed a duty of care by the hospital and by the individual staff delivering care. The question then is whether that care has been delivered negligently. Ask yourself: What would a reasonable ward manager do in this situation? What guidelines, protocols or evidence can you produce in justification?

TENSIONS BETWEEN ROLES OF NURSE AND MANAGER

As ward manager, you will be liable as a nurse for your personal nursing actions and as a manager you will be liable for your managerial actions. Tensions can arise between the two roles. For instance, pressure on beds might mean early discharge of a patient. As a nurse you recognise that discharge is not in the patient's best interests but as a manager you are under pressure to maintain the service and know that the patient being admitted is in greater need of the bed. If the patient discharged early suffers harm, whether the nurse manager was negligent in some way or not might depend upon whether evidence can be shown that the discharge was in accordance with ward or hospital guidelines and the proper procedures were followed.

You have a responsibility to address factors that might result in poor patient care. These factors may include:

- incompetent or inexperienced staff whether members of your team or the wider interdisciplinary team
- poor skill mixes
- lack of permanent staff
- inadequate resources
- unethical or illegal practice
- bullying.

If you don't address these factors, in law you may be seen as adopting these bad practices and so become liable yourself.

STAFFING SHORTAGES

Sometimes it is impossible to get sufficient qualified staff for a shift. This may be an ongoing problem on your ward. Ensure a proper record is made, submit the appropriate critical incident form and work with senior managers to find ways to address the problem. If a patient inadvertently suffers harm in that situation, you will be able to show that as a reasonable, responsible ward manager you met your duty of care.

In one case involving a short-staffed neonatal intensive treatment unit (ITU), a nurse accidentally put a baby's feed into the tube going into the lungs not the stomach. Care of all the patients was shared amongst all the staff rather than adopting a named nurse approach. The nurse was cleared of negligence since it was held that a responsible nurse with her training in the same situation would have made the same mistake. It was held that it was the fault of the hospital which had done little to address this long-standing situation. These days, the ward manager would be expected to show proper delegation of tasks, risk monitoring and appropriate actions addressing and reporting staff shortages.

SENDING STAFF TO OTHER WARDS

You may be asked to send staff to help on an understaffed ward. You need to consider whether this will put any of your patients at risk. Your duty is towards your own patients. You may find that staff asked to go to another ward refuse to do so. Listen to the reasons they give, and ensure you are not asking them to undertake any responsibility for which they do not have the knowledge or skills. It is better to find out why they refuse to go and identify what would help the situation.

VICARIOUS LIABILITY

Usually, if fault is established, the employing hospital is vicariously liable for the actions of their employees, which means that they pay the compensation to the victim. However, they can claim all or some of that compensation back from the employee as described earlier in the scoliosis patient case. Ensure that you have insurance at least through union membership.

EXPANDED ROLES

Nurses are constantly expanding their roles. Your role as manager is to ensure that changes in practice are properly implemented. One trust agreed that midwives could top up epidurals if trained and assessed as competent by anaesthetists. Over the years, without the trust realising, this slid into midwives showing other midwives without any formal assessment of competency. An error was made resulting in injury to a patient. It was held that the midwife was acting outside her scope of practice. Furthermore, the trust could have said that she was 'on a frolic of her own' and expected her to pay compensation to the patient out of her own resources.

DUTY TO REPORT CONCERNS

Occasionally, a hospital is held to have primary liability. In other words, the hospital's own negligence is the cause of harm. In one case, a hospital decided to employ only one obstetrician at night even though maternity services were on two sites. Lack of timely care meant a twin boy was left brain-damaged even though all the staff present had acted entirely professionally and competently. If a strategic decision by your hospital could put patients at risk, you have a professional duty to report concerns.

BE CLEAR ABOUT YOUR LINE MANAGER'S ROLE

Your role is to support and develop your team. In turn, your manager's role is to support you and assist in your development. It is not your role to support your manager. If they need support, they should get this from their own line manager or mentor and not burden you with their problems. You have enough of your own. Don't take on your manager's problems as well. You may, however, need to encourage your manager to seek help. You may also have to report concerns about your manager as part of fulfilling your own legal and professional obligations. In any situation like this, always make sure you report your concerns in writing.

SHADOW YOUR MANAGER

It is a good idea to ensure you understand what your manager's role entails and the sort of problems they have to endure. One way to find out would be to spend some time shadowing your manager. Ask to accompany them to a couple of meetings so that you can see for yourself what the job is like and the pressures they are under.

'ACT UP' IN YOUR MANAGER'S ABSENCE

When you are more experienced, ask to 'act up' for your line manager to cover for annual leave. Make sure you get someone to 'act up' for you too. 'Acting up' in someone's absence does not mean carrying on doing your own job as well as covering theirs. 'Acting up' gives you a good insight into the other person's job. Make sure you have full responsibility for decision-making and full access to the tools to do the job, e.g. their email, post, agendas for meetings and what you are expected to contribute.

Make sure you have full handover before your manager goes on annual leave and give a full debrief on their return. You need to know what you did well and what you could have done better. It is the best way to learn from the experience. (Do the same for any staff who 'act up' in your absence.)

BUILD UP A GOOD WORKING RELATIONSHIP

Concentrate on building up a good working relationship with your manager. You need to understand their management style, including their preferred mode of communication. You also need to have a good insight into their priorities as well as their stresses and pressures. Part of your role is helping your manager to achieve organisational priorities. Make sure you work with them and not against them. If you do not agree with their decisions, say so. But make sure you put across your reasons and offer alternative solutions.

Be helpful but not adversarial. A good healthy working relationship is one in which either of you can challenge the other's decisions constructively without anyone feeling threatened in any way. Always show others that you and your manager work well together and communicate regularly. If people see any stresses and strains in your working relationship it will reduce their confidence in your management. They need to know that you are both in control.

You need to be able to decipher whether your manager is being reasonable. If you think your manager is not doing things right or is being a bit too bossy, how do you know if that's normal? How do you know that the reason you are not getting the right resources is because they are not putting your case forward in the business plan? The only way you will know is if you understand what their role is. You can also find out from your colleagues (other ward managers). If you maintain good communication with others you can compare and contrast the role of their managers with yours.

Building up a close working relationship with your manager is so vital for success in your role that this book contains a whole chapter on the subject (see Ch. 12). Knowing their role is the first step to achieving this aim.

REMEMBER YOU ARE THE PATIENTS' OVERALL ADVOCATE

Advocacy is not just about ensuring the patient has the right information and support, it is about influencing a third party on behalf of patients (Teasdale 1998). Your role is to influence others to provide a high standard of care.

PATIENTS FEEL VULNERABLE

In 2003, an article was published in the Telegraph newspaper that outlined people's fears about being a patient (Sergeant 2003a). It struck a chord with many people who are genuinely worried if they or one their family get sick and have to go into hospital. It began with the statements: 'Who is in charge of my health? Who is responsible and accountable for what? These are the questions that many patients are asking with increasing panic'.

The article sparked quite a response from various organisations including the RCN and Kings Fund who pointed out the many improvements that are being made, including the modern matron role. It was also pointed out that despite the pressures, most nurses are doing their best to give the highest standard of care under the circumstances (Kings Fund 2003). But what about the role of nurse managers in all this?

It's interesting to note that the article in the Telegraph was an edited extract from a report published by the Centre for Policy Studies entitled 'Managing not to Manage' (Sergeant 2003b). Amongst other things it claimed that all people wanted was for 'someone to get the lavatories cleaned, to see old people are eating properly, to supervise the training of junior nurses . . .'. The ward manager's role is key to ensuring that these aspects are managed properly and the appropriate resources are available.

PATIENTS NEED STRONG LEADERSHIP AT WARD LEVEL

There has been a huge cry to 'bring back the matron' without realising that matrons are not ward managers. What people are really saying is that they want strong leadership at ward level. They want someone to ensure that they get good care and that the level of care they get will not depend entirely on whichever individual they get to look after them. They want someone in charge who is able to make decisions and challenge poor practice, including government targets. They want someone to acknowledge when mistakes are made, ensure they are rectified and that something is done to ensure those mistakes don't happen again.

Patients are vulnerable and have no 'voice'. When a person becomes ill they become disempowered and are at the mercy of those assigned to care for them and the doctors assigned to treat them. Your role as the ward manager is to coordinate the health care team so the patient receives the best care.

It is not appropriate when a patient or relative makes a complaint to refer them to the complaints department or patient advice and liaison service (PALS) or anyone else for that matter. It is the ward manager's role to make sure the problem is sorted out in the first instance. In order to act as your patients' advocate, you need to make time to be able to direct the care process. You cannot direct others if you are taking the same caseload as your staff. If you allocate yourself an equal number of patients as the rest of your staff, you are not managing. It indicates that you are not in control. Patients and relatives need to see that you are in control. They need reassurance that someone is:

- directing the team of nurses
- coordinating the doctors and other health care professionals
- challenging decisions that may not be appropriate
- ensuring that the focus on government targets is not detrimental to the quality of their care
- protecting them from individual incompetence.

But most of all they want to be reassured that someone is in charge of the ward and that someone has the time and experience to ensure that they are getting the right care. They want someone to be their overall advocate.

DON'T TAKE ON OTHER PEOPLE'S PRESSURES

The role of ward manager is probably one of the most highly pressured jobs within health care. You are responsible for the provision of patient care on your ward 24 hours a day, seven days a week. What's more, most of the care is given through others. That is a huge responsibility. In any other profession, senior managers are responsible for their area between the hours of 9 am–5 pm, and they are rarely responsible for the care and treatment of vulnerable people. Your workload is probably far greater than most senior managers within health care. So don't take on their pressures too.

Many people working in health care seem to be always busy. Being busy all the time means they are not in control of their work. They have either taken too much on or are unable to prioritise their workload. They may not be competent or experienced in certain areas so their work takes twice as long as it would others. The work is controlling them. Bear this in mind when you are asked to take on a project or do a piece of work for someone else.

Don't take on other people's projects, unless it is something you wish to take on to learn and develop in your role. An example is the current Essence of Care benchmarking project in England. Essentially this is an audit tool to help you identify and make improvements to your area. Use it as such. Don't start becoming involved in endless discussions about other people's problems in the subgroups. Some nurses use these group meetings for general talking. Use a benchmarking group to gain ideas and share good practice. If the group is not doing that, either change the way it is being chaired or do not attend. Don't waste your time fulfilling other people's objectives for them.

BE WARY OF NONCLINICAL MANAGERS

There are many nonclinical managers within health care. This is not such a bad idea in principle. Certain jobs need to be undertaken by nonclinical managers in order to allow clinical managers the freedom to fulfil their clinical priorities. However, some take on projects that necessitate clinical involvement in order to achieve their outcomes. Many of these managers are fairly astute. Without the clinical knowledge themselves, they will recruit those who do have the knowledge onto their working group. This is fine if you are expected to contribute your specialist opinion. It is not fine if you are coerced into undertaking work to contribute to the project. If the work required does not fit into your ward objectives, you should not be agreeing to do it. If you can justify that the piece of work they have asked you to do is worth doing, you must then decide what current work you will give up in order to take on this project work. That is unless you do not have enough work to fill your time already!

Don't be coerced into taking on extra work when you already have enough to do. By doing this you are trivialising the rest of your work. You probably want to give the impression that things are fine and nothing is too much for you. You want to be able to contribute. What you are really saying is: 'What I currently do is worth nothing compared to the work that you do'.

The message is simple; don't waste time fulfilling others' goals at the expense of your own. That is not to say you should ignore the pressures that others have. Just don't make them yours.

DON'T ALLOW OTHER PEOPLE'S EMERGENCIES TO BECOME YOURS

Some managers will call meetings at a moment's notice and expect all to attend. Don't fall for this one. Always clarify what the meeting is about first. Make an informed decision. If you have something more urgent to attend to, say so. Do not attend and then whinge. You made the choice.

When a senior manager calls for an urgent meeting, they may not realise that what you had planned is even more urgent. Nonclinical managers are not always aware of the importance of some of the things you do. Don't take on their pressures without making them aware of your own.

BALANCE YOUR CLINICAL WORK WITH ADMINISTRATIVE DUTIES

When you become a manager, you automatically take on a good deal more paperwork. This is one reason why you need to reduce your clinical time. A good ward manager will balance their clinical and administrative duties. If you do not manage this properly, you will end up either as:

● part of the 'numbers', catching up on paperwork at the end of your shift, or
● an office manager, who becomes 'out-of-touch' with patient care or 'the real world'.

The key is to take control of these two aspects of your workload. As the ward manager, you should be allocating yourself the equivalent of one day per week for administrative work. Some call this the 'management' day. I have always thought this rather odd. Does this mean that they do not manage the rest of the time?

With any manager's role comes a fair bit of paperwork. You need to allocate yourself time away from the clinical area to go through it. Some argue that there is not enough money in the budget to do this. If this is the case, it is your fault for not having taken action to ensure it is in the budget. You therefore have two choices:

1. Work with your finance advisor to get this time added to your budget. This can be done either by putting it through as business case or rearranging your staffing levels within the current year's budget.
2. Find some quiet time each day to spend an hour or two in the office. For example, you could work the mornings clinically and take one to two hours each afternoon in the office during the early–late shift overlap.

Do not take the work home. Taking work home with you because you do not have time during your working day is a bad habit to get into. You are not running your own business and having the satisfaction of earning more money with all the extra effort you put in.

If you are working extra hours either at work or home, that is your own decision, nobody else's. You have not been asked to do it and you are not paid for it. Therefore it is not being recognised by your employing organisation. Reprioritise your work to fit into the 37.5 hours per week that you are paid for (see Ch. 2).

REDUCE YOUR PATIENT CASELOAD

If you take on the same number of patients as each of your nurses on the shift, ask yourself:

1. What is the difference between you and them apart from the fact that your patients are probably receiving care from the most experienced person on the ward?
2. How are you able to really manage your team?
3. How can you ensure constant observation of your staff and daily constructive feedback?
4. How can you maintain an overview of what is happening when you are busy taking on the same workload as the rest of your staff?

By taking on the same workload as your staff, you are in effect demeaning your role. You are working as a staff nurse but with the added responsibility of completing the paperwork. This is not managing at all. You are managing not to manage. It is a trap that many ward managers get into. They feel they are letting down their staff if they do not take on the same workload during the shift. In fact, they are letting down their staff by not taking care of aspects of management, such as ensuring the right budget and staffing levels in the first place.

You need to maintain a certain amount of clinical work in order to maintain your skills and credibility. The answer is to allocate yourself fewer patients. Take half the number of patients as your colleagues. As the ward manager, you are more than just the nurse-in-charge of that shift. You need to take a longer-term view than just managing the shift. Your role is to ensure the right systems and processes are in place to enable your staff to carry out their duties to the best of their ability. You cannot do that if you are continuously in the numbers and just managing on a shift-by-shift basis.

You have to let go of some of the clinical work and balance it with the administrative side. It will help you ensure you are in control of your workload and therefore more effective.

BE AWARE OF THE IMPACT OF YOUR ROLE ON OTHERS

Your style of management not only affects the work of those in your team, it also affects other health professionals who have an input into the care of your patients. Try to ensure that the impact is always positive. Wards are often regarded as 'good' or 'bad' depending on who the ward manager is. Make sure people regard yours as one of the 'good' ones.

DOCTORS AND OTHER HEALTH CARE PROFESSIONALS

Make the effort to introduce yourself to all new staff, including doctors and medical students. You may find yourself working alongside them in a few years as consultants or GPs. Introduce a basic introduction package for all new pre-registration house officers (PRHOs). It doesn't take much to point out what the routine is, e.g. how the team nursing works, what is expected of them and what they can expect from you. You and your ward will soon get a good name and doctors will be more willing to help you if you have proved yourself to be helpful and welcoming in the initial stages.

The same goes for other health professionals such as physiotherapists who are rarely based on one ward. Their patients are usually scattered all around the hospital. They soon get to know which are the nice wards and which are not. Don't let your ward be known as the one which everyone dreads going in.

STUDENT NURSES

The way you are perceived in your role is vital to the success of your ward and team. Think back to your student days and your ward placements. What influenced your opinion of the experience? I'll bet that nine times out of ten, it was the ward manager. Many students describe their placement experience in terms of what the ward manager was like.

Your influence on others is immense. Be aware that whatever you do or say is under intense scrutiny and will be discussed amongst students back in the classroom. You cannot afford for any students to have 'a bad experience' on your ward. You want your ward to become the one where students are desperate to get a job once qualified.

PATIENTS AND RELATIVES

Patients and relatives will also remember you. They are probably observing you more closely than anyone else. A good habit to get into is to go round and speak with every patient every day, even if it is part of the drug round. With the rapid patient turnover, you cannot get to see all patients admitted to your ward, but you should aim to see as many as possible.

HOSPITAL MANAGEMENT

How you perceive and carry out your role also impacts on your line manager, your general manager and ultimately your chief executive and board of directors. You will leave yourself with no time to take part or challenge management decisions if you spend your time:

- taking on extra duties
- taking the same patient caseload as your staff each shift
- chasing up staff to cover for the day-to-day staffing shortages.

In order to make an impact on the hospital management, you have to involve yourself in the wider organisation and work together with other ward managers to ensure your voice is heard. If you choose to 'keep your head down' and concentrate on crisis management, you have only yourself to blame.

BEYOND YOUR CONTROL?

In 2001, a report was published which examined the stresses identified by ward managers (Allen 2001). The study found that the major source of stress was 'their anxiety about whether, how and by whom their wards and units were to be staffed each day'. It concluded that much of this stress was found to be due to organisational and managerial factors 'which they felt to be beyond their control'. This included patients being in the wrong place at the wrong time, which again 'they identified as an organisational bed management problem beyond their control'.

Ward managers may have allowed these aspects to be 'beyond their control' by concentrating on micromanaging. If you spend all your time managing the details, someone else will make important decisions without your involvement because you are too busy. Ward managers also work very much in isolation from their peers in equal positions. This makes their position weak within the overall organisation.

Don't always accept that there is nothing you can do and don't become a lone voice fighting for your corner in a huge organisation that doesn't have the time or the inclination to listen to you. Making yourself heard is a key managerial skill. It involves being able to prioritise your work better, knowing who's who, what makes your organisation tick and working closely with all the other ward managers. All these factors are included in this book, so your next action is to read through the rest of the book!

ACTION POINTS

- Assess your current role using the questionnaire provided in Appendix 1.1, and identify areas for improvement.
- Clarify your objectives with your manager within three months of starting your job and review them regularly.
- Explore the option of undertaking a clinical leadership or management course.
- Make sure there are specific written guidelines that outline the steps you and your staff should follow in the event of a shift being short-staffed.
- Make sure you have union membership.
- 'Act up' for your manager to cover annual leave, as a learning opportunity.
- Be specific with others about what your role is and is not.
- Ensure there is an induction/information package for all newcomers to your ward, including doctors.
- Allocate the equivalent of one day per week to deal with the administration/paperwork.
- Reduce your patient caseload if it is the same or more than your staff's caseload.
- Read the rest of this book!

References

Allen I 2001 Stress among ward sisters and charge nurses. Policy Studies Institute, London. Online. Available: http://www.psi.org.uk/publications/SCHS/stressward.htm 10 Oct 2005

Cunningham G, Kitson A 2000 An evaluation of the RCN Clinical Leadership Development Programme. Nursing Standard 15(13–15):34–40

Kings Fund 2003 Kings Fund statement in response to centre for policy studies report, managing not to manage: management in the NHS. Online. Available: http://www. kingsfund.org.uk/news/press_releases/kings_fund_36.html 26 Sep 2005

Kings Fund 2005 Leadership development. Kings Fund, London. Online. Available: http://www.kingsfund.org.uk/leadership 26 Sep 2005

Kouzes J, Posner B 2002 The leadership challenge, 3rd edn. Jossey Bass, San Francisco

NLIAH 2005 National Leadership and Innovation Agency for Health Care, Wales. Online. Available: http://www.chl.wales.nhs.uk 26 Sep 2005

Nursing & Midwifery Council 2002 Press Statements 72/2002 and 179/02. NMC, London

Nursing & Midwifery Council 2004 The NMC code of professional conduct: standards for conduct, performance and ethics. NMC, London. Online. Available: http://www.nmc-uk.org 26 Sep 2005

Royal College of Nursing 2005 RCN Clinical Leadership Programme. RCN, London. Online. Available: http://www.rcn.org.uk/resources/clinicalleadership 26 Sep 2005

Sergeant H 2003a I would not trust my dog, let alone my mother, to many nurses. The Telegraph, 29/11/2003. Online. Available: http://www.telegraph.co.uk 26 Sep 2005

Sergeant H 2003b Managing not to manage: management in the NHS. Centre for Policy Studies, London. Online. Available: http://www.cps.org.uk/pdf//pub/399.pdf 26 Sep 2005

Teasdale K 1998 Advocacy in health care. Blackwell Science, Oxford

Trustees of London Clinic v Michael Alan Edgar QBD (19/4/2000, Hidden J) 2001 LTL 25/06/2005

QUESTIONNAIRE TO HELP IDENTIFY DEVELOPMENT NEEDS FOR WARD MANAGERS

Leadership skills

- Does your team have a vision/goal of where you all want to be in a year's time?
- Do you have set objectives/actions that you have identified together to achieve that vision?
- Have you been able to change what is not right/working in your ward/department?
- Have you been able to change what is not right/working in your organisation?
- Have you had discussions with any of the board directors or general managers within the past three months about any issues in your ward/department?
- Are you actively involved in any trust-wide initiatives?
- Have you evaluated whether any recent changes in trust strategy could result in harm to your patients?
- Does your ward/department have a high profile within the trust because of high standards?

Education

- Are your staff fully trained and developed in all aspects of their work?
- Are you able to access all the educational resources you require for you and your staff?
- Do you know what percentage of your staffing budget is allocated for study?
- Do you plan your staff study leave a year in advance based on appraisal and keeping within the study leave limits?
- If yes to the above, do you involve your whole team in this planning?
- Are all your staff assessed against set clinical competencies on a regular basis?
- Do all your staff have a local mentor/facilitator/coach to guide and support their development?
- Do you meet with your link tutor regularly and maintain close relations with the local university?
- Are all your staff up-to-date with their mandatory training?
- Are you making full use of the in-house and external development programmes to aid career progression of your staff?

Management of staff

- Have you had an appraisal/personal development plan agreed within the last year?
- Have all your staff been appraised within the past year?
- Do you know who your human resource advisor is?
- Do you meet with him/her regularly to discuss personnel issues (e.g. sickness/absence, incompetence issues, recruitment)?

- Have you received training and development on staff management issues such as recruitment, policies and procedures, risk management, etc?
- Do you have appropriate development programmes in place for your deputy ward sister/charge nurse?

Management of budget

- Do you know what your budget is?
- Do you know what your budget is in terms of PAY and NON PAY?
- Does your current budget reflect the skill mix required (as identified through a formal skill mix review)?
- Have you had any training and development on managing a budget?
- Do you contribute to the yearly business planning process?
- Do you meet with your finance advisor regularly?
- Are your staff all involved in managing the budget?
- Do you manage your team's annual leave throughout the year so that the ward does not have 'off-duty' problems in the January to March period?
- Do you have adequate resources for your ward in terms of staff and equipment?
- Do you ensure you have spent your ward environment budget appropriately each year and fully involve staff in this decision?

Maintaining clinical standards

- Do you manage to see every patient on your ward every day?
- Are you happy that your staff are delivering care to a high standard every day?
- How would you justify in a court of law the way you allocate workloads and patients?
- Are your staff taking full responsibility for the care of their allocated patients?
- Do you have set standards/guidelines for all specialist procedures on your ward?
- Do you have a system within your ward of regularly reviewing themes from complaints, clinical incidents and local audits?
- Do you have a system of keeping your patients informed about the complaints themes and what you are doing about them?
- Are you happy that all your nurses are confident enough to question inappropriate medical decisions?
- Are you aware of what the drug error rate is in your unit?
- Do you have a plan of action for each serious incident and complaint within your ward/department?
- Do you have a mentor or clinical supervisor to constantly challenge you and enable you to keep up-to-date professionally?
- Have you and your team made any improvements to care using audit or benchmarking tools?

- Have you agreed cleaning standards with your ward domestics, working closely with them to make sure the standards are met?

Communication

- Do you meet with your team regularly?
- Do you open and deal with your email and post on a daily basis?
- Do you appoint someone to 'act up' in your absence?
- Do you keep your matron fully informed of day-to-day operations and liaise on a regular basis?
- Are you fully aware of your responsibilities regarding the Freedom of Information Act and Data Protection Act?
- Does every member of your team have full access to a computer for email, intranet and appropriate research to carry out their role effectively?
- Do you keep yourself and your team fully up to speed about what is going on in your organisation?
- Do you ensure that your voice is heard at corporate level?
- Do you regularly get staff to shadow you when providing highly sensitive/ complex information to patients and relatives?

Management of self

- Are you able to be a role model for your staff by working 37.5 hours per week and taking your meal/coffee breaks?
- Do you plan your work at least a week in advance rather than just getting through everyday crises?
- Do you have a mentor who provides support as well as challenges you in your professional role?

Please note: This questionnaire is designed simply as an aid to stimulate thoughts and is not meant to be prescriptive or an exhaustive list of tasks that should be undertaken. You may find it helpful to identify those sections where there are mostly 'no' answers and think about what you can do to improve your skills in these areas.

CHAPTER 2

DEFINE AND PRIORITISE YOUR WORKLOAD

Define your workload   26

Plan and prioritise   28

Organise your office   28

Keep everything you need to do on one list   28

Ensure the office environment is in good order   29

Control your diary   30

Prioritise your 'to-do' list   30

Don't keep rewriting your list   31

Set yourself time limits   31

Take your break   31

Pencil in your diary   31

Book all annual leave in advance   32

Keep up with your emails   32

Delegate your emails to someone else in your absence   32

File emails   33

Using emails as an essential time management tool   33

Cut interruptions   33

Ward rounds   33

Let your staff know what you are doing in the office   34

'Open door' policies don't work   34

Don't waste time with unnecessary reading   34

Journal articles   35

Hospital newsletter and internal bulletins   35

Keep up-to-date with the internet   36

Reduce your meetings and get the best out of those you do choose to attend   36

Don't allow your clinical expertise to be abused   36

Meetings should be used for disseminating information   36

Avoid being kept waiting for appointments or meetings   37

Getting the best from meetings   37

Chair meetings effectively   38

Learn to let go through delegation   39

Getting your nursing staff to delegate appropriately to health care assistants   40

Are you still doing the job you were promoted from?   40

Delegating to your deputy   41

How to delegate   41

Be proactive   41

Under-promise and over-deliver   41

Don't put things off   42

Ask for help   42

Keep the paperwork aspect of your work organised   42

As mentioned in the previous chapter, putting in long hours at work does not necessarily mean you are good at your job. Being busy does not equate with being efficient and effective. It suggests that you are not in control. In order to manage your time more effectively, you need to have control over choosing what you do and how to do it. You also need to be able to choose what not to do. Spend your time accomplishing things, not just being busy. Invest time in planning, organising, rearranging, sorting and most important of all, thinking.

This chapter focuses on how to manage your time more effectively and how to achieve a healthy work/life balance in your role.

DEFINE YOUR WORKLOAD

Most ward managers are employed to work 150 hours per month. It's worth taking some time to write down all the commitments you currently have in terms of hours per month, as indicated in Table 2.1. If the total hours add up to more than 150, it means that you do not have enough time to complete what is required. This indicates that in order to fulfil your workload, you are working more than 150 hours or not fulfilling your commitments. You may be:

- taking work home
- staying late regularly
- not getting things done.

Taking work home or staying late regularly?

If you have decided to take work home or stay on late regularly, this is not an appropriate solution. You are not looking after yourself. You should be well rested, healthy and have a good work/life balance in order to be effective in your role. Plus, it is unpaid work. In other words, it is not recognised by your organisation or your manager. It is also not appreciated by the patients.

Not getting things done?

If the hours add up to more than 150 and you are not physically working all those hours, it means that some parts of the work are not getting done. You are probably finding that you are continually busy but don't seem to be getting on top of things. Things either get missed or get left undone.

Problems occur when you do not formally prioritise what gets done and what doesn't. It is often the case that clinical work takes less priority in order to get through the administrative work. That's a poor way to manage a ward. If you need to spend less time clinically, then plan it. Don't allow administrative work and meetings to take over and leave you feeling continually busy and overloaded. Both you and your staff will suffer.

TABLE 2.1: Defining your workload in terms of hours per month

Description of task	Total hours per month
Meetings	
List the meetings you attend, including all one-to-one meetings	
(if weekly multiply hours by 4, if quarterly divide hours by 3)	
1. e.g. Monthly sisters' meeting 2 hrs	2
2. e.g. Weekly ward team meeting 1 hr	4
3.	
4.	
5.	
6.	
7.	
8.	
9.	
10.	
Emails, voicemail and post How many hours per day do you need for this? (multiply by 20 for the monthly figure)	
Investigating and writing responses to complaints (allow an average of 10 hours' work per complaint)	
Staffing issues (include appraisals, recruitment, etc.)	
Compiling the 'off-duty'	
Risk management and governance issues (average time spent on serious incident investigations, audits, pressure sore forms, etc.)	
Teaching (include preparation time)	
Own study/course commitments	
Regular admin/secretarial work (e.g. photocopying)	
Corporate or university work (e.g. 'block' recruitment, interviewing)	
Clinical (time spent on ward as part of clinical shift)	
Other (e.g. current project work)	
1.	
2.	
3.	
4.	
5.	
Total	

PLAN AND PRIORITISE

Start by removing or reducing tasks in order to bring the total down to 150 hours. The first place to start is with the meetings. Do you really need to attend all those meetings? Choose the ones that are essential for the welfare of your patients and staff.

Do the same with any project work. Only keep the tasks that are essential. Essential work includes:

- doing the 'off-duty'
- dealing with complaints
- dealing with serious incident investigations
- reading and dealing with email, voicemail and post each day
- HR/staff issues.

Non-essential work includes:

- some project work
- some corporate work
- teaching externally to the ward.

It is advisable to meet with your line manager to assist you in making the required decisions.

The next step is to realistically identify how much time you have left to devote to clinical work. It may only be 70–80 hours per month. If that is the case, plan to split it into specific blocks of clinical time. This could be something like four half shifts per week. Devote that whole time to clinical work without going off to a meeting or into the office half way through. Let your staff see that you are in control of your work. Having to keep interrupting your clinical shift to go off to meetings or into the office to catch up on paperwork shows that you are not in control of your workload. It is controlling you. Your staff will respect you far more if they see that you are in charge of what you do.

ORGANISE YOUR OFFICE

Many ward managers have to share their office with others. Some offices double up as changing rooms, coffee rooms and in some cases they are the only place available to meet with relatives. If this is how it is with your office, try and designate at least one third of this room as your personal office space with your desk, computer and chair. Make sure all other chairs, coat hooks, beverages, etc., are kept on the other side of the room. You have the most important job on your ward and it is essential that you have some dedicated office space.

KEEP EVERYTHING YOU NEED TO DO ON ONE LIST

Write everything down on your list such as phone calls you need to make, messages to get back to people, reports to be written, project work, etc. All papers associated with your list should be filed away in your filing cabinet. The list can run into three or four sheets of A4 paper but it doesn't matter, as long as everything is written down in one place. Keeping one list is simple but effective. It serves to greatly reduce your stress and worry by literally taking things off your mind and putting them down on paper. The basic concept is that you can stay on top and in control of all unfinished work, projects, reports and correspondence.

Get into the habit of noting down everything that comes to you via post, email, voicemail, fax or phone on your central list of things to do. File emails and associated attachments on your computer if you need to keep them. Don't print them out. It's a waste of time and takes up unnecessary space on your desk or in your filing cabinet.

Set up an efficient filing system

If there are many files in your cabinet left by the previous post holder and you feel you may need to refer to them at some point, then use different types or colour of label for your own files so you can easily distinguish which are your own.

Never keep copies of documents if you can easily access them somewhere else. If you have a copy within your computer files, throw away the hard copy unless you will be referring to it often.

Start a 'bring forward' file

What do you do with agendas and notes for future meetings? What about the notes you need for an appointment next month? Don't keep them in a pile in your in-tray. You do not have time to keep sifting through it for items. Create a 'bring forward' file. You will need to allocate a whole filing cabinet drawer for this purpose, preferably the one in your desk if you have one. Have a set of hanging files numbered one to 31 and another set of twelve, labelled for each month of the year. Keep the first set of files 1–31 at the front of the cabinet. These are for the current month. The remaining twelve files for each month should be set out in order behind these.

Each time you receive something you need to keep for a future date, file it in the appropriate date, 1st to 31st, if it is required for the current month, or in the file of the relevant future month. At the end of each month, remove the next month's papers and file them by day in the current month, 1st to 31st, then put the empty file of the previous month to the back of the twelve monthly dividers. A 'bring forward' file ensures that:

- you are always prepared
- you are not having to continually sift through piles of paper to find things
- your desk is kept free of clutter
- staff will be able to find things in your absence
- important items can easily be found in your absence.

ENSURE THE OFFICE ENVIRONMENT IS IN GOOD ORDER

Keep your office space neat and tidy with no overflowing papers or post-it notes everywhere. Keep all stationery aids in a drawer, e.g. pens, stapler and paper clips. The only things directly on your desk should be your in-tray, computer screen plus keyboard and telephone. It is not always possible but if you can, keep your printer on a different shelf/desk preferably within easy reach of where you sit.

The location of your desk is very important. Your computer screen should be facing away from the window. Any glare from the daylight on your screen will cause strain on your eyes and headaches. Plants and photographs serve to make your office a nice place to spend your time but keep them away from your desk. Other personal items such as tea, handbags and umbrellas should be out of sight in a cupboard or drawer. Ensure you have adequate lighting. Order a desk light from your stationery budget. They are not expensive. It makes your office more comfortable to be in and is better for reading. And one last very important tip is to always keep a store of printer cartridges. They tend to run out at the most inconvenient moment.

Having an organised office makes you far more efficient with your time. Less time and effort will be wasted looking for letters, documents and emails, and you will be far less likely to forget things.

CONTROL YOUR DIARY

When you are working a clinical shift, you plan what you are going to do after handover but it often changes due to patient need. You expect that to be the case. As clinicians we are used to continually altering our plans because looking after patients is unpredictable work. However, this approach to work is not appropriate when dealing with the administrative side of your role. You cannot afford to spend your day reacting to events and constantly being interrupted. The time when you are not directly involved in patient care should be planned.

PRIORITISE YOUR 'TO-DO' LIST

The easiest way to plan your administrative work is to prioritise your list of things to do. Grade each task 1–3 in order of importance:

1. Urgent – needs to be done by today.
2. Important – if possible get done today but can be left until tomorrow.
3. Can be left until next week.

It does not matter whether you have five or 50 tasks, it will make your life easier if you prioritise things. You can then concentrate on completing all those that are graded at priority 1.

Mark against each priority 1 task approximately how long that task will take. You can see at a glance which tasks will take just a few minutes, such as making a phone call. You can then concentrate on achieving those when you just have an hour or so in the office. Tasks such as reading or writing a report can be left for when you have a longer time slot.

DON'T KEEP REWRITING YOUR LIST

Put a line through when you have completed a task rather than just putting a tick against it. This gives a greater sense of achievement. Administrative work does not give the rewards that you get from clinical work. Without having a list you get little sense of satisfaction.

Don't rewrite it each day, as this would be too time consuming. Recategorise the remaining tasks at the start of each day or at the end of each preceding day. Keep adding to the list depending on what happens during the day. Just rewrite the list when it starts becoming unreadable.

SET YOURSELF TIME LIMITS

Be realistic about what you can and can't do. Without limits, you end up being overstretched and working longer hours. Allocate a set time for each piece of work. Allow one hour to do an appraisal, for example, or two hours to prepare an important presentation. If the task is not finished by the end of the allocated time, set time for the next administration slot or submit the work as it is. It is no good striving for perfection all the time. Ask yourself, 'will it do?'. Aim to do things well enough. Doing them better than necessary is a waste of your valuable time.

TAKE YOUR BREAK

Don't forget to schedule in your 30-minute lunch break. In many organisations, staff are not paid for their lunch breaks so don't work through them. Taking a proper 30-minute break will ensure you are appropriately refreshed and your batteries are recharged for the afternoon. You also need to set an example to your staff. If they know you take a proper lunch break they will follow suit. Eating a sandwich in your office whilst checking through your emails is seen as a poorly organised manager unable to manage their workload. It will make your staff feel guilty for taking their own lunch breaks.

PENCIL IN YOUR DIARY

Always use a pencil to write anything in your diary. Health care is full of people who are disorganised and not in control of their work. As a result, meetings are frequently cancelled and rearranged at a later date. Health care work can be very unpredictable. By using a pencil, you simply rub things out and save the page getting into an incomprehensible mess.

BOOK ALL ANNUAL LEAVE IN ADVANCE

Pencil in your important dates and meetings at the beginning of each financial year. Then book your annual leave. If you can, book it all up for the rest of the year. Plan the time off for you and your family and friends. Many have lost annual leave due to poor planning. Something more important always comes up.

In order to keep yourself healthy and keep work in perspective, try to ensure you do not work more than three months without an annual leave break. It really is very important to be in control of your own time as well as your work time.

KEEP UP WITH YOUR EMAILS

Email now replaces post and should be treated with the same urgency. To keep on top of things, make sure you sift through it each day. Schedule time at the beginning and end of each day.

Don't leave the ward every spare moment to catch up with your emails. It is not good time management. When you are working clinically, you should concentrate on being there for your staff and patients.

DELEGATE YOUR EMAILS TO SOMEONE ELSE IN YOUR ABSENCE

When you are on 'days off' and annual leave, delegate your emails to someone else to deal with. This could be your deputy ward manager, one of your staff nurses or even your ward clerk. It keeps your team informed when you are not there. It is good development for your junior sisters and charge nurses. Not only will they delete all the junk mail, read and answer the basic ones on your behalf, but also they will gain an excellent insight into your role and responsibilities. You must not give out your password, but you can enable certain named staff to have 'proxy access' to your emails. Ask your IT department to help you set this up if you have not already done so.

Confidentiality

If you are concerned about confidentiality, then perhaps you need to look at how you and your colleagues are using the email service. For a start, you should never use your work email account for private or personal emails. As a general rule, all your emails should come as no surprise if another member of your team gains access to them. Remember the golden rule: 'No email is ever confidential'. Ensure all your team are aware of this. If you need to discuss confidential information, it should be done face-to-face or on the phone but never written on an email.

FILE EMAILS

Don't get into the habit of printing off emails. File them in your computer as you would a piece of paper. Always use the organisation's shared drive to file emails away. This is the disk that is backed up each day centrally, therefore if your computer fails in some way you will not lose all your files. If you are saving your files on your personal computer (i.e. c:/drive), you risk losing them.

USING EMAILS AS AN ESSENTIAL TIME MANAGEMENT TOOL

Always use email in preference to the phone whenever you can. It saves a lot of time. Nowadays, if you phone you rarely get the other person and end up leaving a voicemail. They then call you and leave a voicemail and this can go on for quite some time.

Emails are an incredibly efficient way of working. They save much time but it does depend on the user. You should have a system with emails as you would with post. If you open post, then leave it in your in-tray, it will get forgotten. The same is for emails. If, for example, you get an email reminding you of a report you are supposed to be working on but haven't started, don't leave it in your in-box. Like the opened envelope left in your in-tray, it will get left. Add the task within the email to your 'to-do' list, then either delete or file the email.

Don't allow email to become another interruption to your working schedule by silencing the beeper that sounds every time you receive an email.

CUT INTERRUPTIONS

It is generally accepted that the ward manager or nurse-in-charge of the shift deals with all the queries and any tasks that are not directly patient related. When you are working clinically, you learn to deal with constant interruptions, but you cannot work like this when managing the paperwork side of your role.

When you plan time in your weekly diary for office work, you need to arrange cover on the ward. You cannot be in charge on the ward and working in the office at the same time.

WARD ROUNDS

Make sure you do a ward round every day. Most ward managers have some way of getting around to speak to all the patients and staff during the shift. This is often incorporated as part of the drug rounds, doctors' rounds, bedside handover or even a round of making beds. Making time to do this every day helps reduce those constant interruptions when you do eventually go into the office.

LET YOUR STAFF KNOW WHAT YOU ARE DOING IN THE OFFICE

Your staff need to respect that you must have uninterrupted time to deal with your administrative work. Let them know what you are doing. If you say you are shortlisting candidates for interviews, compiling next month's 'off-duty' or writing a business case for more equipment, they will understand why you need the time. If you say that you are going to the office 'to catch up on things', it doesn't sound quite so important. Health care professionals see office work as unimportant compared to direct patient care, so make sure your staff are aware of exactly what you are doing rather than just calling it 'general paperwork'.

'OPEN DOOR' POLICIES DON'T WORK

Close your office door and tell people that you will accept interruptions for emergencies only. When you are in the office:

1. If someone comes to your door asking 'Have you got a few minutes?', make a point of glancing at your clock or wristwatch before answering. Tell them exactly how much time you have or are prepared to give them. If you are in the middle of something, say so: 'I'm just finishing off a report; would you mind coming back at 4 o'clock when I can give you my full attention?', or 'I've got five minutes now if it is urgent, but if it can wait until 2 pm I'll have more time for you'.
2. Don't offer beverages to anyone who drops in unannounced. It indicates that you have plenty of time for tea and a chat.
3. Indicate the interruption is over by standing up. If they have not taken notice, show them to the door. Keep smiling throughout so the person does not feel awkward.
4. Don't make your office too welcoming. Do not have your desk facing the door. This encourages people to come in and interrupt you. Keep another chair appropriately placed in the room but well away from your desk. This deters visitors from staying too long.
5. Don't answer the phone whilst you are in the office. Leave it on voicemail and allow 10 minutes at the end of your office session to go through your voicemails. Make sure your voicemail message indicates how you can be contacted in an emergency (preferably by pager).

DON'T WASTE TIME WITH UNNECESSARY READING

Reading can be very time consuming. Some health care documents can be long and complex. In addition, keeping clinically up-to-date involves a lot of time not only reading but also searching for the relevant information. Learning the techniques of scanning and speed-reading can be extremely helpful for all managers.

Scanning

The NHS in particular is adept at producing massive documents, many of which you know you should read but know you will never really have the time. It is also difficult to know whether the document is important enough to be read or not. A good technique to use in these cases is to scan such documents. Get a feel for the content without reading it through. It saves you a lot of time and energy. With every new document, all you need to do is read:

● the title
● the introduction or executive summary
● the subheadings and the first and last sentence of each paragraph or section
● the conclusion.

Scanning can be applied to any sort of document. Try not to read any document or letter without scanning it first.

Speed-reading

The average reading speed is around 250 words per minute. You can achieve double or quadruple this amount after one day's training. It is worth investing in a short course, which usually consists of one to two days. The basic technique is not to understand the actual words but to see the whole picture or concept of what is being said. You don't need to read each word to do this. The technique involves skimming across the page focusing on the main words in the sentence, not on the ones in between. That way, you can skim across paragraphs very quickly.

It takes some practice to do this but can save a huge amount of time. Writing down key points from the document as you go also helps you to understand and remember what you have read.

JOURNAL ARTICLES

Don't keep piles of journals. You will rarely, if ever, refer to them. If you do need to refer to a journal article, you can access them through the library. It is easier to scan through journals. Add a file in your filing cabinet labelled 'Reading material'. If you see an article of interest, rip it out and add to your reading material. Throw the rest away.

HOSPITAL NEWSLETTER AND INTERNAL BULLETINS

Leave any current information such as the hospital newsletter or internal bulletins on the coffee table in the staff room (even if it is the same room as your office). Renew them each week. It will help keep your staff up-to-date as well.

KEEP UP-TO-DATE WITH THE INTERNET

All ward managers should have full access to the internet. Make full use of it. The worldwide web is the quickest and easiest way of accessing information and keeping you up-to-date. Make it a habit to access the NHS website each month. The following websites are useful for regular quick updates:

> http://www.dh.gov.uk – The Department of Health's website. You can also access the Chief Nursing Officer's website from here.
> http://www.nhs.uk/england – This provides information about the NHS in England.
> http://www.show.scot.nhs.uk – This is the official website of NHS Scotland.
> http://www.wales.nhs.uk – The official website of NHS Wales.
> http://www.n-i.nhs.uk – The official website for Health and Personal Social Services in Northern Ireland.

Your hospital intranet site will keep you updated with what is going on in your organisation.

As a ward manager, you need to keep abreast of the ongoing changes both clinically and managerially. Being politically aware about what is going on in your own organisation and in the NHS overall helps you to ensure your patients receive the best from the system.

REDUCE YOUR MEETINGS AND GET THE BEST OUT OF THOSE YOU DO CHOOSE TO ATTEND

Break the habit of going to meetings just because they are in your diary. Meetings take up an awful lot of time in public service organisations. Some managers spend so much time dashing from one meeting to the next that they leave themselves with little time in which to do any work.

DON'T ALLOW YOUR CLINICAL EXPERTISE TO BE ABUSED

For each and every meeting, ask yourself 'Is it really necessary to attend?'. Health professionals are sometimes invited to meetings because the person in charge of the project is not clinical and needs help and advice. Watch for these people. Some will use you and get you to do the work for them. Beware of helping others to achieve their goals/targets whilst falling behind on your own.

MEETINGS SHOULD BE USED FOR DISSEMINATING INFORMATION

Meetings should be used for bringing together the right skills and experiences to be able to make informed decisions and changes. A meeting is not required simply for information-giving. There are far more efficient ways of giving information such as memos, email, communication books and the hospital intranet. The purpose of meetings should be to involve, not to inform.

AVOID BEING KEPT WAITING FOR APPOINTMENTS OR MEETINGS

If you have to meet regularly with someone who is often late, ask them to come to you in future so you avoid wasting your time waiting. When the person arrives after keeping you waiting, ask them to wait for you while you finish what you are doing. If a regular meeting always starts late, get there on time and leave a note saying what time you left and where you can be contacted. This is a somewhat diplomatic way of getting your point across. It works very well with one-to-one meetings.

GETTING THE BEST FROM MEETINGS

Whether a meeting works or not depends entirely on the person running it. Few people have training in how to run a meeting. The following steps are important for successful meetings.

Step 1: Ensure the purpose has been specified
All regular meetings should have terms of reference (see Appendix 2.1). These make it clear what the meetings are for and the way in which they will be run. If any of the meetings you attend do not have written terms of reference, you should question why the meeting is taking place. Sometimes meetings are held when the distribution of a memo or email would suffice.

All one-to-one meetings should also have a specific purpose. 'To discuss the incident' is not specific enough. You need to have an outcome such as 'To identify what actions need to be taken following the incident'. Ensuring you have a specific objective stops you wasting valuable time discussing issues without achieving anything.

Step 2: Prepare
Notify the person running the meeting in advance if you have an agenda item and send them any supporting papers. Do not wait to raise it at the meeting as 'any other business' (AOB). AOB should be for urgent matters only. Read the minutes or action notes at least one day beforehand. This ensures that you are familiar with what happened last time and remember what you had agreed to do. It also gives you time to prepare your feedback about your actions if required. If you are not sure about any items on the agenda, ring up beforehand and ask. You cannot prepare or contribute if you do not understand what it is about.

Let people know if you cannot make it, will be late or have to leave before the end. It is considered very rude to not turn up to a meeting without sending your apologies. Send an appropriate substitute if you can, and if you do, ensure that person is fully conversant with what the meeting is about and why they are there.

For one-to-one meetings, send any items you wish to raise by email in advance. This saves time and gives the other person time to prepare too.

Step 3: Know how to handle a poorly chaired meeting

This can be difficult to do without challenging or criticising the chair's competence. However, you can help to steer them in the right direction, with questions such as:

1. Do you mind if we quickly run through the purpose of the meeting so I can be clear in my mind?
2. Can you summarise that last point for us please?
3. Last time we had the meeting, we took the current list of delayed discharges as a starting point. Perhaps it might be helpful if we took that approach again.

CHAIR MEETINGS EFFECTIVELY

The role of the chairperson is to act as the 'group facilitator'. This includes:

● enabling everyone to contribute or have their say
● ensuring the group comes to a decision or sets actions
● keeping to time
● utilising the best of the skills and experience in the room.

Before you chair any meeting, make sure you prepare beforehand:

1. *Familiarise yourself* with the agenda and previous minutes before the meeting.
2. *Sort out the room* to enable you to start on time and reduce interruptions, e.g. silence the phone, put a sign up outside the door and arrange the chairs.
3. *Send out the agenda and minutes* to reach individuals one week before the meeting if it involves people from other areas. This will not only remind them that the meeting is taking place but will also stimulate them to finish (or start!) the actions they agreed to undertake at the last meeting. Put these details up on your staff noticeboard or communication book if the meeting is for members of your team only.
4. *Start the meeting on time.* If someone comes in late, keep going. Acknowledge them with a nod only. Don't start again, that's their problem. If they sit down and ask where you are at, explain that you will not hold everyone up by going through things again. They will just have to pick things up.
5. *Get everyone to quieten down and then welcome them.* Check that everyone has seen the agenda and minutes. Quickly run through the agenda to remind everyone what they are there for. Introduce any outside speakers and confirm their place on the agenda. Ask for any items under AOB.
6. *Keep the discussion on track.* If you find that people are becoming sidetracked, bring them back by saying something like 'This is a useful

discussion, but we need to concentrate on the main issue. We can agenda that particular issue for future meetings'.

7. *Control interruptions.* Your role is to ensure everyone has the opportunity to contribute. Deal with interruptions quickly or you will lose control of the meeting. Say something like 'Wait a minute, let X speak first, then we'll come back to your point . . .'.

8. *Observe everyone in the room.* Make sure that all have a chance to speak. Notice and act if someone is trying to speak but keeps being interrupted, or if someone looks bored or not in tune with what's going on. Notice if someone is aggressive, angry or upset. Say things like 'OK, you've had your say, I think it's time to let someone else speak on this issue . . .' or 'What do you think, Wendy?' or 'Simon, you appear to be a bit perturbed about this, am I right?'.

9. *Deal with conflict* by pointing out what is happening and saying something like 'Can we get back to the issue on the agenda please?'. Usually that will stop the situation. If not, call for a break. Aggressive behaviour needs to be pointed out. Acknowledge the person's point of view but point out that this sort of discussion is not appropriate and can be finished outside the meeting.

10. *Ensure everything runs to time.* All agendas should be timed. Preferably, the meeting should last an hour. No meeting should go on for more than two hours at the very most. If a discussion starts getting lengthy or going round in circles, summarise where you are at and ask where you want to go from here.

11. *Summarise* the outcome/decision at the end of each agenda item and who agreed to do what. This confirms the message for everyone and makes it easier for the person taking notes.

12. *End the meeting on time.* Thank everyone for coming and their contributions and confirm the time and place of the next meeting.

13. *Produce action notes* with a named lead and the agreed timescale, either as part of the minutes but highlighted in bold or as a separate action plan with headings 'Decision', 'Action', 'Who By' and 'Date'.

14. *NEVER take notes and chair the meeting at the same time.* Always appoint a minute or note-taker at the beginning of each meeting if you have no administrative support.

LEARN TO LET GO THROUGH DELEGATION

Delegation is not about dumping the job onto someone else. Nobody likes working for someone who gives them all the rotten jobs. Delegation is about giving someone the responsibility and authority to carry out some work for you that is geared towards aiding their personal development.

Do not delegate jobs where failure to deliver would cause immense problems and don't delegate jobs that may be beyond the person's skills and abilities. The basic rules of good delegation are to:

- present the task as an opportunity or challenge
- ensure the individuals are fully aware of what is required of them – a written brief is usually advisable
- identify areas where they will need support or further training
- ensure or give the individuals the appropriate authority to carry out what is required to complete the job
- agree timescales
- give feedback to enable them to learn from the process.

Remember that you still take full responsibility for the completion of the job. When you ask someone to do something for you, you are delegating not abdicating your responsibility.

GETTING YOUR NURSING STAFF TO DELEGATE APPROPRIATELY TO HEALTH CARE ASSISTANTS

The changing workforce today means that a greater number of nursing duties are being delegated to health care assistants (HCAs). Some nurses have difficulty with this concept and resort to delegating tasks such as doing the observations or emptying catheter bags. This is not true delegation. These nurses are compensating for their fear that nobody can do the job as well as they can. Proper delegation means giving responsibility for the whole patient care, not individual tasks to complete the overall picture. The nurse should continue to oversee the patient care and take responsibility for it.

HCAs cannot learn and develop if their work is based on delegated tasks. In the long term, delegation of patient-centred care instead of task-centred care will help develop the skills and competencies of HCAs. Nurses need to feel confident in their skills to be able to trust them with the increased responsibilities. However, if they do not practise true delegation, how will HCAs develop the required skills? (See also p. 91.)

The art of true delegation is to enhance a person's development. Delegation is probably one of the most important skills that both you and your staff should develop.

ARE YOU STILL DOING THE JOB YOU WERE PROMOTED FROM?

It is not uncommon for ward managers to find that they are still doing many aspects of their old job in addition to their new responsibilities. Just because you are good at your job of being a clinical nurse does not mean that you should continue to take a patient caseload each shift. You are now in a position in which you oversee patient care rather than actually carrying it out yourself. Your priority has now changed to ensuring your staff have the appropriate skills to be able to deliver that same high standard of care.

It is difficult to let go but if you want to develop in your role as ward manager, you cannot do so unless you let go of your old role.

DELEGATING TO YOUR DEPUTY

A major aspect of your role is to ensure your deputy develops the appropriate skills to be able to replace you in times of annual leave, sickness and when or if you leave your job. As with your staff, don't delegate parts of a project in the form of tasks, delegate the whole project. If you are going to delegate the investigation of a complaint or serious incident, for example, don't ask them just to investigate and report their findings to you. Give them the responsibility and authority to deal with the whole thing including writing the patient response or incident report. Your role will be to provide support, advice and guidance throughout, if required.

HOW TO DELEGATE

When delegating a task, make sure the person understands what is expected of them. Get them to repeat it to you. Write down the objectives to ensure you agree what needs to be done, the limits, and ensure the other person has full authority and training if required for carrying out the task.

Delegate gradually. It is not appropriate to ask a new staff nurse to write a business case for a new electrocardiogram (ECG) machine, for example. However, you could approach it in a less daunting way:

> 'Susan, Paul was going to write the business case for the ECG machine which has to be in next Friday but, as he is going on annual leave next week, would you mind working with him on this? Spend some time with him tomorrow afternoon, see what he has done so far and get him to explain the process with you. I'd like you to have a go and see if you can get a draft to me before the Friday deadline so that I can go through it with you.'

Take a back seat while they are carrying out the work, making sure they know you are happy to support them if needed. Praise them if they are successful. If the task has not been completed to the correct standard it is usually because the person has not fully understood what was required of them. Always give constructive feedback; that is, praise them for things done well and identify areas for improvement if they had to do a similar task in future.

BE PROACTIVE

UNDER-PROMISE AND OVER-DELIVER

A reputation for delivering on time earns you the reputation of being dependable. The only way you can do this is to ensure that you are not over-optimistic when setting deadlines. If you are asked to investigate and report on a serious incident within 48 hours, say you will need five days in order to interview everyone, then set about getting the report done over the next two to three days. If you hand it in on day 3, people will be impressed. Whereas if you had agreed to try and do it within 48 hours and then handed it in on day 3, your work would have been late. Setting a longer deadline date also reduces the pressure when you have any unforeseen setbacks.

Do the same when promising things to your team. If you say you should hopefully have the 'off-duty' done by Tuesday, your staff will be expecting it done by then. They will not be happy if you produce the final 'off-duty' on Thursday. However, if you say you will have it ready after the weekend and then produce it on Thursday, your staff will be under the impression that you are incredibly efficient.

DON'T PUT THINGS OFF

Avoid putting tasks off because you believe they will be difficult. They often turn out to be easier than you think. Even if they are not easy, if you start early, you have the time to spend sorting out the difficulties. You can also renegotiate the deadline if necessary.

Always begin reports early. Write an outline to start you off for reports, complaints responses and serious incident investigations (see Ch. 12). This will help guide you and stop you worrying about what needs to be done. If you don't do this immediately, you will find yourself putting it off by finding more important things to do, like welcoming interruptions to your office! The more you put things off, the more you worry about them and it becomes a vicious circle. Life is too short to spend worrying about things.

ASK FOR HELP

Ward managers tend to work in isolation and are often expected to get on with things. Remember that you have been trained clinically and all this managerial and paperwork stuff is new to you. It all needs to be learned through experience. And you cannot learn if you struggle to do everything by yourself. You'll pick up bad habits, which can then become normal practice.

If you have been delegated a piece of work to do and don't know where to start, go back to the person who delegated it and ask. If you get stuck half way through the piece of work, go back and ask again. It doesn't matter if you feel a fool. Who cares? Next time you do a similar piece of work you will have learned through previous experience rather than struggle all over again.

KEEP THE PAPERWORK ASPECT OF YOUR WORK ORGANISED

Keeping the paperwork side of your job organised will make you feel as if you have more control over your work. Your aim is to complete as much work as possible in your 7.5-hour day, then when you go home you have earned the right to relax and do your own thing with your family and friends. The important thing is to have the time out of work for you. 'You work to live, not live to work.'

ACTION POINTS

- Define your workload and liaise with your manager to review it if you find that your commitments add up to more that 150 hours per month.
- Organise your office space and write everything you need to do on one 'to-do' list.
- Reprioritise your 'to-do' list each day.
- Book all your annual leave for the coming year. Try not to leave more than three months between each one.
- Allocate a set time each day to deal with your emails and post, ensuring that someone has proxy access to deal with them in your absence.
- When doing office work, ensure that you are not interrupted and keep your staff informed about the work you are doing.
- Do not bother to read all documents. Scan or speed-read them.
- Cut out all unnecessary meetings that do not benefit you, the team or your patients.
- When delegating work, ensure it is always a learning opportunity. Make sure your staff do the same.
- From now on, always make sure you under-promise and over-deliver.

EXAMPLE OF TERMS OF REFERENCE FOR A MEETING

Delayed discharge meetings

Terms of reference

Purpose:

To reduce the number of delayed discharges by making improvements to the overall patient discharge process.

Terms:

- Members of the meeting include the following list. Those who cannot attend are required to send an appropriate representative from their area.
- If a member misses more than three meetings in a row, the group will automatically assume that person has resigned.
- Agenda items to be with the secretary five days before the meeting date.
- Meetings will be held on the first and third Monday of each month, starting promptly at 2 pm and finishing at 3.30 pm.
- Latecomers will be expected to enter quietly and not attempt to interrupt the group by making apologies. The meeting will not be interrupted to update latecomers.
- Anyone who needs to leave early must make this known before the meeting starts.
- The first agenda item is to collate any other business (AOB), which is for emergency or short information items. The only points allowed under AOB will be those that were raised and agreed at the start.
- The second agenda item will always be to check the progress of action points from the previous meeting.

CHAPTER 3

CREATE A POSITIVE WORKING ENVIRONMENT

Have a plan 46

Team objectives 47

Communicate effectively 47

Know your team well 47

Set meaningful objectives with your team 48

Finding out what your team wants 48

Developing a team action plan 49

Be a good listener 49

Do you focus on understanding what people are saying? 50

Feedback with sincerity 51

Thanking staff at the end of the shift 51

Use general feedback as an opportunity for others to learn 51

People receive feedback even if you do not give it 52

Know your staff well 52

Focus on strengths not weaknesses 53

Devote equal time to every member of your team 53

Be involved in all appraisals 53

Never talk disapprovingly of others 54

Your manager(s) 54

Talking about others achieves little 54

Look for the positive in others 55

Get your staff to take more responsibility 55

Allow your staff to do more for their allocated patients 56

Have a system for dealing with patients' visitors 56

Make your ward welcoming 56

First impressions always count 57

Be careful with patient confidentiality 57

Deal with conflict 58

Disciplinary action 58

Don't allow disagreements to get out of hand 58

Bullying or harassment 59

Not all conflict is detrimental 59

Implement clinical supervision 59

Why have clinical supervision? 59

All your staff should have access to someone more experienced 59

Clinical supervision courses 60

What motivates a person to come to work? The answer is obvious; money. There are very few jobs where people would turn up for work if they were not being paid. However, what motivates a person to do well and want to achieve more when they are at work? More money perhaps! But people who enter the caring professions have not done so to earn lots of money. (If they have, it was rather a foolish decision!) They have entered the profession for a different reason; to be able to make a difference to people's lives. So why have so many become so demotivated? The answer is easy. They feel less able to make that difference in people's lives.

Poor leadership leaves teams feeling low in their ability to achieve anything. Work is unsatisfying and frustrating. When individuals feel unempowered, they tend to lose confidence in themselves and lack self-esteem. Much of the psychological research and theory shows that increasing people's self-worth and confidence in achieving things at work are great motivators. Teams rarely motivate themselves. They need good strong leadership. As their manager, what you need is a plan . . .

HAVE A PLAN

Any group of health professionals working together can be described as a team. However, to be able to work together effectively and make the most of each other's skills, they need to be motivated. Your job is to create a motivating environment to enable your team to flourish. Take a good look at your team now:

1. Are there any problems with lateness and/or sickness?
2. Are any of your staff displaying inappropriate or unprofessional behaviour (e.g. flouting the uniform policy, sloppiness, defensiveness or uncaring attitude)?
3. Are there problems with some members of the team who don't get on?
4. Are there individuals who persistently moan about things?
5. Are problems continually being discussed without any effective action ever taken?
6. Are they not particularly bothered about what is going on elsewhere in the organisation?
7. Have any cliques formed within the team?

If you answered yes to any of the above questions, then action is needed to transform your working environment into a more healthy and motivated one. Inappropriate behaviour tends to proliferate in poor working environments.

Tackling individuals about these problems will not make much difference unless you set objectives with your team, communicate effectively and ensure you know each and every individual in your team well. These three elements are mentioned in most leadership and management textbooks, but tend to be submerged in various models, theories and jargon.

TEAM OBJECTIVES

What are your team's aspirations? What do your staff want your ward to look like this time next year? You probably know what you want and where you are heading, but have you any idea what your team want? Have you sat down with them all and asked them?

Some ward managers will say how they share their vision and goals with their team and keep them fully informed. This is a very 'top down' transactional approach. It would be far better to work with your team and establish some clear goals about what you want to aim for together. You may think that your main aim is to ensure patients get good quality care with proper discharge planning, but the main aim of your team could be simply to get home on time and stop having to stay late after each shift to get the evaluations done. This is not going to make for effective team working. For a team to cooperate with each other and work hard, you need to know and agree what your priorities are.

COMMUNICATE EFFECTIVELY

Some think that being an effective communicator is to keep the team fully informed through regular meetings and perhaps using a communication book, which staff have to sign to prove they have read it (and to cover themselves from staff saying 'no-one told me'). This is effective information-giving, not effective communication. Effective communication should be two-way and that involves really hearing what others have to say and giving feedback.

Spend time listening to what your staff have to say. This sounds easy but it isn't. People tend to take the easy way out and give advice, opinions or relate a similar experience of their own and say what they did. It's a way of getting out of having to really listen to what they have to say.

In addition to listening effectively, try and ensure that everyone receives regular feedback on how they are doing. Tell your staff when they have done something well and when they have not. It does not take as much time as listening but reaps massive rewards in terms of staff performance.

KNOW YOUR TEAM WELL

Once you know the individuals in your team, you can enable them to work on their strengths and to be aware of each other's weaknesses. Try not to focus on improving a person's weaknesses unless it involves clinical competencies that need to be met. Focus on their strengths; that way they can only get better. Everyone has different strengths they can contribute to their team.

Focus on these three issues

Make it your personal plan from now on to focus on the above three issues. Don't waste your energy on motivating individual staff. It takes up too much time and energy to motivate each individual and will rarely work if you do not have a motivating environment. Focus instead on creating a positive working environment, which is the essence of being a good leader.

SET MEANINGFUL OBJECTIVES WITH YOUR TEAM

Some managers have spent many hours with their staff facilitating discussions about their values and beliefs. From these, they would produce a written mission statement or ward philosophy. It used to be the 'fashionable' thing to do. The ward philosophy would then be laminated and put up on the wall at the entrance to the ward. Did anyone ever read these woolly statements? Most staff have far better things to do.

However, your team do need to work towards some common goals or objectives in order to be able to work well together and work hard. These objectives should reflect their views on what constitutes a good working environment, and ultimately good patient care.

FINDING OUT WHAT YOUR TEAM WANTS

It is a good idea to set objectives each year with the team. Ideally, it would be nice to get all the team together at once, but impossible when you have to cover a ward 24 hours a day, seven days a week. So conduct two separate meetings with half the team attending the first one and half attending the second one. It is important that every single one of your staff is involved, so even three or four meetings may be necessary to allow for sickness, annual leave and emergencies.

At each meeting, ask your staff where they all want to be as a team in a year's time. Ask them which aspects of work they are dissatisfied with and what would they want to change. Values and beliefs will automatically be discussed and debated as your team aim to clarify what their mutual goals are. Remember to really listen to what they are saying and try not to impose your views. You may get a list looking something like the following:

- to get off work on time each shift
- to have enough pillows for all the patients
- to reduce the paperwork required on admission
- to stop being hassled by matron and bed manager about the bed state
- to know more about what is going on in the rest of the organisation
- to get more staff on the team
- to have food available when patients return from surgery or get cancelled
- to be able to get proper breaks off the ward at night.

Be careful to make sure the goals are congruent with the organisational goals. If, for example, your team would like to set up a postdischarge telephone helpline for patients and it is not part of your organisation's contract with the purchaser, then it cannot be part of your yearly objectives (although it could be an objective to add to the business plan next year).

You may prefer to start your meeting by getting the group to brainstorm ideas about what they want. Write each point up on a whiteboard or flipchart, then discuss and agree which are the top three to four priorities. Or you could ask everyone to identify his or her own personal three priorities and get each one of them to put a mark against each of their three priorities on the whiteboard or flipchart. Once everyone has done this, you should be able to see at a glance what the team's top priorities are, i.e. the main three to four points with most marks against them.

DEVELOPING A TEAM ACTION PLAN

Once the main objectives have been agreed, your next step is to agree actions to achieve them. If, for example, the team's main objective was to get off work on time at the end of each shift, possible actions could include:

- reviewing the handover system to make it shorter, e.g. taped handover
- giving health care assistants (HCAs) more training to take on extra roles
- changing the times when routine work is undertaken
- reviewing the system of organising patient care.

Make sure that the meeting is solution-focused, not problem-focused. If you allow the team to focus on the problem, discussions tend to go around in circles and can easily devolve into whinging sessions. By looking at possible solutions, you are focusing their minds on what they can do, not what they can't.

Ensure the actions are SMART, i.e. Specific, Measurable, Achievable, Realistic and have a Timetable. The final agreed action plan should then be reviewed regularly with the team together. Some of the objectives can even be incorporated into induction programmes and performance appraisals.

Having a set vision of where you and your team want to be in a year's time is crucial to effective team working. It is an essential but frequently overlooked part of good leadership.

BE A GOOD LISTENER

Few health care professionals have had specific training in listening skills. Most will be familiar with the skills of active listening such as paraphrasing. It's usually pretty obvious when someone is using a specific technique. Sometimes rather than getting someone to talk, it can end up achieving quite the opposite. People may think they are being manipulated. Staff need to be sure that you really empathise with what they are saying.

DO YOU FOCUS ON UNDERSTANDING WHAT PEOPLE ARE SAYING?

Sometimes when listening to others we do not really hear what they are saying. While the person is speaking, we tend to:

- think about a similar experience that we have had ourselves
- try to see things from our own point of view
- think of answers or suggestions.

We then spend time relating our own similar experience, telling them our opinion or giving advice based on what we think is going on. In essence, we have not really listened to them at all. Take a look at the following example of a conversation between a staff nurse and ward manager:

> 'Sister, can I have a word with you? I'm having a problem with the porters. They are being a real pain at the moment. They are reluctant to take our patients to x-ray. The x-ray porter is on long-term sick leave and they say they are not x-ray porters.'
> 'I've had this problem before. I called the head porter and he sorted it. Try him and see what happens.'
>
> One week later:
> 'I called the head porter last week like you said, and he said he would speak to them, but nothing seems to have changed. They still won't listen to me.'
> 'I think they are just being obstructive. Leave it to me, I'll go and speak to them.'

You probably recognise these types of responses. The ward manager is well intended, but is basically interpreting what the staff nurse is saying and giving advice based on her own previous experience ('I've had this problem before') and opinions ('I think they are just being obstructive'). She has not really listened so cannot really understand what the issue is. Now consider the following scenario:

> 'Sister, can I have a word with you? I'm having a problem with the porters. They are being a real pain at the moment. They are reluctant to take our patients to x-ray. The x-ray porter is on long-term sick leave and they say they are not x-ray porters.'
> 'You sound really frustrated.'
> 'Yes I am. I've tried talking to them but they just ignore me. I'm not sure if I'm going about it the right way.'
> 'How do you mean?'
> 'Well, I do have a tendency to apologise every time I call them. I feel as though I'm asking them to do me a personal favour, but it is their job.'
> 'You mean perhaps you are asking them too nicely?'
> 'Yes, I suppose I am really. Perhaps I should be just a bit more assertive and direct when I call them, rather than beginning with an apology.'
> 'That might be an idea. Is there anything you would like me to do?'
> 'No, not yet. I'll try and be a bit more direct from now on when I call them to transfer my patients. If it doesn't work, I'll let you know.'

By spending just a little more time trying to understand what the staff nurse is saying, the ward manager has been able to find what the real issue is. Giving advice won't help matters unless you find out what the problem really is. It only clears up what appears on the surface. In the first scenario, the staff nurse would have been left frustrated and probably with reduced confidence. Before being given a chance to go through the issue, the ward manager is taking the issue off her hands and dealing with it herself. If the staff nurse had a problem with assertiveness, the first approach would only serve to exacerbate that problem.

Try and spend just a little more time listening to your staff. It will not only help you to really understand the problem, but also, when given the opportunity to explain things staff will often come up with the answers themselves during the process. By really listening, you are being both influential and transformational.

FEEDBACK WITH SINCERITY

THANKING STAFF AT THE END OF THE SHIFT

Some managers will say they always thank their staff at the end of each shift, but giving out a general thank you to everyone is not particularly sincere. What is it specifically that they have done which you are thankful for? Giving general thanks is not genuine praise. It will not improve people's performance. It simply acknowledges their presence. One might as well be saying 'Thank you for turning up today!'. General praise can be rather patronising. The manager is saying that everyone has done well but what about the one or two who have not? There will always be some people who have worked harder than others. They have not been genuinely appreciated. They will feel that their hard work has obviously gone unnoticed if those who did not work so hard are included in the general praise.

Be genuine

People need genuine feedback to know what they are doing well and which areas need to be improved. And they should not have to wait until their appraisal to find this out. Make it an aim to provide some sort of feedback to each member of your team on a daily basis. If a member of your staff spotted a patient deteriorating and took corrective action, for example, then tell them, 'Well done. I'm impressed with the way you handled that. You did well to lay the patient flat immediately and increase the fluids before calling the SHO'.

If you give feedback like this, your staff will know what they did well and ensure they do it next time. Just saying 'well done' generates very little in terms of improving performance.

USE GENERAL FEEDBACK AS AN OPPORTUNITY FOR OTHERS TO LEARN

Try to ensure you give positive feedback in front of others. It not only makes the person feel good, it helps the rest of the team to improve their performance too. They are learning what they should be doing themselves in such circumstances.

You also need to ensure members of your staff know when they have not done so well. But never criticise! You want to keep your staff motivated. Always remember the golden rule: With any feedback, whether negative or positive, the person receiving it must leave you feeling good about themselves.

Negative feedback

Treat negative feedback as an area for improvement but make sure it is sandwiched within lots of positive feedback. For example, 'Well done. You did well to lay the patient flat immediately and increase the fluids before calling the SHO. It might be worth remembering next time to ensure you chart the observations before calling him, but I am impressed with the overall way you handled the situation'.

The person receiving such feedback will make a mental note to chart the observations down in future but the most important thing is that their self-esteem remains intact.

It's your role as a leader to increase the confidence and self-esteem of each and every member of your team. They will end up a lot more motivated. You know yourself how good you feel when you receive constructive feedback. When giving any type of negative feedback, make sure that:

1. *You are objective, never subjective.* In other words, stick to the facts and leave out any personal opinions. Saying, for example, 'You don't seem to be prioritising your work as well as you could be' will be far more effective and less damaging than saying: 'Your work is sloppy and unprofessional'.
2. *You listen carefully and try to enable the person to come to their own conclusion about what they can do to improve.* You can give them information and share ideas but if you get them to think of the answer, they will be more likely to put this into action.

PEOPLE RECEIVE FEEDBACK EVEN IF YOU DO NOT GIVE IT

If you do not give regular feedback, your staff will be left to guess what you are thinking. They will note your body language, listen to gossip or look to others less experienced for feedback, which may not be appropriate. Be proactive and make sure all feedback is given in a positive manner.

KNOW YOUR STAFF WELL

Aim to have an individual knowledge of each and every member of your team that you work with and directly supervise. Recognise the strengths each person brings to the team. If there is someone in your team who is really popular and networks well, for example, ensure that person represents your team on important groups within your organisation. They can tell everyone about the good practice on your ward and at the same time bring relevant information back to your team. It does not just have to be you or your deputy who attend meetings. Use the talents of others to the team's advantage.

FOCUS ON STRENGTHS NOT WEAKNESSES

If you enable the individuals in your team to develop their strengths, you will consistently improve the whole team. Focusing on a person's weaknesses only serves to demoralise and reduce self-esteem. Some say that weaknesses should be seen as 'areas for improvement'. However, if you put too much focus on improving weaknesses, a person's strengths may not be used to their full potential. Their strengths become weaker, and their weaknesses become stronger. The result is that the person becomes average. You end up with a team of nurses turning out average work. Work on the individual strengths within the team and you will have a better than average team.

DEVOTE EQUAL TIME TO EVERY MEMBER OF YOUR TEAM

Try and treat each of your staff fairly. When you first become a manager, you may notice that your staff fall into one of two groups. The first group are those that are naturally enthusiastic and motivated. They are generally ambitious, love their job and want to get on. Staff that fall into the second group are those that fulfil the basic requirements of their job but are unwilling to take on any additional responsibilities or get involved in any new initiatives.

It is easy to fall into the trap of devoting more time and effort to staff in the first group. These people want to get on so you naturally feel they deserve more of your attention. You could not be more wrong. If you do this, you run the risk of creating resentment and ultimately you are discriminating against the other members of your team. It is advisable to ensure that all receive an equal share of your time and resources.

In the same way, try to ensure that you do not personally put extra time and effort into helping a member of your staff who needs additional education and supervision. Allocate one of your senior staff to assist. Doing it yourself will only take your attention away from the rest of the team. You may be the most skilled and experienced member of the team but it does not mean that you are the only one who can deal with problems. Your role is to empower others to do so. That way, you will ensure that they become more skilled and experienced.

BE INVOLVED IN ALL APPRAISALS

Make sure you are involved and sign off all performance appraisals for your team. This does not mean you have to do them all. That would not be a good use of your time. You just need to make sure that you are continuously aware of where your staff are heading in terms of career development and where their strengths and weaknesses lie.

The development needs of your staff are paramount. Sending them away on courses is a very small part of their development. Being aware of their needs and strengths will ensure that you are able to build on them on a day-to-day basis during the working shift.

NEVER TALK DISAPPROVINGLY OF OTHERS

It doesn't matter how much someone frustrates, annoys or upsets you, try not to let your team see this. They will not respect you for talking about others in such a manner. Losing the respect of your team will make your job a lot harder than it already is.

YOUR MANAGER(S)

Be careful about using the term, 'The management'. You are part of 'The management'. You shouldn't create the impression that it is 'us and them'. If you say things like 'I can't let you do that because the management won't let me', you create the impression that you are weak and have no influence.

If you feel your own line manager is not particularly good at their job, keep that frustration to yourself. Your team need to feel confident in you and the rest of the organisation. They need to feel that you are influential and that together, you and the organisation have their best interests at heart. Work it through with your mentor if you just feel the need to moan and whinge about any managers. Talk to your spouse, partner or friends with no professional connections. Just keep it out of the work environment. The informal 'grapevine' in large public organisations means that very little remains confidential for long.

TALKING ABOUT OTHERS ACHIEVES LITTLE

You will always have colleagues, managers and even friends who do not do their jobs properly, behave in ways you don't like, or are unable to manage their priorities, thereby creating more work or problems for you. That's life! But moaning about it is not going to make life any better. It achieves nothing. If you find yourself moaning about others, make yourself stop and think, 'What can I do about it?'. Then take action. If you can't think of an answer, then don't moan. It's a waste of your precious time. People see those that moan and whinge as idle and petty. It gives the impression that they do not have enough work to do. That is not the impression you want to create.

It is also a cardinal sin to talk about a member of your staff with another, either in confidence or in front of others. If any members of your team hear you making disparaging remarks about one of their colleagues, all they will think is 'What is being said about me when my back is turned?'. You risk losing their trust in you.

LOOK FOR THE POSITIVE IN OTHERS

Make it your mission to always see the positive in people. Don't dwell on the negatives. If you hear members of your team talking negatively about their colleague, either:

1. *Turn the conversation around by mentioning the individual's positive aspects.* It usually has the effect of making the negative talker feel guilty and they tend to stop, or
2. *Ask them, 'Have you told x how you feel?'.* More often than not, they will not have done so, and again it will usually stop the moaning. They will understand that what you are really saying is, 'If you can't tell this person to their face, then it's not very nice to talk about it behind their back, is it?' but in a nice kind of way!

As their leader, you are your team's role model. If you are consistent in your manner and are never seen to moan or talk disapprovingly of others, your team will take note and follow in your footsteps.

GET YOUR STAFF TO TAKE MORE RESPONSIBILITY

Empowering staff is not as easy as it sounds. You have to be very confident in the skills of your team. It means that you can no longer have full knowledge of what is going on. When you have overall 24-hour responsibility for the welfare of the patients on your ward, it is difficult to devolve responsibility to others. But in order to allow the individuals to flourish in your team, you have to let them learn from their experience, including their mistakes. There are still some wards where the nurse-in-charge has a list of things to do for the patients, such as:

● following up the consultant ward round
● calling up the social worker to sort out some delayed discharges
● ensuring wound swabs/urine samples are taken
● ensuring preoperative patients are all prepared for theatre.

This is a very top-down approach. The nurses who have been allocated their patients, either through patient allocation, team nursing or primary nursing should be wholly responsible for everything to do with their patient on that shift. If a patient's discharge needs sorting it should be by them and nobody else. The role of the nurse-in-charge is to assist them should they need it. If there are things to be sorted from ward rounds, for example, it is the patient's nurse who should be dealing with these things, not the nurse-in-charge.

'Nurses only have time to do the basic care'

Some managers say their nurses don't have the time to sort out things like the patient's discharge because they need the time to care for the patient. However, sorting out things like social work referrals, discharge arrangements or implementing changes from the ward round is all part of caring for the patient. Spending the shift undertaking delegated nursing tasks rather than having responsibility for total patient care is very unsatisfying. Doing it day in and day out is boring and will produce apathy in your staff. In this case, care is not patient-centred. It is centred with the nurse-in-charge.

ALLOW YOUR STAFF TO DO MORE FOR THEIR ALLOCATED PATIENTS

Giving full responsibility for all aspects of the patient's care is the only way your staff will learn and develop. It is also highly satisfying and motivating to be totally in charge of all care for a group of patients.

The role of the nurse-in-charge should be to support and coordinate the team, not take over or delegate parts of the care. Staff who are given full responsibility for a group of patients are far more satisfied in their work than those who are expected to carry out only the basic nursing tasks for their patients. The latter is not team nursing or patient allocation, it is task allocation, and is very demotivating. But you have to trust your staff and that is not easy. You have to trust that they will sort out the patient's discharge arrangements, take that urgent wound swab, speak to the relatives, etc. You also have to support them when they make mistakes. The key is to ensure you support them to learn from their mistakes and for you or the nurse-in-charge to be available and help out when needed. Your staff are more likely to develop and flourish in such an environment.

HAVE A SYSTEM FOR DEALING WITH PATIENTS' VISITORS

Being the relative of a patient is an incredibly anxious and stressful experience. To leave your loved one in such a vulnerable state in the hands of strangers in a strange environment is not easy. But to enter that environment and see one or two nurses rushing around looking hassled and overworked does not inspire one's confidence. Worse still, having to wait for ages to grab someone's attention only to get answers like 'sorry, she's not my patient' or 'I've just come back after days off' or 'he hasn't had his bath/wound dressed/drip changed because we are too short staffed' is not very encouraging. And people wonder why relatives get so angry and demanding!

MAKE YOUR WARD WELCOMING

Hospitals are unfamiliar environments to most people. Entering a ward can be an unnerving experience. Few wards indicate where visitors should go or to whom they should speak. Nerves are easily frayed and tempers easily lost. You do not want to expose your staff to any unnecessary abuse or harassment.

Don't blame the relatives; firstly look at your environment. Imagine being a stranger entering the ward. Is it indicated clearly where you should go and to whom you should speak to?

You may have an information/photo board at the entrance to the ward, showing who your staff are, what their uniforms mean and perhaps even how they are split into smaller teams. But is it clear which nurses are looking after which patients? If you have divided your staff into two teams such as red and blue, which are the red and blue beds? How can the relatives match the two? Do you have boards by the beds indicating which nurses are looking after the patients that day? If you don't, relatives will continually ask, causing unnecessary interruptions for your staff. If you make as much information as possible available at a glance, it will serve much to appease your visitors.

FIRST IMPRESSIONS ALWAYS COUNT

You want the visitors to be content that your ward is well run and their relative is in safe hands. Despite the advent of primary nursing, team nursing and increased responsibility of staff nurses, relatives still see the ward manager, sister or charge nurse, as the one who should know everything. It's advisable to ensure that the nurse-in-charge is available at visiting times. It saves so much angst. If they ensure they are around to talk to visitors and answer any queries, it will reassure people that they are in control of their work and do not look like they cannot manage the demands. You need to give the impression and reassurance that the patients on your ward are in safe hands.

Obviously times have changed and you cannot know everything about every patient on your ward. The turnover of patients is too fast nowadays. However, you should know the basic details such as the patient's name and why they are in hospital. Refer them to the appropriate nurse looking after the patient if further information is required. If the member of staff looking after the patient is an inexperienced nurse or an HCA, then stay and support them in giving the information.

BE CAREFUL WITH PATIENT CONFIDENTIALITY

Care plans and evaluations left at the end of patients' beds are left open to the perusal of visitors. If possible try and leave them with the patient at the head of the bed or in their locker. Keep all records behind the reception desk if the patient is not in a position to keep them confidential, e.g. confused patients or those just returned from surgery.

Use your common sense with regards to the Data Protection Act. There is little wrong with patient name boards at the head or end of the bed. The risk of not having one is far too great in terms of mixing up patients' treatments. Just don't add the little extras like 'diabetic' for everyone to see. That would be breaking patient confidentiality.

DEAL WITH CONFLICT

No matter how happy or motivating you make the working environment, you will always come up against difficult people and difficult situations. Never ignore these situations or you will allow them to blow up out of all proportion.

Whatever preventative steps you take, arguments may still occur between visiting relatives, health professionals and within your own team. The main rule is to take the argument away from the patients. If you catch staff or doctors having arguments or heated discussions in front of patients, take them elsewhere immediately and explain that the behaviour will not be tolerated on your ward. Support your staff in doing the same thing. They also need to gain the skills in dealing with conflict and not shy away from it.

DISCIPLINARY ACTION

Make sure you know your organisation's disciplinary policy. This outlines what constitutes unacceptable behaviour and the steps to take when such behaviour is displayed (see Ch. 4). Don't threaten disciplinary action. Disciplinary action can only be taken after a formal investigation.

If someone's behaviour is unacceptable under the terms of the disciplinary policy, seek advice from your human resources (HR) department about instigating a formal investigation. It is advisable to ensure you are familiar with what sorts of behaviour are not acceptable according to your organisation's policy. As the manager, you will have to make instant decisions in such situations. It is best to make sure that you have the appropriate knowledge to do so.

DON'T ALLOW DISAGREEMENTS TO GET OUT OF HAND

There are still wards and departments in which some health professionals within a team do not speak to each other or don't get on. Allowing these situations to continue has major knock-on effects:

1. It reflects badly on the ward manager who has allowed it to get out of hand.
2. It has a detrimental effect on the rest of the team who end up having to take sides.
3. It affects the standards of patient care because people are not working together.

Don't allow it to happen on your ward. If you have a situation like this and feel unable to handle it, get help. Don't bury your head in the sand. You must do something about it. Not only that, you must be seen to do something about it. No team will respect a leader who cannot handle conflict. If you do not feel you have the skills, find someone who does and get them to support you through the process.

BULLYING OR HARASSMENT

If any of your staff are bullying or harassing others, you must also take action. It should not be tolerated under any circumstances. If you have a situation where someone like the bed manager or a consultant is behaving aggressively towards your staff, it is your duty to protect them. Consult your bullying and harassment policy and involve HR right from the beginning.

It is usually advisable in the first instance to help and support the individual to deal with the situation themselves. If you take over immediately, it may only serve to reduce their self-esteem even further. To be able to confront someone who is bullying or harassing them with your full support may give the individual a greater sense of satisfaction and self-worth. If it does not work, at least they will know they have tried.

NOT ALL CONFLICT IS DETRIMENTAL

Conflict at work is not always such a bad thing. In fact, if everyone insisted on smoothing things over and continually compromising their work in order to avoid causing fuss or arguments, things might never change. Maintaining the status quo is not always the best option. Encouraging people to speak up and confront people or situations that may be harmful for the patients should be encouraged. However, it's imperative to ensure your staff have the skills to do so (see Chs 12 and 13).

IMPLEMENT CLINICAL SUPERVISION

WHY HAVE CLINICAL SUPERVISION?

Nursing care and clinical treatments are continually changing and being updated. Unfortunately, getting a diploma or degree does not give nurses skills for life. A lot of nursing skills can only be gained through experience. Skills such as dealing with bereaved relatives, counselling a person prior to disfiguring surgery or teaching a newly diagnosed diabetic how to give their own injections can only be perfected through practice. But they can only be perfected if the nurse has someone more experienced to help them reflect on their current practice.

ALL YOUR STAFF SHOULD HAVE ACCESS TO SOMEONE MORE EXPERIENCED

In an ideal world, a clinical teacher would be available at all times on the ward to work with individual staff to give advice, guidance and support, and ensure that they reflect and learn from their daily work. However, this is not an ideal world, so the next best thing is to ensure all your staff have access to a more experienced member of staff whom they can learn from. It doesn't matter what you call it – mentorship, coaching, facilitation or clinical supervision. Some nurses become too focused on definitions about what clinical supervision is or isn't and what the different models are. Does it matter? In essence, all members of your team should have access to a more experienced member of staff regularly to help them reflect and learn from their everyday experiences.

The most obvious and inexpensive way to do this is ensure that each junior staff nurse is matched up with a more experienced senior staff nurse, *who is not a direct assessor or allocated to do their performance appraisal.* If the junior member thinks that what they are going to say may influence their performance appraisal, they may be reluctant to be open about their practice.

If you operate team nursing, it might be worth considering allocating each junior nurse a more senior nurse from the opposite team. That way at least there will be more chance of the two of them working the same shifts.

One-to-one or group supervision?

One-to-one clinical supervision is ideal but expensive. If you are allowing an hour per month for each individual member of your staff to have clinical supervision, it can prove to be very costly unless they can find time during the shift to go off somewhere quiet for an hour. A less expensive way of ensuring your staff are learning from their experiences is through facilitated group supervision, in other words, having someone to facilitate a small group of staff to reflect and learn from their experiences together. Even if the group just go through one issue from one member of the group, the whole group are reflecting and learning from their colleague's experience.

CLINICAL SUPERVISION COURSES

Whether you decide on one-to-one or group supervision, you will need to ensure that the senior members of your team have the appropriate facilitation skills to help others to reflect and learn from their practice. Most organisations offer short courses on this type of training. It's well worth the investment.

As health care professionals your staff have a duty to continually update themselves by reflecting and learning from their experience. As their manager, you have a duty to provide the right conditions for doing so.

ACTION POINTS

- Use your next few team meetings or arrange a couple of away-days to identify your priorities as a team and agree specific team goals to achieve over the coming year.
- From now on, each time a member of staff comes to you with a concern, take time to really listen before giving advice.
- Give some specific feedback to each member of staff that works with you on your shift. Do this every shift.
- Each time you find yourself moaning or whinging about something or someone, stop yourself and concentrate on finding a solution to the problem.
- Consider how your team are allocating patients. Are all staff being given the opportunity to have full responsibility for their patients?
- Put up an information board for visitors at the entrance to the ward or review the one you have to ensure it is clear where to go and who to see.
- Read your local disciplinary policy to ensure you are familiar with what your organisation defines as unacceptable behaviour.
- Find out what training is available for the senior members of your staff to develop their clinical supervision skills.

CHAPTER 4

MANAGE AND TREAT YOUR STAFF WELL

Get to know your HR advisor 64

Arrange regular meetings 64

Learning from experience 65

Involve HR at the informal stage 65

Get to know each other's teams 65

Write everything down 66

Keep file notes 66

Keep meeting notes 67

Keep a communication book or folder 67

Make appraisals work 67

Why do we need appraisals? 67

Why some people don't like appraisals 68

Formalising what is already known 68

Five steps for a successful appraisal 68

Adapt the form to the appraisal, not the appraisal to the form 69

Know how to handle unacceptable behaviour 69

Guidelines for carrying out the first meeting 70

Don't allow the behaviour to continue 71

Deal with poor performance 71

What exactly is incompetence? 71

Procedure for incompetence 71

Know when and how to discipline 72

Minor breaches of conduct 72

Major breaches of conduct 72

Actively manage sick leave 73

Fit for return to work after short-term sick leave? 74

Deal with long-term sick leave 75

Dealing with unauthorised absence 76

Ensure all staff have appropriate training, development and support 76

Induction 76

Ward-based teaching 76

Mandatory learning requirements 77

Learning from experience 77

Link lecturer 78

Inform and involve your team 78

Information from meetings 78

Involvement in making
decisions 79

Business planning and
recruitment 79

Planning the team's study
leave 79

Investigating complaints 80

**Implement
self-rostering 80**

Self-rostering is easier in small
teams 80

Advantages of
self-rostering 81

Set 'off-duties' 81

Managing staff is an important part of the ward manager's role. It entails keeping them informed, involved and empowered to make decisions for themselves. It also includes dealing with inappropriate or unacceptable behaviour from individuals. Unacceptable behaviour is any behaviour that disrupts your team and/or is detrimental to the welfare of the patients. It also includes behaviour that is unlawful or unethical.

Any inappropriate behaviour that disrupts others should be 'nipped in the bud'. Allowing it to continue would affect staff morale. You owe it to the rest of the team to deal with any individual behavioural issues swiftly and proactively. Don't bury your head in the sand. Don't blame others, e.g. 'human resources told me I couldn't do that!'. Know your policies and know how to use them, and most of all, involve the human resources (HR) team as early as possible.

GET TO KNOW YOUR HR ADVISOR

Good staff management is of such great importance to health care organisations that each deploys an entire HR department to ensure that their staff are managed and treated appropriately.

Managing staff is a skill that is mainly learned through experience, but you do have an allocated HR advisor who is there to help and guide you. Part of their role is to make sure you adhere to your organisation's policies and procedures which set out how your staff are expected to behave. These policies and procedures also outline the steps you should take when staff behaviour becomes unacceptable.

ARRANGE REGULAR MEETINGS

It is wise to build up a professional relationship with your HR advisor right from the start, rather than wait until you need them to help you sort out a problem. Meet them regularly, once a month or so, to go through any issues and potential problems, and to keep them up-to-date with how your team are getting on. They will become familiar with how you run your ward and the sorts of problems you are dealing with on a day-to-day basis. If you have to deal with a major disciplinary matter, it is much easier to take advice from someone you know and trust rather than someone you have hardly met.

In addition, if your HR advisor is called to help deal with a staff issue whilst you are on days off or annual leave, they are more likely to be aware of the background to the problem and be able to give appropriate advice. By keeping your HR advisor informed, you can also rest assured that your senior staff will be well supported in your absence.

LEARNING FROM EXPERIENCE

Like you, most HR advisors are also learning from each new experience. If they do not have experience of a particular problem, they do have direct access to the HR director for advice and guidance. They also gain experience of issues from other departments such as disciplinary hearings, which they can share with you. Having insight into general HR issues will help you deal with future problems as and when they occur.

INVOLVE HR AT THE INFORMAL STAGE

Don't wait to inform your HR advisor of a problem until the point where you feel it needs to be dealt with on a formal basis. This is often too late. They need to be involved at the informal stage.

Most policies set out what to do at the informal stage. If you do not deal with the problem informally as set out in the appropriate policy, you will not be able to proceed to the next stage if the situation does not improve. Your HR advisor is there to support and guide you through all stages when dealing with a staff problem, not just at the final formal stages.

GET TO KNOW EACH OTHER'S TEAMS

Invite your HR advisor to help you with interviewing staff. Involve them in your team meetings where you set goals together and devise action plans to deal with ward issues. They will note how you are leading your team and share your good practice with their colleagues. It will help increase the profile of your ward within the organisation.

When you do meet your HR advisor, try and make sure you go to see them in their department rather than have them come to see you all the time. You will become familiar with how the HR department works and who are the major people to know, including the reception staff. It helps to know who does what and to be able to greet them on first name terms. This improves access when you really need them. It also helps you to know the different skills and attributes everyone has in the team. You can then contact them directly for help rather than just to blindly phone the HR department.

WRITE EVERYTHING DOWN

KEEP FILE NOTES

Try and get into the habit of keeping brief notes of face-to-face meetings or phone conversations and file them away (preferably on your computer to save space in your filing cabinet). This saves so much time in the future when trying to recall what was said, where and when. Keeping notes before incidents happen will also help enormously. It is too late afterwards to remember that you had several conversations with a person who denies that you mentioned something. If you kept file notes, they will aid you in remembering what was said and when, rather than hazy details.

The file notes can be kept either in the person's personal file or a file of your own. They can help months or even years later when an incident involving a member of your staff occurs and you are asked if it was a problem earlier.

Don't focus on negative events

Don't just note negative things that may be useful if an incident occurs subsequently. It is also helpful to make file notes whenever a member of staff does something positive and is praised for doing so. All the file notes you keep about staff will be a useful aid when you come to doing their appraisal as well as any future references.

File notes save time

It can be difficult to fit the writing of file notes into a busy schedule but once you get into the habit you will find that they save you time. Keep notes throughout your day. Make a file note of any meetings you have had either with staff as a group or in one-to-one meetings. Keep the file notes short and to the point. Briefly note any actions agreed. These notes can prove useful as the basis for the next meeting or review of progress.

What you can and can't include in file notes

Never write down anything derogatory or subjective, and never write down anything that you can't justify or substantiate at a later date. The Data Protection Act and Freedom of Information Act give all staff certain rights to see any documents within their organisation that have their name mentioned (Information Commissioner 1998 & 2000). If you keep any notes about anyone, they should never contain anything that you would not want the person to see.

Be open and honest with your staff. Show them the file notes you make, or at least let them know that you will make a note of the conversation you have just had. The file notes enable you to:

- carry out better performance appraisals
- provide an accurate recording of events months or even years later if required
- write informed references for your staff

- provide information that would help in future decision-making
- remind you of previous events
- help you to review progress of certain behaviours or events.

KEEP MEETING NOTES

When you attend any meetings, keep brief notes and share them with your team. Leave them on the coffee table in the staff room before filing them away every few weeks. Keep notes of all your own team meetings. You do not have to keep formal minutes. Minutes of meetings can be seen as stuffy and boring. Write up some brief notes, which serve simply to keep your staff informed.

KEEP A COMMUNICATION BOOK OR FOLDER

This is an ideal way to keep your staff informed. Print off any important emails, new policies or procedures or any written communication that you receive which may affect them. Don't put in everything you have received. Your staff do not have the time or the inclination to sift through loads of papers full of jargon. Highlight any pertinent bits, particularly on minutes of meetings.

Asking your staff to sign the book when it has been read is a rather top-down approach and not a very transformational way of working. If you make sure the information is relevant to their day-to-day practice and highlight the relevant parts in any long documents, there is little chance your staff will not be motivated to read it.

MAKE APPRAISALS WORK

Don't take on too many appraisals. Some ward managers take it upon themselves to carry out appraisals on every single member of their staff. This is not appropriate and is certainly not an effective use of time. It allows little space for staff to develop their skills in this area, and is a very top-down approach. It is advisable to stick to a select few, such as:

- your deputy ward manager(s)
- one or two more experienced senior staff nurses
- the ward receptionist.

The deputy ward managers should formally appraise the senior staff nurses. The senior staff nurses should formally appraise the junior staff nurses and so on.

WHY DO WE NEED APPRAISALS?

The purpose of formal appraisals is to enhance a person's development and skills to ensure they are meeting the goals of the team and the organisation. It is not meant to be a list of the individual's personal wants and needs. You should not be agreeing personal development plans or granting courses of study that are not congruent with the goals of your team or the organisation.

The NHS is now using the knowledge and skills framework (KSF), which was brought in with the new pay banding process (Department of Health 2004). The KSF provides a set of competencies, which identify the knowledge and skills that individuals need to apply in their post. An individual's personal development plan should therefore be based on three very important documents:

1. The objectives of the organisation.
2. The objectives of your ward team.
3. The KSF assessment tool (if working within the NHS).

WHY SOME PEOPLE DON'T LIKE APPRAISALS

Some people groan when you mention performance appraisals. This is usually because they have had bad experiences of them in the past. The one thing that managers often do badly with appraisals is they take too long. If you are giving feedback to each and every one of your staff on a regular basis (see p. 51), then you should need no more than one hour to carry out a performance appraisal. If more than one hour is needed, then there is something wrong with the process. It indicates that you are not spending enough time listening to your staff or giving regular feedback in between appraisals.

FORMALISING WHAT IS ALREADY KNOWN

An appraisal is not the time for discussing anything new. It should just be a formal confirmation of what both parties already know and have discussed on previous occasions. The appraisal is the end of a continuous communication process that includes the manager giving regular feedback on the person's performance. When you give constant feedback during the year, the appraisal will be easy to do and comfortable.

Never postpone or cancel an appraisal unless absolutely necessary. It can be incredibly damaging. It gives the impression to your staff that their appraisal is not important. To them, it is very important.

FIVE STEPS FOR A SUCCESSFUL APPRAISAL

Step 1: Self-assessment by appraisee
A few weeks before the appraisal, ask the appraisee to write down what they would like to discuss and the objectives they would like to agree at appraisal. Most organisations provide a self-assessment form with questions to help stimulate their

thoughts. Make sure you let the appraisee know that their notes will be discussed with your line manager.

Step 2: Meet with your own line manager

Review the self-assessment form with your line manager to ensure the objectives are congruent with the organisation's objectives. They will also be able to give advice about where else the appraisee can go for guidance and support in meeting the objectives.

Step 3: Carry out the appraisal

Your organisation will provide a form to assist with the process. If possible, try to ensure you complete as much of the form as you can with the appraisee as part of the review rather than writing it up at a later date. It will save you a lot of time. Another good idea is to encourage the appraisee to write up the notes afterwards.

Step 4: Agree the final appraisal document

Agree the notes with both the appraisee and your line manager. All three of you should sign the final document.

Step 5: Set a date for review

Mark in next year's diary when the next appraisal review is due. You may also want to set a date half way through the year to review the person's progress towards their objectives.

ADAPT THE FORM TO THE APPRAISAL, NOT THE APPRAISAL TO THE FORM

Try not to focus too much on the actual form. It should be used as a guide. You don't have to fill in all the boxes. Adapt the form to the appraisal. Don't fall into the trap of adapting the appraisal to the form. Everyone is different and each appraisal will be different. If you focus on just filling in the form, the process becomes a waste of time. Your role is to help your staff remove the barriers to achieve success. Focusing on form-filling is not being a good role model.

KNOW HOW TO HANDLE UNACCEPTABLE BEHAVIOUR

If a person's behaviour starts affecting others in the team and reducing morale, it becomes unacceptable. You need to take action quickly.

First, identify the problem behaviour. Once you have done this you can identify which organisational policy applies to the situation. Is the person reporting in sick too late? This would be managed by referring to the sickness/absence policy. Is the person incompetent? This would be managed by the competence or capability policy (sometimes called the poor performance policy). Are they being negligent or perhaps even malicious? In this case, you would refer to the disciplinary policy. It is always wise to liaise with your HR advisor to ensure you consult the appropriate policy.

Second, make sure you address the problem behaviour early and when you are not angry. Never allow your feelings to colour your input or behaviour. If you are very angry or irritated, it is usually better to talk at a later time when you have calmed down. This makes sure that you can think and speak objectively and rationally.

Arrange to meet with the person as soon as possible. Leaving it will only add to their worry (and yours) and may cause them to become defensive and upset. Liaise with your HR advisor before the meeting to ensure the correct policy/procedure is being used, including union guidelines. Be clear about if and when you can issue verbal or written warnings.

GUIDELINES FOR CARRYING OUT THE FIRST MEETING

1. Don't set an open-ended meeting. It could go on for hours, especially if the staff member denies their behaviour is unacceptable. Set a time limit on the discussion, and stick to it.

2. Ask them to go through with you their version of the events or incidents in question. Take the time to listen. Try to see their point of view and do not be defensive.

3. Once you have listened to their version, you can then give your assessment. Refer to facts only, not opinions. Respect their right to disagree with your assessment of the situation, but remember you're the boss.

4. Keep the discussion focused on their behaviours. Don't let them blame personality or another person's actions. An example would be to say, '. . . that may be true about Jane, but we are here to discuss your behaviour and how it is impacting on the rest of the team'.

5. Summarise the discussion and the agreed actions clearly and succinctly at the end of the meeting.

6. Ensure the meeting is documented. Write up your notes in a factual, concise manner, listing the desired behaviours, policy or procedural references, and agree an action plan (including any training needs) with a clear timetable.

7. Both you and the employee must sign all documentation. Even if this is just a quick 10-minute discussion where the person agrees verbally to improve their behaviour, it must be documented.

8. Always try to end these meetings on a positive note. Remember the rules about giving feedback: positive, negative, and then positive (see p. 52).

9. It is very important to make sure you follow up the meeting. Arrange a date for review of progress. Hopefully the problem will be resolved and you will be able to give positive feedback.

DON'T ALLOW THE BEHAVIOUR TO CONTINUE

Do not allow the member of staff to continue to practise unacceptable behaviour. If it does continue, go on to the next step of the policy. If you do not, the behaviour will only continue or worsen and the rest of your team will lose respect for your management abilities. They may even adopt such inappropriate behaviour themselves having seen that one person has got away with it. 'Nip it in the bud' and you will maintain a well-balanced team who respect your ability to manage situations rather than allowing them to get out of hand.

DEAL WITH POOR PERFORMANCE

WHAT EXACTLY IS INCOMPETENCE?

Before you label a member of your staff as incompetent, first ask yourself, 'How do I know that they are incompetent?'. In other words, what criteria are you measuring them up against? Personal opinion is not sufficient. While you may think they are incompetent, another person may not.

Competence should be assessed with reference to the knowledge, skills and aptitudes required for the job you employed someone to do. In other words, you need to have very clear competencies or standards against which you can assess your team's performance. An individual cannot be deemed incompetent if:

- their job description has recently changed
- new systems or technology have been introduced
- they are newly appointed.

These are factors beyond their control and it is your job to ensure appropriate support, training and development are given to meet the appropriate competencies or standards.

Other causes of poor performance

If the person's incompetence is due to ill health, you would need to follow the steps outlined in the sickness/absence policy. If it is due to laziness, negligence or general unwillingness to carry out duties properly, then it is usually appropriate to follow the disciplinary procedures for misconduct. Always ask your HR which policy is the most appropriate for your individual situation.

PROCEDURE FOR INCOMPETENCE

Most competence or capability procedures begin with an informal stage where you are required to meet with the member of staff to clarify their role, what is expected and agree a plan with a timetable to achieve the standards. Any training or retraining needs should be established and agreed.

If this fails, progression to the formal stage is indicated. This usually consists of a formal meeting with the member of staff, often with a trade union representative and an HR representative. A further plan with a timetable is then agreed. If it fails again, a further meeting may be agreed with a further plan but this time with a warning that failure to meet the objectives could lead to dismissal.

Throughout the whole process, full consideration should be given to:

● doing everything you can to encourage improvement
● appreciating the level of improvement attained throughout the process
● identifying and dealing with any extenuating circumstances
● identifying the possibility of transferring to a different department where the skills are more matched to the role
● the overall attitude of the employee.

The capability/competency policies vary between organisations. It is wise to ensure you are familiar with your local policy before taking any steps to deal with a member of staff thought to be incompetent in their role. And remember to involve your HR advisor at the earliest possible stage. It may prevent the need for formal action.

KNOW WHEN AND HOW TO DISCIPLINE

Never take any action under the disciplinary procedure until you have sought advice from your HR advisor and your line manager.

MINOR BREACHES OF CONDUCT

Some organisations recommend in their disciplinary policy that you use a structured meeting or review in cases of minor breaches of conduct or performance. Using this approach you can give a verbal warning, and it is good practice to make a file note of the conversation and agreed outcomes. Examples of cases that you could deal with on an informal basis include:

● failure to carry out reasonable instructions
● unauthorised absence
● persistent poor timekeeping
● poor adherence to the uniform policy.

MAJOR BREACHES OF CONDUCT

The disciplinary policy is one of the few policies where often the first step is to undertake a formal investigation. This is usually undertaken by someone other than the line manager who is not directly involved in the matter. The formal disciplinary procedure may be used for incidents such as:

- physical or verbal assault
- corrupt practices such as gambling or private trading on the premises
- fraud, e.g. falsely claiming unsocial hours payments
- turning up for work drunk or under the influence of drugs
- negligent behaviour, which seriously threatens the health and safety of others
- malicious damage
- theft
- sexual or racial harassment.

Disciplinary action can only be undertaken once a formal investigation of the incident has been carried out. In some cases, the police will also need to be involved. Suspension from duty may be necessary but this is not a disciplinary action and does not imply guilt or misconduct. Its purpose would be to investigate the full circumstances of the allegation being made. Never suspend a member of staff without consulting HR and your senior manager first.

Because the nature of the incident is usually extremely serious, the disciplinary procedure does not consist of a series of meetings like most other policies. It consists of one disciplinary panel, which is brought together to consider the results of the investigation and make a final decision. The panel usually consists of the manager and an HR representative. Other people present will be the employee, their union representative and where appropriate, the investigating officer. Witnesses may be required to attend where appropriate. The outcome can be one of the following:

- an oral warning
- a first written warning
- a final written warning (if this is a repeated offence)
- a dismissal (dismissal without notice will only be used in cases of gross misconduct).

In cases of gross misconduct, the case may also be referred to the appropriate professional body for further investigation. This may result in the individual's removal from the register.

ACTIVELY MANAGE SICK LEAVE

If your team are well motivated, it is less likely that you will have continual sickness/absence problems. If you do, look first at your leadership style and if there is any way that you can improve your teamwork before dealing with the individual.

Most sickness/absence policies clearly lay out the steps that your staff should take when they are sick. This usually entails phoning you or the nurse-in-charge and informing you of:

- the nature of their illness
- when they expect to return to work
- any work issues that need to be addressed while they are away.

They are usually required to keep in touch at regular intervals and give at least a day's notice before return. You should keep a record of all contacts.

FIT FOR RETURN TO WORK AFTER SHORT-TERM SICK LEAVE?

Your job is to make sure that all staff who have been off sick are fit for work on their return and to decide if any special arrangements are needed. This means that you should see every member of staff informally on return even if only one day's sick was taken.

All details should be noted on the person's personal file. Remember that this is confidential information. As their manager, you are entitled to know about the person's sickness but the rest of the team are not. Keep all staff personal files locked away and do not divulge any information to others.

If the individual does not want you to know the nature of their illness, then it's best to ask your occupational health (OH) department to see them to determine on your behalf that they are fit to return to work.

Take action in cases of continual short episodes of absence

Organisational policies on sickness usually advise a referral to the OH team if staff have more than a certain number of absences over a certain time period; more than three episodes within six months, for example.

If you do decide to refer to the OH team, you must tell them the reason for referral. In the referral letter, state clearly what you want to know:

1. Do you want them to reassure you that the person is now fit for work?
2. Do you want to know if the sickness leave they are taking is reasonable for their condition?
3. Is the sickness liable to continue?
4. If they consider it excessive, what is a reasonable level of sickness for their condition?

Check your organisation's sickness/absence policy. It will outline the steps to take if you have a member of staff who continually takes an unacceptably high amount of sickness despite being declared fit for work by the OH department.

What further action can be taken?

The procedure usually starts with a meeting to establish the reasons and set targets. If these are not met, the next step is often a formal meeting. This meeting may result in:

● a further period of monitoring
● a further referral to the OH department
● consideration of a transfer
● a formal caution for a period of around six months.

If attendance does not improve, the next stage may lead to a final formal caution for a period of around twelve months. If the behaviour continues after this stage, many policies will then give you the final option of dismissal after a further review.

As a ward manager, you do not have the authority to terminate the employment of your staff. This responsibility lies with your own line manager whom you should fully involve at this stage.

DEAL WITH LONG-TERM SICK LEAVE

Long-term sick leave is dealt with very differently. Long-term sick leave is often defined as leave consisting of four weeks or more. There is very little you can do when a member of staff has taken long-term sick leave, but you must make sure that the OH department are fully aware and involved.

Whatever the reason, don't forget about someone who is on long-term sick leave. Keep in constant contact. If you cannot keep in contact by letter or phone, you can visit them as long as you have given them prior notice. You are still their manager and therefore have concern for their welfare.

Don't allow long-term sick leave to affect the rest of your staff

Do not just make do with bank/agency nurses day after day. Can you open up the post as a secondment for another nurse who wants to gain further experience in your specialty? Can you employ another nurse full time in their place using finances from elsewhere within your directorate? If so, speak to your manager. You could also liaise with HR to see if it is possible that this person can be employed elsewhere, such as administration, whilst unable to return to clinical duties for a while. Explore all options involving all departments. Do not cope without that member of staff and let the rest of the team suffer.

Fit for return to work after long-term sick leave?

Always involve the OH department before allowing a member of staff to return to work following long-term sick leave. A decision needs to be made in conjunction with the returning nurse and the OH department as to the terms of their return. They usually have one of four options:

1. Return to the same job as before.
2. Return to the same job but with a graduated return, i.e. part time and then full time.
3. Return to the same ward but with modified duties.
4. Return to a different job, on health grounds.

If the OH team determines that the person will be unable to return to work at all, their employment may be terminated, e.g. retirement on grounds of ill health.

DEALING WITH UNAUTHORISED ABSENCE

It is important to take immediate action in any cases of unauthorised absence. If a member of staff does not turn up for work and has made no contact at all, do everything you can to find out where they are. Get someone to physically go around to their home if necessary. Your first major concern is for their welfare. If they are fine, you can deal with it informally depending on the reason. An odd occasion of oversleeping would not warrant formal action, but it would involve a meeting with the person on return.

If you feel they were neglectful you do have the option of deducting their pay for those days in which they were absent (deducting pay is done by completing a form which you can get from your HR or finance department). In more persistent or major cases of unauthorised absence, the disciplinary procedure may be instigated.

ENSURE ALL STAFF HAVE APPROPRIATE TRAINING, DEVELOPMENT AND SUPPORT

All development needs including courses and training should be formally identified through the appraisal process. You only have a certain number of study days to allocate to your team over the year. Use them wisely.

INDUCTION

Staff induction is the most important teaching package you can have, yet one that is so often neglected. Every new staff member should have the time and opportunity to familiarise themselves with both the organisation and the workings of the ward.

There is no formal requirement as to the length of induction but it would be wise to allocate around two weeks at the beginning, during which the new person is supernumerary.

Following this, you would need some sort of package detailing the clinical competencies that need to be met. For newly qualified staff, a six-month preceptor package is ideal. Many organisations now run a central preceptorship programme. For those working in the NHS, all other competencies can be assessed using the KSF appraisal tool.

WARD-BASED TEACHING

Regular ward-based teaching sessions are a must but don't just think up subjects randomly. Use your regular meetings to assess the learning requirements of your staff. Asking staff what teaching sessions they would like is insufficient on its own. Use your regular reviews of the complaints and incidents, etc., to provide information about what your team need. Try to involve the whole team in making such decisions, not the requests of individuals.

A teaching programme devised by one or two members of staff without the full involvement of the rest of the team will not be very motivating. Few will turn up. Some external speakers such as nurse specialists find that few people turn up to their teaching sessions. This may be because they have not ascertained that staff feel it is something they need or tailored the actual session to what they say they need.

MANDATORY LEARNING REQUIREMENTS

Fitting in mandatory training is every ward manager's nightmare. The subject list is becoming huge. There are a number of things you can do to accommodate these, which include:

1. *Using the induction programme.* Fit all mandatory training requirements in the two-week induction period for all new staff. This negates the need for anything else for a whole year. It will save a lot of study leave especially if you have a fairly high turnover of staff.
2. *Asking for shorter sessions.* Work together with your ward manager colleagues and your organisation's training and development team to devise sessions that cover mandatory elements in a shorter time span. For example, there is no reason why cardiopulmonary resuscitation (CPR), manual handling and health and safety training cannot be given in three two-hour afternoon sessions or altogether on one day rather than three separate days.
3. *Using the link nurses.* Have link nurses for the mandatory training subjects where possible. Giving an individual member of staff study leave to train as a CPR trainer or manual handling trainer will negate the need for your staff to leave the ward for training. In other words, you could bring the training in-house.

LEARNING FROM EXPERIENCE

Courses and study days are not the only methods of learning. One of the best ways of learning is through experience. However, without the appropriate support and guidance systems in place, staff will not learn as much as they can from their experiences. Most people will know of someone somewhere who has had many years of experience but still does not seem to know much or do their job very well.

Your job as the ward manager is to make sure systems are in place to ensure your staff gain as much learning from their experience as possible. Make sure that every member of your team has some sort of mentor or clinical supervisor. This should be someone who is more experienced than them, but does not necessarily have to be more senior. It's up to you whether you allow individual staff to choose or whether you allocate a mentor or clinical supervisor. This more experienced person should be able to work with them or at least meet with them once a week to help them reflect and learn from their day-to-day experiences.

LINK LECTURER

Most wards have a link lecturer from their local university. Your organisation will have paid the university for this service. It's up to you to make the best use of their skills. Work closely with them and identify together how you can best utilise their time. Most should be able to work on your ward with a student or staff member for around three half shifts per 'off-duty'. Or you may prefer your link lecturer to provide clinical supervision for small groups of your staff, on a weekly or fortnightly basis.

Unless you are proactive and build up a good professional relationship with your link lecturer, you may end up receiving the bare minimum from them. Remember to give something back too. There is no reason why you or your team cannot provide input into work at the university for your link lecturer. The more helpful you are to them, the more helpful they will be in return.

Do not teach at the university just because you or individual members of your team are interested in the subject or just because you have been asked. In other words, do not allow your services to be abused. Your first and foremost concern is to your ward team. Teaching at the university as a favour for your link lecturer is beneficial in the long run but teaching on an ad-hoc basis is not. It will be just another thing that takes you away from the ward and is not your priority.

INFORM AND INVOLVE YOUR TEAM

If people are given a say about the way they do their work, receive adequate information and support, and are fully engaged in any organisational changes, they are more likely to maintain high levels of health, wellbeing and performance (Health & Safety Executive 2004). In other words, you will have fewer problems with sickness absence, high staff turnover and poor performance

Be completely open and honest with your team about everything that is going on. Generally the only part of your job that you need to keep confidential is staff personal details. Question any manager that says 'don't tell your staff until we say so'. Unless it involves private and personal staff details, nothing should be confidential.

INFORMATION FROM MEETINGS

When you attend the meetings held by your line manager or nursing director, let your staff know of all decisions that have been made and any information you have gained. Just giving your staff the minutes to read through is not enough. They do not know which bits are important and may not understand or be bothered to read through the jargon. Highlight the parts that are pertinent to them. Clarify for them what the decisions mean.

INVOLVEMENT IN MAKING DECISIONS

Keeping staff informed about everything to do with the ward is essential, but even more important is getting them involved. Be honest. If you are unsure how a future change is going to affect their jobs then say so, but make sure you involve them in the process of finding out.

Try not to make all managerial decisions by yourself. Involve your team. One good example is when deciding what to do with the £5000 ward environment fund (currently only available in England). Get your staff together to say what improvements they think should be made. Devise a list of all their suggestions and using either the 'three-point priority system' (see p. 49) or general discussion, you can all agree on the best way of using the funds.

BUSINESS PLANNING AND RECRUITMENT

Involve your team in the business planning process each year and in monitoring how the budget is being spent.

Review your budget statement with your staff each month. When a member of staff leaves, review with your team what the role should be and what should be put in the advert. Identify who wants to be involved in the interviews and whether the selection process should involve a presentation. This is a far better way of treating your staff than just informing them that your budget is overspent or you are recruiting another member of staff.

PLANNING THE TEAM'S STUDY LEAVE

When deciding each year how to allocate your study leave for the team, involve them in that decision too. List all the courses that staff would like to undertake in the coming year. Add up all the study days these will cost the team. Let them know how many study days you have to allocate over the year (usually around 2% of your budget, see p. 115) and decide between you who and what takes priority.

Your staff will be far more motivated if they can see the restrictions you are working to. Understanding why the decision needs to be made leaves them a lot less willing to find someone to blame if they cannot have all the study leave they would like.

INVESTIGATING COMPLAINTS

Investigating and writing a response to a complainant is an excellent learning experience not only for the person you delegate the investigation to, but also to the whole team. Share the results of the investigation and the difficulties you had during the process. Show them the final response letter and ask if they all agree with what you are saying. This not only gives them an insight into the problem, it keeps them involved. It shows that you truly value your team and their opinions.

IMPLEMENT SELF-ROSTERING

By having shared goals and an action plan, you are well on the way to ensuring your staff work better together. Getting them to appreciate each other's needs is another hurdle. One way you can do this is through self-rostering. Self-rostering does not mean having everyone writing down when they want to work and whoever gets there last gets the worst shift pattern! It also does not mean having everyone fill in their requests on a draft 'off-duty' plan. Self-rostering is about giving your staff the flexibility to cover the ward in their own way instead of your way.

SELF-ROSTERING IS EASIER IN SMALL TEAMS

Don't implement self-rostering for the whole team to do at once. It will not work. There is no way you can get them altogether for a start. There are far too many of them and you cannot leave the ward without cover. The ideal way to self-roster is within teams.

Many wards nowadays are divided into two or three teams. Give each team their part of the 'off-duty' and ask them to sort it out amongst themselves to cover their patients on a 24-hour basis. They will soon become more aware of each other's needs and more willing to give and take. They will be more aware of who needs to work with their mentor and who needs time off to take their kids to football practice every Thursday evening. They will have to decide among themselves who is more deserving of the weekend off. They will have to choose between the one who wants to go to the wedding or the one who wants to go to a concert. Leaving it for your staff to decide amongst themselves in small teams makes them appreciate each other's needs far better than if the decision was left to you.

If you are restricted to having one senior staff nurse on per shift from either team, it may be easier to get one team to do their part of the 'off-duty' first, then the next team to devise their part around it. They can swap over next time to make the process fair. It ensures that there is always an appropriate senior member in charge per shift.

The Department of Health produced some handy guidelines for team-based self-rostering in 2003. They are worth a perusal (Department of Health 2003).

ADVANTAGES OF SELF-ROSTERING

There are many advantages to team-based self-rostering. The benefits for staff include:

● having more control over their working lives
● linking start and finish times to travel restrictions
● covering for each other to fit in with family care arrangements
● opting for fewer longer shifts or shorter split shifts to cover for each other
● more control to be at work for individual work commitments, e.g. link nurse meetings or patient case conferences
● more control in planning team activity.

SET 'OFF-DUTIES'

Another option of giving staff more autonomy in their shift pattern is to have a master 'off-duty'. This is where each member of staff has a set line within the 'off-duty'. You can then give your staff the option of swapping lines or individual shifts between themselves to meet their personal requirements. This is less flexible but could be a good starting point rather than going for complete self-rostering straight away.

ACTION POINTS

● Arrange regular meetings, every month or so, with your HR advisor to discuss any day-to-day problems or potential problems and give them a general update.
● Start keeping brief file notes of day-to-day meetings and phone conversations.
● Set up a communication book/folder for staff if you do not have one already.
● Delegate appraisals to staff ensuring they have the appropriate skills to do so, and make appointments in your diary for those you need to do yourself.
● Read through and familiarise yourself with your sickness/absence policy, competence/capability policy and disciplinary policy.
● From now on, make sure you see every member of staff on return from sick leave and make a brief file note if you don't already do so.
● Set dates for monthly staff meetings to review the budget, complaints, serious incidents, etc., and involve your team in any decisions.
● Set up a two-week induction package for all new staff (include all mandatory sessions for the year), and review ongoing teaching packages with your team.
● Consider the implementation of self-rostering to get your staff to be more considerate of each other's needs.

References

Department of Health 2003 Working lives: programmes for change: team-based self-rostering. DH Publications, London. Online. Available: http://www.dh.gov.uk/assetRoot/04/03/50/32/04035032.pdf 28 Sep 2005

Department of Health 2004 The NHS knowledge and skills framework (NHS KSF) and the development review process. DH Publications, London. Online. Available: http://www.dh.gov.uk/assetRoot/04/09/08/61/04090861.pdf 28 Sep 2005

Health & Safety Executive 2004 Management standards for work-related stress. HSE, Suffolk. Online. Available: http:// www.hse.gov.uk/stress/standards/pdfs/shortguide.pdf 28 Sep 2005

Information Commissioner 1998 The Data Protection Act. HMSO, London. Online. Available: http://www.informationcommissioner.gov.uk 28 Sep 2005

Information Commissioner 2000 Freedom of Information Act. HMSO, London. Online. Available: http://www.informationcommissioner.gov.uk 28 Sep 2005

CHAPTER 5

MAKE SURE CARE IS PATIENT-CENTRED

Maintain your clinical skills   84

Learning from experience   84

Textbooks and journals   85

Clinical supervision   85

Learn through teaching others   85

Ensure that all patients have a full assessment and care plan   86

Which model?   86

Standardised care plans   86

Accountability   87

Care plans as teaching tools   87

Care plans as communication tools   87

Be clear about what health care assistants can and cannot do   88

Decisions should be based on individual ability   88

Empower HCAs to care   88

Eliminate long handovers   89

Office handovers   89

Bedside handovers   89

Combination handovers   90

Confidentiality and bedside handovers   91

Use task-orientated care only when appropriate   91

Delegation of care   91

Delegation of tasks   91

Task allocation is incompatible with the nursing process   92

Work towards primary nursing   92

Primary nursing vs patient allocation   92

Primary nursing vs team nursing   92

Primary nursing in practice   93

The best method of care for your ward   93

Make sure patients are informed   93

A 'welcome' information board   94

An information board for comments and suggestions   94

Information sheets and leaflets   94

Improve care through audit and benchmarking   96

Falling standards   96

Use audit tools wisely   96

Benchmarking   97

Don't accept poor standards of care when short-staffed   98

Stop coping   98

Show your staff how to prioritise and document their decisions   98

Take the lead on ward rounds   99

Ensure the patient is involved in discussions   100

Clarify anything that the patient does not understand   100

Contribute to decision-making on the patient's behalf   101

Communicate any changes or decisions to the rest of the team   101

Use ward rounds as a learning opportunity   101

Many ward managers will say that the care they provide on their ward is patient-centred, but is it really? If your team still undertake drug rounds at set times or carry out observations at set times, then the care is not patient-centred. It is centred around staff routine. Truly patient-centred care means that care is centred around the patient's needs, not the staff's needs or ward routines.

The only way you can provide truly patient-centred care is to ensure that there are systems and processes in place to find out what your patients really need and then to base your care around those needs. This chapter takes a look at those systems and processes required to maintain a high standard of patient-centred care.

MAINTAIN YOUR CLINICAL SKILLS

Keeping up-to-date clinically is essential for the ward manager role. You cannot maintain high standards of care without having a thorough knowledge of your specialty. You need an in-depth knowledge of your subject to be able to act as a role model for others. You also have to protect the patients from others who are less experienced, including junior doctors.

Having defined your workload (see Ch. 2) you may find that you can spend only four half-days a week on the ward in a clinical capacity, so you should make the most of this time.

LEARNING FROM EXPERIENCE

Make it your mission to learn something new on each and every shift. Keep a notebook specifically for that purpose. Choose something you encounter during your work such as a new condition, new drug or new procedure. If there is nothing new, then find out more about something that is not new. Take 10–15 minutes out during or between shifts to look it up. Use a textbook or access the internet. If you take just a little time out every day, you will become far more knowledgeable without having to spend hours in the library or taking yet another formal course of study. Never become complacent. There is always something new to learn. Your confidence will grow as you become more of an expert in your field.

You should also have a thorough knowledge of all the main drugs used in your specialty. When you are giving patients their medications, make sure you know why the patient is taking them, how they work, what their common side effects are and any contraindications. The British National Formulary (BNF) is only adequate for looking up a drug quickly during the drug round, but the information is brief and covers all uses of the drug whereas a textbook will explain the uses of drugs in context with the specialty in which you work.

TEXTBOOKS AND JOURNALS

Make sure you have full access to appropriate up-to-date textbooks on your specialty. Keep them in your office for you and your staff to refer to when necessary. You can source funding for textbooks and journals through:

● your stationery budget
● ward funds
● one of the hospital charities, e.g. League of Friends.

Subscribe to your specialist professional journal and keep the most recent copy on the coffee table in the staff room. It's a simple way of enabling both yourself and your staff to keep up to date.

CLINICAL SUPERVISION

Find yourself a clinical supervisor, someone who is more experienced and expert than yourself. One of the main consultants or senior registrars linked with your ward is a good option. A good clinical nurse specialist or nurse consultant could also be a good option, or perhaps the link lecturer may be suitable. You do not have to make it too formal. The aim of clinical supervision would be to:

● stop you picking up bad habits
● challenge and make you think more deeply about certain areas of practice
● ensure you are learning from your experiences
● get advice and support.

Having an appropriate clinical supervisor is essential for you to help maintain your professional competence and credibility.

LEARN THROUGH TEACHING OTHERS

Invite staff or student nurses to shadow you regularly for a shift. This not only gives them valuable experience but their enquiring minds will help stimulate your thinking and question your practice. Giving regular teaching sessions also keeps you 'on the ball'. Teaching is a valuable learning experience for the teacher as well as the student.

It is a huge pressure for you to feel that you have to know everything but if you make sure you learn something from your experience every day, it soon accumulates.

ENSURE THAT ALL PATIENTS HAVE A FULL ASSESSMENT AND CARE PLAN

Care planning is an essential part of patient care, but in times of staffing shortages or increased workload it becomes low on the priority list for some. Yet without a specific document outlining the plan of care, important issues are likely to be missed. Care planning provides a guide to all who are involved with the patient's care, including temporary staff.

It is essential that all patients are fully assessed using an appropriate nursing model, not a tick sheet. The written plan of care should be based on that assessment. This may seem basic but it's still known for some patients to be discharged without having had a nursing assessment or written plan of care throughout their hospital stay.

Care plans save so much time, particularly if you have to use bank and agency nurses regularly. They ensure handovers are safe and efficient. Staff do not have to keep explaining what needs to be done for the patient if it's written in the care plan. Bank and agency nurses don't have to keep interrupting other staff during the course of their shift to ask questions about their patients' care.

If a patient does not have a care plan, nurses have little defence against allegations of negligence. Legally, it will be assumed that the nursing care was not planned if there is no evidence of a care plan.

WHICH MODEL?

'Roper's' model still appears to be the most popular method in the UK as it incorporates all activities of daily living (Holland et al 2003, Roper et al 1996). However, it really doesn't matter which nursing model you advocate for use on your ward. You just need to have some sort of assessment system in place that identifies the patient's nursing requirements, followed by a written plan of care.

STANDARDISED CARE PLANS

Standardised care plans save time but try to ensure that your staff adapt them to the individual patient. Sometimes with standardised care plans, staff get used to seeing the same old thing. As a result, you may find that they tend not to read or refer to them. If you specify to your staff that they must write the patients' individual needs on the care plan in addition to the routine predicted needs, it will increase the likelihood of them being read.

Some nurses are under the misconception that writing the patient's name under each problem heading is individualising the standardised care plan. This is unnecessary and serves no useful purpose other than to waste precious time. The patient's name only has to be written once on each sheet of paper.

ACCOUNTABILITY

As the ward manager, you are responsible for ensuring the *systems* are in place to:

● enable your staff to devise a full nursing assessment and care plan for their patients
● ensure that every single patient in your ward receives a full assessment and care plan.

The registered nurses in your team are responsible for the *content* of the assessment, care plan and subsequent evaluations. The Nursing and Midwifery Council (NMC) Code of Professional Conduct clearly states for nurses that, 'You must ensure that the health care record for the patient or client is an accurate account of treatment, care planning and delivery . . . It should provide clear evidence of the care planned, the decisions made, the care delivered and the information shared' (Nursing & Midwifery Council 2004; Standard 4.4).

Get your team together and use their skills and experience to decide on which model is the most appropriate for assessing and planning care for the type of patients you have on your ward. If they have taken part in choosing which model to use, they are more likely to be willing to use that model in their day-to-day practice.

CARE PLANS AS TEACHING TOOLS

Make sure your staff write clear care plans. The goals and actions should be specific and measurable. For example, a goal for a postsurgical patient such as 'to prevent a chest infection' is not specific. A goal such as 'to remain free from chest infection as evidenced by T < 37°C, WBC between 4–11, lungs clear on auscultation and negative sputum culture' is a lot more meaningful. When care plans are used this way, they can also be invaluable teaching tools.

CARE PLANS AS COMMUNICATION TOOLS

The ultimate purpose of the care plan is to inform everyone in the team of the patients' care needs. Any nurse coming back from 'days off' or annual leave and unfamiliar with the patient should be able to find all the information they need in the care plan. If there is no care plan, they will waste unnecessary time trying to find out.

To condone the non-use of care plans on your ward equates to allowing poor standards of communication and patient care. Lack of care plans increases the risk of untoward incidents and unintentional neglect.

BE CLEAR ABOUT WHAT HEALTH CARE ASSISTANTS CAN AND CANNOT DO

The role of the health care assistant (HCA) in supporting registered nurses has always been a contentious issue. The main concern is usually around the nurses' accountability for the actions of HCAs. The NMC Professional Code of Conduct states clearly that it is up to the individual nurse delegating the task to decide in each situation whether the HCA has the appropriate skills and competence:

> 'You may be expected to delegate care delivery to others who are not registered nurses or midwives. Such delegation must not compromise existing care but must be directed towards meeting the needs and serving the interests of patients and clients. You remain accountable for the appropriateness of the delegation, for ensuring that the person who does the work is able to do it and that adequate supervision or support is provided.'
> (NMC 2004; Standard 4.6)

HCAs are as much part of the team as registered nurses. Unfortunately, there are some managers who insist on having separate handovers for registered staff, and some that don't include HCAs in the handover process at all. Handovers should include the whole team. The registered nurses and HCAs can then plan the care of their patients together.

DECISIONS SHOULD BE BASED ON INDIVIDUAL ABILITY

Leave it up to the individual registered nurses in your team as to what they can and cannot delegate. Your role is to help and guide the nurses in making that decision. There is probably no reason why an HCA at NVQ level 3 standard with several years' experience could not update the care plan of a patient if the registered nurse they are working with feels they have the skills and competence to do so. However, it must be checked and signed by the registered nurse, who will remain accountable for what the HCA has written. If that nurse is not confident in the HCA's ability to do this, then it should not be delegated. Leave it up to your staff nurses to make that decision.

A blanket management decision saying that all HCAs who have attained NVQ level 3 standard can write care plans is not appropriate. The registered nurses need to be able to assess each person on their merits. They cannot be expected to take accountability for the actions of an HCA whom they feel does not have the appropriate skills. As a general rule, the registered nurse may delegate a task to an unregistered nurse only if they are confident that the patient will receive as high a standard of care as if they undertook the task themselves.

EMPOWER HCAs TO CARE

Delegating tasks creates a 'them and us' atmosphere. With the emphasis on achieving competencies for NVQ levels 2 and 3, HCAs are becoming more highly skilled. Rather than delegate a series of tasks to HCAs, it is now more appropriate to delegate a small caseload of patients with supervision. This maximises the use of their skills and abilities by enabling them to carry out the care as prescribed in the care plans. It enables HCAs to use their initiative rather than complete a set of delegated tasks. The registered nurses remain available to assist in areas where the HCAs do not have the competence to carry out a nursing task.

HCAs should also be included in all team and decision-making processes. At the time of writing this book, HCAs are not a regulated profession but plans are underway to ensure that they will be in the near future. Once HCAs become a regulated profession, there will be a lot less pressure on the rest of the team with regards to accountability issues.

ELIMINATE LONG HANDOVERS

If handovers are continually taking much more than half an hour, then perhaps you and your team need to revise the way they are carried out. Precious time for patient care is being lost. Long handovers cause resentment among staff hanging on for a well-earned break or waiting to go home.

The shift handover is a crucial period for maintaining communication and continuity of care. The importance of getting the system right should not be underestimated.

OFFICE HANDOVERS

Advantages
Office handovers can be quick and effective if carried out properly without devolving into lengthy discussions about each patient. They avoid the risk of being continually interrupted by visitors, other health professionals or the patients themselves. There is also minimal risk of other patients and visitors overhearing confidential details.

Disadvantages
The problem with office handovers is that the patient is not involved at all. The handover may not always be based on the plan of care, which stays by the patient's bedside. When shut away in the office the reporting nurse may become judgemental, giving the next shift's nurses preconceived ideas about the patients they are about to care for. In addition, office handovers used alone can become very lengthy, especially if the nurse who does the first few patients then has to go and find the relevant nurse to hand over the next few patients and so on.

BEDSIDE HANDOVERS

Advantages
Bedside handovers allow for greater patient involvement. Patients have the opportunity to contribute. The nurse taking over for the next shift can put a face to

the name and remember more easily who is who without having to resort to the piece of paper in their pocket. It also negates the need for the nurses to visit all the patients after handover to introduce themselves and familiarise themselves with their care plans.

Disadvantages

The problem with bedside handovers is that in some areas they have devolved from a 'bedside' handover to an 'end of bed' handover. This rather impersonal approach is similar to some doctors' rounds where the patient care is discussed between health professionals without the participation of the patient. The only patient involvement is through unavoidable eavesdropping. It can also be difficult to maintain patient confidentiality with 'end of bed' handovers.

COMBINATION HANDOVERS

A combination of office handover based on 'name, age & diagnosis' followed by a bedside handover using the care plans can be the most efficient and effective process of handing over between shifts. The first part in the office should be kept brief. The receiving nurses would then divide up into teams to receive a full handover by the patients' beds, but only for the patients they will be looking after. This keeps the handover focused and relevant. It maintains the advantages of each method and reduces the disadvantages.

Ways of reducing the length of handover over all include:

- handing out printed versions with the patient's name and bed number to each nurse coming on duty
- using taped handovers (this is especially useful when nurses come on duty at different times)
- ensuring the handover is based on the patient's care plan
- nurses to only receive detailed handover for the group of patients they have been allocated to care for
- the system of allocating nurses to patients ensures that, as far as possible, the same staff care for the same patients each shift.

There have been some studies and general debate about the effectiveness of nonverbal and taped handovers (e.g. Kennedy 1999, Prouse 1995) but beware of using these methods as the only means of handover. A report produced by the Health and Safety Executive into effective shift handover studied five major disasters, including the Piper Alpha disaster, which were caused by faults in the shift handover system (Lardner 1996). The report concluded that effective shift handovers should:

- be conducted *face-to-face*
- be *two-way* with both participants taking joint responsibility for ensuring accurate communication
- use verbal *and* written means of communication
- be given as much time as necessary to ensure accurate communication.

CONFIDENTIALITY AND BEDSIDE HANDOVERS

Make sure that your staff maintain confidentiality when handing over their patients by the bedside. The nurses should preferably sit down with the patient and discuss the care plan together. This helps to prevent others overhearing. If the patient has visitors, the handover can be carried out quietly and confidentially between the team elsewhere.

It is advisable not to leave the care plans at the end of the patients' beds for anyone, including visitors, to pick up and read. Leave them *with* the patient at the head of the bed or in their bedside locker. If the patient is confused, or unable to look after their care plan for some other reason such as postsurgery, the care plan should be kept somewhere safe such as by the nurses' station.

USE TASK-ORIENTATED CARE ONLY WHEN APPROPRIATE

Many nurses say their chosen method of nursing care delivery is patient allocation, team nursing or primary nursing. Few would admit to carrying out task-orientated care. Yet in reality this is what is happening in many areas. Take the expression, 'You do the "obs" and I'll do the drugs'. Does that sound familiar? It is so easy to fall back into task allocation without realising it is happening. Task allocation is sometimes necessary if the workload increases unexpectedly or in times of acute nursing shortage. If it is a shared decision, there is no problem with this approach. It can be necessary in times of severe nursing shortages.

DELEGATION OF CARE

Whatever model of nursing care delivery you use, the overall responsibility for the patient's care should be assigned to registered nurses only. However, with the increasing reliance on HCAs, nurses tend to delegate tasks rather than sharing the responsibility. Apart from giving out medications, HCAs who are trained to NVQ level 2 or level 3 standard are often competent to implement most of the care that a nurse can. As long as the patients have clear and up-to-date care plans, there is no reason why HCAs cannot be allocated the overall care of patients under the supervision of a registered nurse. They can make their own decisions as to what gets done and when. Many wards managers now take this approach. Resorting to task allocation tends to induce apathy and reduce team morale.

DELEGATION OF TASKS

If you have HCAs who have not attained their NVQ qualification and the associated competencies, task allocation may be the most suitable way of allocating the workload. After all, the registered nurses are ultimately accountable for patient care. When you increase the areas of practice for untrained personnel (i.e. multiskilling) you must ensure they have undergone 'rigorous training and competency assurance systems' to reduce risk (Horbury & Wright 2001; p. viii). If you have not done this, then task allocation may be your only option until you get the appropriate systems in place.

TASK ALLOCATION IS INCOMPATIBLE WITH THE NURSING PROCESS

Although task allocation can be deemed appropriate in some circumstances, it is better to aim for a more patient-centred delivery system. The emphasis on tasks removes the notion of individualised patient care. It is therefore incompatible with the nursing process. This probably explains why in some areas it is considered unimportant for patients to have care plans. If the patients do not have care plans and care is centred on achieving tasks, the bulk of the responsibility lies with one person; the nurse-in-charge. This is not an ideal situation. Working towards a primary nursing model is a much fairer system for all your staff.

WORK TOWARDS PRIMARY NURSING

To be able to admit a patient, plan their care and look after them every time you are on duty, through to their discharge, is a very satisfying experience. People take pride in their work. In primary nursing, the primary nurse does not necessarily have to care for their own patients during their shift. They can delegate to other nurses or HCAs, who can also care for the patient when the primary nurse is on days off. The primary nurse carries responsibility for writing the care plan and ensuring that long-term goals are met, rather than just the short-term goals during the span of one shift.

PRIMARY NURSING vs PATIENT ALLOCATION

The main problem with patient allocation is that nobody takes responsibility for the whole patient care package. Who is responsible if a patient's discharge was not planned and implemented effectively during their stay? Who is responsible if a patient's condition deteriorated over three days and nothing was done? If nurses care for a group of patients on one shift, then another group on the next shift, they will not only have less responsibility but also less pride in a job done well.

PRIMARY NURSING vs TEAM NURSING

In theory, team nursing is a little better than patient allocation. The team leader is the person who takes responsibility for each patient in the team from admission through to discharge. In practice, this does not always happen. Some wards simply split the number of beds into two or three groups and allocate a team of nurses to each area. Each team leader than allocates patients to the team members after handover. It then becomes patient allocation but within smaller teams. However, team nursing can help in areas where there are fewer registered nurses.

PRIMARY NURSING IN PRACTICE

In theory, primary nursing sounds perfect, but when you are 'running on bank and agency' almost every shift, it is not always feasible. Primary nursing requires each primary nurse to have associate nurses who care for the patient in their absence. It is something that could be quite difficult to organise on an 'off-duty' when you do not have your full staffing establishment.

THE BEST METHOD OF CARE FOR YOUR WARD

A simpler way to ensure nurses take more responsibility is to establish a form of primary nursing based on the organisation of care that you already have in place in your ward. You just need to establish a system whereby the nurse who undertakes the initial patient assessment and care plan will be the patient's main nurse throughout their stay. If they are coming up for days off, it's up to them to ensure that another nurse will take on that responsibility for the next few days instead. The primary nurse does not necessarily have to be allocated the patient to care for on every shift (although it is the ideal option). They just need to be the 'named nurse' responsible for ensuring the patient receives the appropriate care, by regularly reviewing the care plan and delegating as necessary.

Accept that the system will not be perfect and you will not be able to ensure it is fully implemented for every single patient who comes to your ward. Fluctuating staffing levels, increased patient turnover and the continual moving of patients from one ward to another makes it extremely difficult to run any model of nursing care effectively. The best you can do is to aim for your patients to be content in the knowledge that there is a specific individual who is responsible for their care from admission to discharge.

MAKE SURE PATIENTS ARE INFORMED

There are three good systems you can introduce to keep the patient and their relatives informed:

1. A 'welcome' information board.
2. An information board for comments and suggestions.
3. Information sheets and leaflets.

A 'WELCOME' INFORMATION BOARD

Use this board to inform new patients and relatives when they first come to be admitted or visit. Some suggestions include:

- a welcome sentence in large print
- directions on where to go and who to report to
- a photo and information on who the ward manager is and their role
- a photo and information on who the matron is, their role and contact details
- an explanation about who is who and how to identify staff by their uniforms
- which team or individual staff are looking after which bed numbers (remember you cannot put patient names on the board)
- the ward layout, including the bed numbers and where they can find the toilets (including directions for visitors' toilets)
- a sentence asking if there is any further information currently not up on the board which they would like to see.

AN INFORMATION BOARD FOR COMMENTS AND SUGGESTIONS

Keep a suggestions box with paper and pen nearby. Ask the patients and relatives to write down their comments or suggestions for improvement and put them in the suggestions box. Put extracts of these up on the board accompanied by a written response. Renew them each month. This may help prevent your staff being hassled for things. If, for example, one of the bathrooms is out of action, you can put up a written response on the board saying that the estates department are aware but there are problems with the plumbing that will take around two weeks to fix. This will stop patients and relatives continually complaining to your staff.

When you first put up the board, you will probably get very few or no suggestions. One idea to start the process would be to put up some examples. If, for example, you are continually being asked about the short visiting times, write up a response to a sample comment card explaining why you have had to restrict the visiting times. Magazines use a similar approach to attract people to read about certain issues. People are more likely to read a problem page to find the answer to an issue, rather than read an article on the subject.

INFORMATION SHEETS AND LEAFLETS

Ensure you have as much written information as you can available for patients. Coming into hospital is such an overwhelming experience for some that they rarely take in all that is being said.

First, ensure that there is some sort of leaflet or information sheet for when they arrive onto your ward which explain things like what the staff uniforms mean and where to get a cup of tea. Many hospitals provide this information in leaflet form. If not, it would not take long to compile your own local one. Second, make sure patients have a leaflet explaining their condition or the investigations or surgery they have come in for. It's advisable not to devise leaflets of your own without first looking up to see if there are any other sources you can tap into. There are many good websites that produce information leaflets, which you can download or adapt for your own area, such as:

> http://www.patient.co.uk – This has over 600 leaflets on health and disease, including tests and investigations.
> http://www.medinfo.co.uk – This site provides information sheets for patients on common conditions and drugs.
> http://www.prodigy.nhs.uk – This site is aimed at health care professionals providing advice, information and useful links as well as downloadable patient information leaflets.
> http://www.pharmweb.net – This site contains useful links to various specialist websites about drugs and conditions.

Producing your own information for patients and relatives

If you wish to produce your own patient information sheets or leaflets within the NHS, there are specific guidelines which you must adhere to regarding the presentation and the need for the appropriate NHS logo and colour. Your organisation's communications department will have the appropriate information. A dedicated website has also been developed in each of the four countries of the UK to guide you in developing patient information sheets and leaflets (Department of Health 2005, Department of Health and Social Services in Northern Ireland 2005, NHS Scotland 2005, NHS Wales 2005). These give guidance on how to improve written patient information and provide templates to help you.

The main things to remember when writing your information sheets or leaflets are:

1. Present all information in at least 12 point font, preferably bigger.
2. Try not to use words of more than two syllables.
3. Keep the sentences to no more than 15–20 words long.
4. Make it personal by using 'we' and 'you'.
5. Explain any instructions, e.g. if you tell them not to drive for two weeks after the operation, explain why.
6. A question and answer format tends to be more favoured by patients.
7. Cover only one investigation or condition per leaflet.
8. Encourage your staff to write the patient's name on the information sheet as it will make them more likely to read it.

The NHS toolkits recommend that every leaflet your ward or department produces should have the following consistent features:

Front cover:

- your NHS logo
- title of leaflet
- your ward, department or directorate.

Back cover:

- website address (if you have one)
- date of publication
- leaflet code
- copyright note of your organisation.

Never produce patient information without having it endorsed by your organisation. If you do, you could become personally liable for the information given, particularly with regards to clinical advice.

IMPROVE CARE THROUGH AUDIT AND BENCHMARKING

FALLING STANDARDS

There's no question about it; basic standards of patient care have fallen in certain areas over the past ten years or so. Many nurses will be familiar with some of the following contributory factors:

1. Student nurses used to work on the wards as part of the 'numbers'. Now they do not.
2. All registered nurses had to go through four rigorous assessments to ensure their knowledge, skills and competence in aseptic technique, giving out medications, total care of the patient and being in charge of a shift. Now they do not.
3. The patient throughput and workloads have greatly increased. The staffing budgets have not always increased in line with this.
4. Many nurses, once qualified, would stay working in the clinical area. Now they do not.
5. Hospitals used to prepare the food and employ cleaners as part of the team. Now they do not.

It really is not surprising that certain standards of care are not as good as they could be. But using an audit tool to confirm these poor standards is not hugely helpful on its own. Having to undertake audits can just add to the ever-increasing workload. Some nurses groan whenever auditing or benchmarking of care is mentioned. However, most of the standards are simply common sense and it's a sad reflection on our current care provision that such tools are needed at all. They cannot be ignored and you have to ensure that standards on your ward measure up to standards throughout your organisation. Just make sure that you focus on making the identified improvements rather than filling in the paperwork.

USE AUDIT TOOLS WISELY

Audit tools that measure care include the Essence of Care benchmarking standards (Modernisation Agency 2003) and the Fundamentals of Care performance standards (Welsh Assembly Government 2003). They can be lengthy documents that take ages to go through, but only if you allow them to be. The key to using them appropriately is not to concentrate too much on ensuring all the right boxes are filled in. Don't allow these documents to become yet another huge piece of paperwork that takes you away from your patients. Keep the focus on patient care.

If you are asked to audit an aspect of care, don't do it immediately unless you have something to gain from the results. Your team are there to provide care, not to spend their time filling in audit forms.

BENCHMARKING

Benchmarking takes the process of auditing one step further. It's a process of comparing audits from different areas. The idea is that all areas make improvements to attain the same standards as the one that had the best audit results.

The Essence of Care benchmarking tool in England gives the opportunity to audit up to nine aspects of patient care in your ward (Clinical Governance Support Team 2005). They are:

1. continence, bladder and bowel care
2. personal and oral hygiene
3. food and nutrition
4. pressure ulcers
5. privacy and dignity
6. record keeping
7. safety of clients with mental health needs in acute mental health and general hospital settings
8. principles of self care
9. communication.

Each aspect of care is made up of various factors. The idea is that you and your team get together and assess your work against these factors. You can grade your area from A (best practice) to E (worst practice). You decide between you what you think indicates best practice. Once you have done this, you can get together with other wards and departments and compare each other's results. Those who marked themselves at A or B can share any good practice. Those who marked themselves at D or E can take action to improve their own service to match the departments at A or B level. The meetings stimulate lots of debate as to what constitutes best practice. The toolkit comes in very handy at this stage because it gives statements and ideas to stimulate your thinking (Modernisation Agency 2003).

Try and keep the benchmarking meetings to an hour or less. It would be counterproductive to spend hours in meetings debating your work rather than actually being out there and doing it (that is unless you have extra funding in your budget to cover benchmarking work).

DON'T ACCEPT POOR STANDARDS OF CARE WHEN SHORT-STAFFED

Nurses have an amazing ability to cope when short-staffed. The trouble is just that; they cope. And it's tiring work covering the workload of absent staff as well as your own day after day. It can only lead to exhaustion and increased sickness levels, which just serves to make matters worse. It will not come as a surprise to any nurse to learn that the main source of stress in nursing is high workload coupled with staff shortages (Williams et al 1998).

In the long term your role is to ensure your staffing levels match the workload through:

- effective rostering (including study and annual leave)
- being fully involved in the business planning process, so that more staff are added to the establishment if there is an overall increase in workload
- taking extra initiatives to recruit and retain staff
- managing staff sickness.

However, there will be shifts when you have staff sickness, vacancies or unexpected increases in workload and are unable to 'fill' with bank or agency staff. Carrying on and coping on these shifts is still unacceptable.

STOP COPING

When a shift is short of staff and/or the workload for that day has increased unexpectedly, some adopt the attitude that the team have no other option but to just cope and get on with it. This is not appropriate and an example of poor leadership. Good leadership is ensuring that staff spend time at the beginning of the shift planning and prioritising the work that needs to be done, and making conscious decisions about work that will be left undone. For example, if you have two staff down on an early shift (and there are no bank or agency staff available), the rest of the team should not try to get all the work done and resign to accepting incidents where care is substandard. Phrases such as, 'it can't be helped, we were short-staffed' or 'I didn't get round to doing that because it was so short-staffed this morning' are not acceptable. Poor staffing is no excuse for poor care.

SHOW YOUR STAFF HOW TO PRIORITISE AND DOCUMENT THEIR DECISIONS

When your team have exhausted all other avenues of getting staff they must sit down and prioritise. At times like these, you still have to assert some control over your workload. Get your team to decide together at the beginning of the shift:

- which aspects of the work are essential, e.g. food and fluids, medications
- which aspects can be done to a lesser standard, e.g. hygiene, rehabilitation activities
- which aspects can be left undone until the next shift or next day, e.g. making beds, certain wound dressings, rehabilitation activities, further admissions.

These decisions should be made together, documented and the appropriate line manager informed. Don't allow the decision to remain at ward level. The rest of your organisation must be aware of the pressures that your team are under on that shift at the time. Raising the issue at a meeting afterwards is too late, and just telling people about the situation is insufficient. The documentation should include:

- the reasons for short-staffing (e.g. sickness)
- what steps you have taken to try and get further staffing (e.g. other wards, line manager, bank/agency)
- what your team have prioritised during that shift as essential and nonessential
- other actions (e.g. asked bed manager to hold admissions until next shift, etc.).

An email will suffice as evidence that it has been documented. Keep a copy of the email.

If your staff do not prioritise and document their decisions

Trying to do everything and accepting that whatever you don't get round to doing gets left, is an unsafe way of working. Important care may be missed. Make a conscious decision about leaving nonessential care. Patients will not suffer if their beds are not made. If staff have the time to make beds, they cannot complain that they have no time to provide adequate care. Few patients will suffer if they are not assisted to have a wash in the morning. Patients can wait until the afternoon to be assisted with a wash, or even go without, if the situation is explained. Daily observations can be left for the next shift, etc.

You owe it to your staff to empower them to make these decisions in times of acute staffing shortages. Your role as a manager is to provide your staff with 'adequate and achievable demands in relation to the agreed hours of work' (Health & Safety Executive 2005; p. 3). You would be failing in your duty as a manager if you allow your staff to continue to cope in times of acute staffing shortages without giving them authority and skills to prioritise, document and inform the appropriate senior managers of their decisions.

TAKE THE LEAD ON WARD ROUNDS

The main role for nurses taking part in ward rounds is to act as the patient's advocate by:

- ensuring the patient is involved in the discussions
- clarifying anything that the patient does not understand

● contributing to decision-making on the patient's behalf
● communicating any changes or decisions to the rest of the team.

Attending ward rounds is not just about taking notes and passing the information on to the rest of the team. If that's all that were needed, you could get one of the junior doctors to hand over the list of changes afterwards, and need not attend at all.

Ensure it is the patient's own nurse who attends the ward round

In days gone by, it was always the ward manager or nurse-in-charge that attended the ward round. Some consultants today still expect that to be the case but times have changed. Nurses no longer care for patients through the delegation of tasks from the nurse-in-charge. Nurses are now responsible for the full care of their patients, which means that they are the best people to attend the ward round.

With today's high turnover of patients and increasing patient dependency, the nurse-in-charge cannot be expected to know every detail about every patient on their ward. The role of the nurse-in-charge is therefore to ensure that the nurse who attends the ward round is the patient's own nurse, and only to take over when that nurse is unavailable.

ENSURE THE PATIENT IS INVOLVED IN DISCUSSIONS

Some health care professionals, including doctors, have a tendency to stand at the end of the bed to discuss the patient's treatment and care without including them. In any other situation, this would be considered quite rude but often the patient is too ill and too vulnerable to do anything about it. The nurse can ensure their patient is included by going to sit with them at the bedside. The rest of the ward round members would then have to turn towards the patient when liaising with the nurse. It's a simple and easy way of ensuring the patient is involved.

CLARIFY ANYTHING THAT THE PATIENT DOES NOT UNDERSTAND

When anyone starts using medical or technical terms, asking the patient if they understand is not always sufficient. Being surrounded by a group of doctors and other health care professionals can be quite overwhelming. In these circumstances, it is difficult for patients to ask the right questions. Your role is to assist their understanding, rather than just checking it. It would be far more useful for the patient if you asked them, 'would you like us to explain what the term x means?' rather than 'do you understand?'.

CONTRIBUTE TO DECISION-MAKING ON THE PATIENT'S BEHALF

Your team spend more time with the patients than other health care professionals so are usually more aware of their needs than the rest of the ward round. It is therefore only natural that they should contribute to all the decision-making. Part of your role as ward manager should be to spend time developing the skills and confidence of your staff to enable them to speak up on behalf of the patient. Decisions should only be made with full contribution from all members of the multiprofessional team.

Observe the patients' body language

Be wary if your patient is being given too much information. They may not be able to take it all in. As their advocate, it's up to you to recognise the signs. Are they looking nervous? Are they looking away from the person speaking to them? A simple question such as, 'are you alright?' or 'would you prefer to discuss this part of the treatment at a later date?' should be sufficient for the patient to be able to speak up. 'Patients should be given the sense of freedom to indicate when they do not want any (or more) information: this requires skill and understanding from healthcare professionals' (Kennedy 2001; Recommendation 16).

COMMUNICATE ANY CHANGES OR DECISIONS TO THE REST OF THE TEAM

In some wards, the nurse-in-charge attends the ward round then goes round to the patients' allocated nurses and explains what decisions were made about changes in care. This is simply duplicating work and wasting precious time. It makes a lot more sense for the patient's own nurse to attend the ward round. This nurse would note any changes or decisions in the patient's care plan at the time of the ward round. The information should then be passed to the next shift through the routine handover. Only information affecting the management of the ward would need to be passed to the nurse-in-charge, such as a change in the patient's discharge date.

USE WARD ROUNDS AS A LEARNING OPPORTUNITY

Whenever you can, have a junior member of staff or student accompany you on the ward round to appreciate the art of communication. It enables them to understand that attending a ward round is far more than just taking notes. Have them observe the techniques you use in acting as the patient's advocate. Take time after the ward round to discuss what they have learned. You can send your staff on any number of communication courses, but you can't beat learning through observation and experience.

ACTION POINTS

- Get yourself a notebook specifically for your own learning and note something in it each day to keep yourself up-to-date.
- Make sure your team are aware that full assessments and care plans are mandatory for all patients admitted to your ward.
- Include HCAs in handovers, decision-making processes and planning care if you do not already do so.
- Review your handover system if it is taking too long.
- Review the system you use for organising patient care, if it does not ensure that one registered nurse is responsible for a patient's care from admission through to discharge.
- Put up information boards at the entrance to your ward to welcome all visitors, give appropriate information and invite comments/suggestions.
- Use audits and benchmarking to improve care but don't allow them to become paper exercises.
- Give your staff the skills and authority to prioritise and let go of nonessential tasks in times of acute staffing shortages.
- Develop the skills of your staff in acting as the patient's advocate during ward rounds.

References

Clinical Governance Support Team 2005 Essence of Care programme. Online. Available: http://www.cgsupport.nhs.uk/Programmes/Essence_of_Care_Programme/ 25 Nov 2005

Department of Health 2005 NHS identity. Online. Available: http://www.nhsidentity. nhs.uk 10 Oct 2005

Department of Health and Social Services in Northern Ireland 2005 Corporate identity for the Northern Ireland departments. Online. Available: http://www.northernireland.gov. uk/identity 10 Oct 2005

Health & Safety Executive 2005 Tackling stress: the management standards approach. HSE, Suffolk. Online. Available: http://www.hse.gov.uk/stress/standards/pdfs/ shortguide.pdf 10 Oct 2005

Holland K, Jenkins J, Solomon J et al 2003 Applying the Roper–Logan–Tierney model in practice. Churchill Livingstone, Edinburgh

Horbury C, Wright M 2001 Development of a Multiskilling Life Cycle Model. HSE, Suffolk. Online. Available: http://www.hse.gov.uk/research/crr_pdf/2001/crr01328.pdf 10 Oct 2005

Kennedy J 1999 An evaluation of non verbal handover. Professional Nurse 14(4):391–394

Kennedy I 2001 Learning from Bristol: the report of the public inquiry into children's heart surgery at the Bristol Royal Infirmary 1984–1995. Online. Available: http://www. bristol-inquiry.org.uk/final_report 10 Oct 2005

Lardner R 1996 Effective shift handover – a literature review. HSE, Suffolk. Online. Available: http://www.hse.gov.uk/research/otopdf/1996/oto96003.pdf 8 Oct 2005

Modernisation Agency 2003 Essence of Care: patient-focused benchmarks for clinical governance, DH Publications, London. Online. Available: http://www.modern.nhs. uk/home/key/docs/Essence%20of%20Care.pdf 10 Oct 2005

NHS Scotland 2005 The NHS Scotland identity. Online. Available: http://www.show.scot. nhs.uk/nhsscotlandci 10 Oct 2005

NHS Wales 2005 NHS Wales identity guidelines. Online. Available: http://www.wales. nhs.uk/documents/nhs-guidelines-e.pdf 10 Oct 2005

Nursing and Midwifery Council 2004 The NMC Code of Professional Conduct: standards for conduct, performance and ethics. NMC, London. Online. Available: http://www. nmc-uk.org 8 Oct 2005

Prouse M 1995 A study of the use of tape-recorded handovers. Nursing Times 91(49):40–41

Roper N, Logan W, Tierney W 1996 The Elements of Nursing: a model for nursing based on a model of living. Churchill Livingstone, Edinburgh

Welsh Assembly Government 2003 Fundamentals of care: guidance for health and social staff. Welsh Assembly Govt, Cardiff. Online. Available: http://www.wales.nhs. uk/documents/booklet-e.pdf 10 Oct 2005

Williams S, Mitchie S, Pattoni S 1998 Improving the health of the NHS workforce: the report of the partnership on the health of the NHS workforce. The Nuffield Trust, London

CHAPTER 6

GET YOUR BUDGET RIGHT

Know what your budget is   106

Are you managing or just monitoring?   106

Your staffing establishment   106

Matching the 'off-duty' to your staffing establishment   107

Prioritise PAY   107

The importance of good 'off-duty' management   107

Share staff with another ward   109

Be flexible   109

Go through your budget statement each month   110

Checking through the columns   111

Involve your team   111

Manage annual leave   112

Spreading annual leave throughout the year   113

Getting staff to take annual leave   113

Manage your allowance for unplanned absence   113

Sickness levels   114

Maternity leave   115

Other leave   115

Plan your study leave allowance   115

Other sources of funding   116

Mandatory training   116

Get your staff involved in NON PAY   116

Pharmacy/drugs   117

Medical supplies   117

Stationery   117

Ward environment budget   117

Be more active in the business planning process   118

The business plan   118

How to write a business case   119

Don't do anything without identified funding   119

Get it in writing   120

Meet regularly with your finance advisor   121

If you manage a ward or department, then you also manage a budget. Don't let others manage it for you. You are the most appropriate person to ensure this money is used appropriately and effectively. Only you understand what the needs of the patients are on your ward, and the demands on your staff. Only you can decide on the different mix of bands and skills required within your team. And only you have an idea about the amount of equipment and consumables required.

Some ward managers say that their clinical duties are more important than the budget, but it is the budget that determines what you can and cannot do clinically. How well the budget is managed directly affects how good the care is on your ward.

KNOW WHAT YOUR BUDGET IS

It costs around £500 000 per year to run a ward. The amount obviously varies depending on the number of beds and specialty. Most ward managers claim they manage a budget but few can say what their budget is when asked. Do you know what your budget is? It is very important you are aware of how much money you are responsible for, and where and how it should be spent.

The actual figure will be shown on your monthly budget statement. It is the total amount at the bottom of the column marked 'ANNUAL BUDGET'. It is usually around £500 000 but can be anything from £300 000 to over £1 million depending on how many beds you have, the sort of patients admitted to your ward and the type of treatment required. The budget is often much more than £1 million for areas such as intensive care units and accident and emergency departments. As a result the management of these budgets is often (or should be!) devolved down to team leaders.

ARE YOU MANAGING OR JUST MONITORING?

Having such a large amount of money is quite a responsibility but some make the mistake of assuming that checking through the monthly statements is all that's required. This is not managing the budget, it's simply monitoring it.

Actively managing a budget entails:

- planning how next year's budget will be spent
- keeping to specific guidelines for allocating annual leave, sickness and study leave allowances
- performing regular skill mix and workload reviews
- being fully involved in the yearly business planning process, which includes identifying cost pressures and service developments and writing business cases where necessary.

YOUR STAFFING ESTABLISHMENT

Staffing costs should be regularly revised following any changes in workload. There are several off-the-shelf models currently in use for reviewing skill mix (Hurst 2002). These models calculate the patients' care requirements in terms of staff numbers and band mix. The measurements determine the ideal numbers and types of staff required per shift or the ideal numbers per group of beds, e.g. one nurse to eight beds.

Currently, many nurse managers use their own in-house criteria to determine their staffing numbers such as:

● no less than two registered nurses per shift
● no less than three staff on nights
● one extra registered nurse each shift for 'theatre days', etc.

The nurse manager's intuition and common sense with regards to staffing requirements is often far better than any skill mix review.

MATCHING THE 'OFF-DUTY' TO YOUR STAFFING ESTABLISHMENT

Your staffing establishment is worked out by your finance advisor using information from your 'off-duty' numbers (i.e. the minimum staffing levels required per shift that either you have identified personally or through a formal skill-mix review). It is essential that the minimum staffing levels on your 'off-duty' match the numbers in your staffing establishment. If you do not know for sure, ask your finance advisor to work it out for you.

Each directorate usually has a dedicated finance advisor. It is their job to work with you to ensure the budget is right for your needs. It is your job to maintain regular contact with them. If you do not, who is it they are getting their information from? And how accurate is that information?

PRIORITISE PAY

Your budget is made up of two parts:

1. PAY – this section reflects the salaries of your staff.
2. NON PAY – this section contains the money for equipment and consumables.

The PAY section takes up the first part of your budget statement. It is the part that you need to concentrate on because it usually comprises at least 80% of your total budget.

THE IMPORTANCE OF GOOD 'OFF-DUTY' MANAGEMENT

If your PAY budget is overspent, it can be due to inefficient 'off-duties'. It costs, on average, around £50 000 per month to staff a ward. In other words, whoever does the 4-week 'off-duty' is responsible for deciding how to spend around £50 000 of your budget. It is a big responsibility so any delegation of the role should not be taken lightly.

To manage the PAY part of your budget effectively, you need to:

● ensure your staffing establishment matches your required 'off-duty' numbers
● manage the 20–23% allowance, which covers annual leave, study leave and unplanned absence such as sick leave
● control agency and bank usage to within the 20–23% allowance.

Staffing establishment

You will probably have set minimum staffing levels for each shift over a seven-day week (Table 6.1). The person who does the 'off-duty' then allocates the staff to meet those minimum levels on each shift. Your staffing establishment (which you should receive with your monthly statement) is worked out based on your set shift requirements (Table 6.2). You must check regularly with your finance advisor that they match up. If you do not ensure that the staffing establishment meets the set shift numbers then you cannot devise the 'off-duty' within budget and are therefore failing to manage it.

20–23% absence allowance

When your finance advisor works out your staffing requirements, they use your 'off-duty' numbers but also put in an additional 20–23% to cover annual leave, sickness/absence and study leave. It means that your final staffing establishment

TABLE 6.1: Example of minimum staffing levels over 7-day week

	Mon	Tues	Wed	Thurs	Fri	Sat	Sun
Early	6	7	6	6	6	5	5
Late	6	6	6	6	5	5	5
Night	4	4	4	4	4	3	3

TABLE 6.2: Example of a ward staffing establishment

Description	Budget (WTE*)	Actual (WTE)
Ward manager (band 7)	1.0	1.0
Sister/charge nurse (band 6)	2.0	1.8
Staff nurse (band 5)	12.0	12.2
HCA (band 4)	8.0	6.0
HCA (band 3)	5.0	7.0
Ward clerk	1.0	1.0
TOTAL	29	29

*WTE, whole time equivalent; 1.00 WTE is full time, <1.00 WTE is part time.

should provide you with enough to cover your annual leave, sickness/absence and study leave requirements and remain within budget.

Sometimes some of this allowance is separated as a separate line within your budget statement and labelled as 'bank/agency costs'.

The additional 20–23% is usually comprised of:

- 13.5% annual leave
- 1–2% study leave
- 5.5–7.5% unplanned absences (e.g. sickness/maternity).

If you do not manage annual leave, sick leave and study leave correctly, you can overspend unnecessarily by as much as 20–23%. Check out with your finance advisor exactly what percentage your organisation adds to cover absence allowance. Without knowing this figure, you cannot manage your PAY budget.

Bank and agency usage

Use bank instead of agency wherever possible. They cost little more than permanent staff. If you are sent an agency nurse because no bank nurses are available, an additional 30% is charged in commission to the agency. This means that for every three shifts covered by agency staff, one shift should remain unfilled in order to make up for the extra cost. Obviously this needs to be handled very carefully because, at the same time, you cannot compromise patient care. Some managers compensate for the extra commission charges by booking agency nurses for a 'half shift' only.

In some organisations, the most popular shifts for bank staff are early shifts. This means that the late and night shifts are covered by agency. It therefore makes sense to compile 'off-duties' to ensure that most late and night shifts are covered by your own staff, leaving the vacant shifts mainly as early shifts. This will ensure that there is a higher chance of getting bank staff rather than agency.

SHARE STAFF WITH ANOTHER WARD

Try and work closely with another ward manager and share staff between your two wards during the hard times. It is advisable to link up with another ward or department with a similar specialty within your directorate for the purpose of sharing staff. You could meet with the manager once per week to go through the next week's 'off-duty'. This enables you to identify areas where resources could be shared and to plan ahead for expected shortfalls.

BE FLEXIBLE

Be more flexible with your staffing establishment. If you are unable to recruit a certain grade of staff into your vacant post, then consider other options. Can you replace with a different grade of staff? Think carefully; perhaps it would be better to employ an available lower grade of staff rather than fill the vacancy continually with bank and agency.

As the budget holder, you do not have to stick to the grades of staff in your budget statement. You can adjust them according to the needs of the ward and what's available so long as you remain within budget. Your finance advisor's role (along with your line manager) is to assist you in doing so and will calculate any differences for you. Liaise closely with your human resources (HR) advisor to ensure you are abiding by your organisation's policies regarding equal opportunities.

GO THROUGH YOUR BUDGET STATEMENT EACH MONTH

The budget statement tells what you have spent. It's like going through your own bank statement at the end of the month. Nothing should come as a surprise. It should confirm what you already know.

The layout of the budget statement varies between organisations. However, the information contained is basically the same. It is usually divided into two parts, PAY and NON PAY, and is best read using the following columns.

Establishment (budget)
This column tells you how many staff you can employ within your budget. (WTE stands for 'whole time equivalent'. 1.00 WTE is full time, and anything less than 1.00 WTE is part time.)

Establishment (actual)
This column tells you how many staff you have in post. The numbers will vary. For example, if you cannot recruit up to establishment in band 6, you can recruit more in band 5 to compensate, as long as the final salary figure remains the same.

Code
This is the finance code given to each particular grade of staff or type of equipment. The first part of the code relates to your ward (usually a 4-digit number). The second part relates to the category of staff or equipment (usually another 4-digit number).

Annual budget
This is usually the last column on the right hand side of your budget statement. The numbers in this column never change. It tells you what money you have to spend over the whole year. You should be very familiar with these figures.

Current month's budget, expenditure and variance
These three columns tell you what you had to spend in the last month (budget), what you did spend (expenditure) and what the difference is (variance). Budget

statements use the word 'variance' which means the 'difference' between how much money you were allocated and what you have spent; in other words, whether you are over- or under-spent. Any money left over (or 'under-spend') is enclosed in brackets.

Year to date's budget, expenditure and variance

These three columns tell you what you have had in your budget so far since the beginning of the financial year (budget), what you have spent in that time (expenditure) and where you are at the moment in terms of overall under-spend or over-spend (variance).

CHECKING THROUGH THE COLUMNS

When you receive your budget statement, the first thing you need to do is check the total amount in the 'year to date' variance column. It tells you how over-spent or under-spent you are at the moment. Remember to concentrate on the PAY section, as this is usually the part where most of your budget is allocated.

If you have an over-spend, take a look at the rest of this column to find out which bit is over-spent. Over-spends should not be a surprise. You know when you have used extra agency to cover high sickness levels or an unexpected increase in workload in the past month. The key to managing your budget effectively is deciding what to do about this over-spend. You should have already warned your general manager and finance manager, and together worked out a plan of action to bring the budget back in line. If not, it is advisable to do so at this point.

You also need to check the first two columns in the PAY section (i.e. budgeted and actual establishment) for accuracy. It is often the case that a 'leavers' form may not have been processed when a member of staff leaves or transfers to another ward. If this happens, your ward will continue to fund their pay until the form is processed.

Overall, your main task with the budget statement is to check for any inaccuracies and identify the main variances. You should then discuss your findings with your financial advisor each month and write yourself a plan of action for the coming month.

INVOLVE YOUR TEAM

Go through your budget statement with your staff regularly. Get feedback from those who have responsibility for aspects of the NON PAY (see pp. 116–117). Discuss and agree actions for both PAY and NON PAY. Sharing the budget statements with your team helps in their development and ensures they appreciate the links between good budgeting and good patient care.

MANAGE ANNUAL LEAVE

The average percentage given for annual leave is usually 13.5%. This equates to around seven weeks per person. Check with your individual organisation what your allowance is. In order to manage this annual leave allowance effectively, you have to make sure that a certain number of staff are on annual leave at any one time. The way to calculate this is to view the percentage in terms of shifts following two simple steps:

Step 1: Add up the number of shifts required to run your unit in one full week (Table 6.3).

Step 2: Convert the 13.5% allowance into shifts per week (Box 6.1).

In the ward x example (outlined in Table 6.3 and Box 6.1), a *maximum* of three people can take annual leave at any one time. However, what some managers do not realise is that this also means there must be a *minimum* of three people on annual leave at any one time too. This ensures that annual leave is spread throughout the year so that adequate numbers of staff are available to work at all times.

TABLE 6.3: Example of adding up the number of shifts per week of 'off-duty'

	Mon	Tues	Wed	Thur	Fri	Sat	Sun	_TOTAL_
Early	6	7	7	7	6	6	6	45
Late	6	6	6	6	6	6	6	42
Night	3	4	4	3	3	3	3	23
TOTAL	15	17	17	16	15	15	15	110

Total number of shifts required to staff one week in ward x = 110

BOX 6.1: EXAMPLE OF HOW TO CONVERT THE ANNUAL LEAVE ALLOWANCE INTO NUMBERS OF SHIFTS PER 'OFF-DUTY'

Total number of shifts on ward x is: 110 shifts

Annual leave allowance on ward x is: 13.5%

Percentage calculation: $13.5 \div 100 \times 110 = 14.85$

14.85 rounded up to 15 means that on ward x: 15 shifts of each week on the 'off-duty' must be allocated as annual leave.

15 shifts equates to three weeks, therefore three staff need to be on annual leave at any one time in ward x, in order to remain within the allocated budget.

SPREADING ANNUAL LEAVE THROUGHOUT THE YEAR

Poor staffing levels between January and March due to high levels of annual leave indicate that the ward manager has not managed their budget properly. Encourage your staff to take annual leave regularly throughout the year and book this at least four weeks in advance of the 'off-duty'. The following guidelines are generally recommended (check with your local organisational guidelines):

1. By June 30 – minimum of one week must have been taken.
2. By Sept 30 – minimum of three weeks must have been taken.
3. By Dec 31 – minimum of five weeks must have been taken.
4. Jan 1 to Mar 31 – maximum of one week of annual leave to be taken.

   A good tip is to keep an annual leave planner on the wall in the ward office with separate annual leave lines for the number of staff who can take annual leave at any one time. Staff can then fill in the slots where they want to take annual leave over the coming year. You can also see at a glance what is happening and be able to intervene. It will stop staff leaving it to the last minute to book and finding out there are no annual leave slots left.

   If any of your staff wish to carry annual leave allowance over into the next financial year, you should clarify first with your financial advisor how you can allow for this within the following year's budget.

GETTING STAFF TO TAKE ANNUAL LEAVE

If your organisation does not have any specific guidelines for booking annual leave, do not enforce local guidelines straight away. If your staff have been allowed to book annual leave when they want and tend to leave it to January–March time without any consideration for the budget, you cannot enforce local guidelines immediately. The best way forward is to ask your team for their views on how to manage the annual leave budget:

1. *Explain the implications to your team.* Let them take on board how important it is that a maximum number of staff should be on annual leave at any one time.
2. *Suggest the guidelines outlined above but do not enforce them.* If your staff are not happy with the suggested guidelines, ask them to find an alternative way to ensure that the annual leave allowance is equally spread throughout the year. That way, your team will become responsible for their part of the budget rather than leaving it all to you.

MANAGE YOUR ALLOWANCE FOR UNPLANNED ABSENCE

You usually have an allowance of up to 7% for unplanned absence such as sick leave, maternity leave, carers' leave, etc. (check what your own organisation allows): 7% equates to around four weeks of unplanned absence per person per year without incurring an over-spend.

Make sure you have systems in place to monitor sickness rates closely. You need to be able to look at trends over time. It is not enough to get a 'feel' for the level of absence. Calculate it at the end of each completed 'off-duty'. In some organisations, the HR team send ward managers a summary of their staff sickness rates each month. If your organisation does not have this system in place, you can easily work it out for yourself using the equation outlined in Box 6.2.

On completion of each four-week 'off-duty', it is advisable to keep and update a continuous record of the team's sickness rates (Table 6.4).

SICKNESS LEVELS

You should be able to demonstrate that you are taking action where sickness levels are high. If the sickness rates go beyond your organisation's target level you need to look at the reasons and take action to reduce them. If the main reason for sickness is due to back problems, for example, then it would be wise to undertake further moving and handling risk assessments, involve the manual handling advisor and invest extra funding into moving and handling training/equipment.

BOX 6.2: CALCULATING STAFF SICKNESS RATES

Number of days lost ÷ number of days rostered × 100 = sickness percentage

Example: If Nurse Smith was rostered to work 20 days during the last 'off-duty' but was off sick for four of them:

$$4 \div 20 \times 100 = 20\%$$

The time lost by Nurse Smith was 20% of her potential working time.

TABLE 6.4: Example of record of staff sickness on ward x at 6 months

Staff	Shifts rostered	Shifts off sick	% Sickness	Episodes
Rose	120	6	5	3
Emma	122	8	6.5	2
Jane	120	2	1.7	1
Susan	119	0	0	0
Amy	120	5	4.2	1
Gemma	121	0	0	0
Dave	120	2	1.7	1
John	100	0	0	0
TOTAL	942	23	2.4	8

Total no. of shifts lost to sickness ÷ Total no. of shifts rostered = 23 ÷ 942 × 100
Total percentage of sickness to date = 2.4%

MATERNITY LEAVE

The percentage for unplanned absence usually incorporates maternity leave. If the maternity leave is particularly high within your department, you need to highlight this with your general manager who will have the authority to transfer funding between departments if necessary.

Some organisations hold the maternity leave budget centrally. If this is the case, you must ensure the allowance is allocated to your budget when affected by maternity leave. This can be achieved through close liaison and monitoring with your finance advisor.

OTHER LEAVE

With the increasing emphasis on family-friendly and flexible working policies, there are now other types of leave that you need to manage carefully within your allowance for unplanned absences. These include paternity leave, time off to attend antenatal classes, adoption leave, carers' leave and compassionate leave. You probably already seek advice from the HR department with regards to granting this type of leave but do you also check with your finance department how much it costs you?

PLAN YOUR STUDY LEAVE ALLOWANCE

You usually have an allowance within the budget of around 2% for covering study leave (some organisations allocate more, some less, so you must check exactly what you have with your finance advisor). Two per cent of 225 (365 days minus annual leave) equates to around five days per staff member per year. This does not mean that each member of your team is entitled to five study days per year. The study leave allowance should be viewed as a total for the whole team of staff. For example, if you have a team of 30 WTE, 2% study leave allowance would give you up to 150 study days per year that can be granted to your team (30 × 5 days = 150 days).

The study leave allowance needs to be planned carefully at around November time in the preceding financial year, taking the following steps:

Step 1: Multiply the total number of your budgeted WTE establishment by the number of study days your organisation allocates per WTE (2.25 days if 1%, 5 days if 2%, 7 days if 3%), which will give the total number of days that can be allocated for study leave over the coming financial year.

Step 2: Identify all the study needs of all staff in your team (via the annual appraisal process) both in terms of mandatory requirements plus professional and personal development needs.

Step 3: Find out exactly what the study leave requirements are for each course that staff members have identified.

Step 4: Total the amount of study leave that your staff will require for the coming year.

Step 5: If the total study leave required is more than the total number of shifts allowed in your budget, priorities have to be made. A good way to decide these priorities is to ask your team. Use a team meeting to get them to decide amongst themselves who gets priority. Facilitate the discussion to ensure it is done in a fair and consistent manner.

It is always advisable to keep a portion of the study leave allowance aside to be used for unexpected courses, workshops or seminars that may arise throughout the year, which would benefit the staff and service. If extra courses come up during the year that do not come within the 2% allowance, replacement costs must be identified from another source, unless the workload means you can 'go down' on numbers.

OTHER SOURCES OF FUNDING

Keep close links with the manager of your trust's training and development department and with your link university. This will help keep you aware of any further 'pots' of money that become available throughout the year (often at the end of each financial year between January and March). Various charities such as the League of Friends will sometimes support staff for training courses. You have to find out where these extra funds are; they tend not to be generally advertised.

MANDATORY TRAINING

Include all mandatory training within your allowance. If you are not careful, mandatory training can use up all your study leave allowance. The staff in the training department may not realise this. It is up to you and your colleagues to point it out to them and present an alternative solution. Some organisations have condensed their training into short two-hour sessions, which can either be put together to cover three to four subjects in one day or held as separate sessions during the afternoon handover period.

Study leave needs to be carefully controlled. Keeping your staff informed and fully involved in the process of allocation helps them to understand the restrictions you are working to and reduces any feelings of resentment about study leave allocation.

GET YOUR STAFF INVOLVED IN NON PAY

The NON PAY part of your budget is usually set out in the second part of your budget statement. The only difference between PAY and NON PAY is that the establishment and WTE columns will remain blank because NON PAY does not involve people. The overall amount you have in NON PAY is usually far less than the PAY section. The list of items may be longer but this does not mean it is more important. It is just easier to ascertain where the money has gone.

NON PAY is your lowest priority but still needs tight control. A good way to manage it is to delegate each budget line to a member of your staff. This will give them a good insight into budget management and helps them to develop budgeting skills with appropriate support. The main ones to delegate are pharmacy/drugs, medical supplies and stationery. These usually have another separate list showing more minute details of the expenditure that your staff can manage, leaving you to concentrate on the PAY budget only.

PHARMACY/DRUGS

The nurse responsible for this budget would probably form close links with the ward pharmacist. Their role would include going through the monthly pharmacy budget in detail and becoming familiar with what is being used, what is needed and any changes that are being made. They would be able to identify any cost pressures (see p. 118) such as new routine drugs introduced during the current financial year that were not originally budgeted for.

MEDICAL SUPPLIES

Most hospitals nowadays rely on a top-up system. Having a member of your team to monitor usage and trends will help keep the stock levels appropriate to what is needed and identify any unnecessary expenditure. They will also be able to liaise with the appropriate company representatives (alongside NHS supplies if working within the NHS) to keep abreast of what's new and perhaps more appropriate for your group of patients.

STATIONERY

The stationery budget is often best delegated to your ward receptionist who is usually the most appropriate person to know what is being used and where to make savings.

WARD ENVIRONMENT BUDGET

In England, all NHS ward managers have a small additional budget of £5000 per year to 'be spent on whatever ward sisters/charge nurses consider will best enhance and humanise patient care or improve the working lives of staff' (Department of Health 2000). Each ward manager is issued with a purchasing card to ensure easy access to this budget (Department of Health 2001).

Try to always involve your team when deciding how to spend this budget. Ask them for their ideas and rationale. Discuss and agree what your priorities are as a team. Doing it this way will motivate and inspire them. Making the decision on your own will not.

Remember that your trust has to find this money from within their current budget. No extra funding came with this initiative when it was introduced in 2000. This means that other departments have to do without in order for you to have this £5000, so spend it wisely.

BE MORE ACTIVE IN THE BUSINESS PLANNING PROCESS

Get involved with the business planning process for your directorate. The budgets are reset each year through the annual business planning process known as SAFF (service and financial framework). It's something with which you should be familiar as the budget holder. Some ward managers are left out of this important process. It's up to you to make sure you get involved. Ward budgets can be inappropriate if someone else is deciding what the ward needs.

The process usually begins around November every year in the NHS when all wards and departments in your organisation have to identify what they need for the next year. The whole process takes up to six months (remember, each financial year is from April to April). The general manager's role is to produce the final business plan at the end of the process, which represents all the wards and departments in their directorate. The final plan outlines to the board what funding is required to manage the service in the coming year. It includes any extra funding required due to changes in the service.

The director of finance together with the other board directors agree how much each directorate will get based on the business plans which the general managers have submitted and the level of funding available. It's the general manager's role to write the full business plan, not yours. You are a nurse manager, not a business manager. However, you do need to contribute to the process.

THE BUSINESS PLAN

Your general manager is usually tasked with identifying the *cost pressures* and *service developments* through all their department leads:

1. A cost pressure is an approved change that has already happened over the past year, which needs funding for the future to *maintain existing service levels*, e.g. equipment that requires updating/replacing or a nationally approved pay rise for staff.
2. A service development is an authorised planned change that will be needed to *improve the quantity or quality of service* in the future, e.g. the implementation of a patient follow-up service or the appointment of a nurse specialist.

The general manager usually has to produce evidence for each item in the form of a business case. This is the stage where you need to ensure you are not left out. If you need something really badly, e.g. another member of staff due to increased turnover of patients, then you have to present a 'business case'. Do this together with your manager and finance advisor who will work out all the costs for you.

If you do not do this, either:

- someone else will do it for you; someone who may not understand the service as well as you and therefore will not present your case so well, or
- your needs will not be added to the overall business plan.

There are usually too many cost pressures and service developments so priorities have to be made. Some will be rejected because there is simply not enough money for them all. If you are not involved and don't get across to your general manager the importance of your needs then you may not get them.

HOW TO WRITE A BUSINESS CASE

There is no point in writing a business case if:

- your manager does not agree and has no intention of agreeing to include it in the overall business plan, or
- your manager feels that the funding could be sought elsewhere.

A business case is simply a way of presenting evidence that the item is really needed. Some trusts provide a business case form to be completed in each case. If yours does not do this, Box 6.3 gives an example of a format you could use. Try and keep it short and concise. One piece of A4 paper will usually suffice.

DON'T DO ANYTHING WITHOUT IDENTIFIED FUNDING

It is imperative that you do not implement anything new at all without the identified funding. As mentioned previously, nurses have a wonderful ability to cope when under-resourced. Unfortunately this leads to more problems than it solves. If you can take on extra work without extra resources, then why would the organisation give you further funding?

If you are already providing an extra service without extra funding, write a business case to get the funding put into the following year's budget. For example, if you have a couple of health care assistants (HCAs) who have automatically been given a pay increase for achieving NVQ level 3, but no budget had been set aside for this, it would be classified as a cost pressure.

In the meantime, look at what service you will cease to provide in order to provide the extra service within budget. For example, you can alter the staffing establishment to meet the extra cost of the HCAs' increased salary. Always involve your finance advisor. Being refused a cost pressure does not give you the automatic

BOX 6.3: EXAMPLE OF A FORMAT FOR WRITING A BUSINESS CASE

Title
Explain as fully as you can within the title. Include the cost here (e.g. replacement ECG machine @ £5000).

Introduction
Give a brief summary of what the problem is, the solution, why and what is the cost.

Background
Explain the background but remember that nonclinical people may be reviewing this so you should assume that they know nothing about it. Explain what the benefits will be and what will happen if you do not get it. Your case will be much stronger if you can relate it to government targets, policy or standards. Also include risk assessment results where possible.

Options
List all the options that could be taken and explain why you have chosen this one. Where applicable, give options of types of equipment you could buy and include a cost–benefit analysis (e.g. what would the more expensive one provide as opposed to the cheaper version?).

Preferred option
State your preferred option and say why. Also list all the items that make up your final cost figure. Don't forget to include time and people. Include any potential savings that could be made (e.g. reduced cost of calling out facilities to fix the ECG machine every few weeks).

What may/will happen if not implemented
Always include this option. Explain what would happen to patient care. Try to talk in numbers as much as possible (e.g. how much it would cost in terms of nursing hours spent going round other wards each day to borrow an ECG machine). Your finance advisor will cost it out for you. How many patients would suffer? How many may have treatment delayed? What care standard will you not meet?

right to over-spend because you have the service anyway. You have to make savings elsewhere within your budget.

GET IT IN WRITING

Never be persuaded to take on any extra workload without extra funding. Don't accept verbal promises of extra funding either. Ensure you have some sort of written confirmation. It's not uncommon for ward managers to open extra beds or be persuaded to provide an extra service on the promise that funding will follow, only to find that the funding never materialises. The new service soon becomes established and cannot be withdrawn or patient care will suffer. Don't let yourself get into such a situation. Becoming wise to the business planning process reduces the risk of being duped into taking on work without appropriate funding.

If it does happen (e.g. your line manager may have agreed on your behalf to a change without realising the extra work involved and it is too late for the decision to be reversed), moaning and whinging will not help. You should take action quickly by identifying which aspects of your existing workload must be cut in order to provide the new service. Let your manager know your decision in writing (email is sufficient). Don't try to cope and allow your staff to become exhausted and stressed by trying to provide extra services without the appropriate resources. To do so amounts to ineffective management.

MEET REGULARLY WITH YOUR FINANCE ADVISOR

It is essential that you meet with your financial advisor regularly to:

1. *Ensure that any inaccuracies in your budget are rectified*. If you have been charged for something that you have not used, it is your financial advisor's job to get the money transferred back to your budget, but you have to identify it first. Unprocessed 'starters' and 'leavers' forms are a common source of inaccuracies that need to be identified and corrected quickly.
2. *Ensure that your staffing establishment always matches the limits set on your 'off-duty'*. This is essential for good budget management. Each time a member of your staff resigns, review the job with your team (see p. 163). Don't always replace 'like with like' as the workload or skill requirement may have changed. Your finance advisor will be able to advise how you could achieve the change within your current staffing establishment but still remain within budget.
3. *Check that you are using bank and agency wisely*. If you are using them just to cover staff vacancies, there should be no over-spend. If you are using bank and agency to cover sickness, there should not be an over-spend unless your sickness levels are above the sickness allowance that was added to your budget.
4. *Calculate and prepare for any predicted over-spends*. Obviously there will be unforeseen costs such as an outbreak of methicillin-resistant *Staphylococcus aureus* (MRSA) or a patient who requires one-to-one care for some time. These types of extra costs are not included within your budget but you do need to monitor them closely. Simply saying 'we are over-spent because it's been busy' is insufficient. It will appear that you are not managing your budget properly. It's far better to report that 'we have a predicted overspend of £6000 this month due to the extra staffing required to special a high dependency patient for seven days because there were no available beds in HDU'. You must see your finance advisor early so they can forecast the extra cost to your budget. You can then work together with them and your line manager to plan how you can get your budget back on line over the rest of the financial year.

5. *Help you prepare a business case should you require more staff or equipment.* You will need your general manager's agreement before you go ahead and compile a business case.

It is the finance manager's role to provide specialist expertise and support you in managing the budget. But they will not come to you. Be proactive. Go to them and seek their advice. They are not clinical and often do not understand the complexities of running a ward. You are not a finance expert and do not understand the complexities of the finance world. Work together and use each other's skills to ensure your budget is managed efficiently and effectively, thus ensuring a high standard of patient care.

ACTION POINTS

- Meet with your finance advisor to find out if your 'off-duty' numbers match the staffing establishment, confirm the percentage of absence allowance and go through your budget statement explaining anything that you do not understand.
- Follow up with regular appointments throughout the year, either monthly or every other month. Go through your budget statement and discuss any problems and any changes you wish to make.
- Convert the annual leave allowance into shift numbers allowed per 'off-duty' and ensure all future 'off-duties' are compiled accordingly.
- Starting from this year, plan your next year's study leave quota in advance with your team.
- If your HR team does not supply you with monthly sickness figures for your team, maintain your own records for now.
- Delegate some NON PAY budget lines to your staff for professional and personal development purposes, and to allow you to concentrate on PAY.
- Have a look at last year's business plan and ask your general manager to go through it with you, explaining anything you do not understand. Get involved with next year's plan and put forward your team's needs.
- Review the budget in all your team meetings. Explain and involve them in issues such as annual leave and study leave allowances.
- Involve your staff in *all* decisions such as who gets study leave and how the ward environment money could be used.
- Don't take on extra work without written confirmation of funding.

References

Department of Health 2000 Guidance: Ward environment budgets. Department of Health, Leeds. Online. Available: www.dh.gov.uk/assetRoot/04/01/46/56/04014656.doc 15 Oct 2005

Department of Health 2001 Empowering nurses and slashing red tape means better care and cleaner wards for patients. Press Release Ref 2001/0359, 31 July 2001. Online. Available: www.dh.gov.uk/PublicationsAndStatistics/PressReleases 15 Oct 2005

Hurst K 2002 Selecting and applying methods for estimating the size and mix of nursing teams. Nuffield Institute for Health, Leeds University. Online. Available: http://www. nuffield.leeds.ac.uk/downloads/nursing_teams.pdf 1 Oct 2005

CHAPTER 7

RESPOND WELL TO COMPLAINTS

Work on the content, not number of complaints   126

Dealing with verbal complaints   127

Dealing with written complaints   127

Take appropriate steps before you investigate   128

Contact the complainant personally if appropriate   128

Write a draft response (before investigating the situation)   128

Investigate sensitively   129

Appoint an investigator   129

Collating the written information   131

Responsibilities for maintaining confidentiality   131

Getting information from the staff involved   131

Know when to stop the complaint investigation   132

When disciplinary action may be necessary   132

When the complainant states an intention to take legal action   133

Consider holding a meeting with the complainant   134

Use meetings with complainants as learning experiences   134

Preparing for the meeting   134

Follow six key steps during the meeting   135

Step 1: Listen attentively   135

Step 2: Empathise   136

Step 3: Explain and apologise if appropriate   136

Step 4: Agree a course of action   136

Step 5: Close the meeting   137

Step 6: Follow up   137

Write a good final response letter   137

If you are stuck for words in starting your letter   139

The apology or words of sympathy   140

Explanation of the facts   140

The plan of action   141

If you are stuck for words in finishing your letter   141

Check the layout is easy to read   142

Confirm the final letter with all staff involved in the issue   142

Follow up the complaint with action   142

Share all complaints with your team   144

Comment cards/information board   144

The main aim of the NHS complaints procedures across the UK is to achieve 'local resolution'. This means that complainants should have their complaint dealt with locally by front-line staff. If they are not satisfied with the written response to their verbal or written complaint, they can take it further to the second more formal stage. There are different procedures for the second stage depending on which part of the UK you work in. It usually involves either asking for an independent review or going straight to the health service ombudsman.

This chapter focuses on the first stage of local resolution. It is the stage you have to follow when a complaint is received. Local resolution consists of either a verbal response to a verbal complaint and remedial action taken, or a written response to a verbal or written complaint. Additionally, or instead, it may consist of a meeting with the complainant followed by a letter.

The information contained in this chapter will help you not only to investigate and respond appropriately but also to do this quickly and efficiently, thus leaving you with more time to spend on making the changes to your services that have been highlighted.

WORK ON THE CONTENT, NOT NUMBER OF COMPLAINTS

Having a higher rate of complaints does not necessarily mean you are providing a poorer service. If you publicise the complaints process widely (which you are required to do as part of the complaints procedure), then you are bound to increase the number of complaints received. This is not such a bad thing. What would be bad is if you continued to receive a high level of complaints about the same issue.

Your highest category of complaints, for example, could be about patients' experiences of poor pain management; therefore you should take action to improve the management of pain for future patients. Action could consist of a number of things such as getting more equipment for self-administration of intravenous pain relief, further training and development for staff or implementing a different pain assessment tool. If, following your actions, the overall number of complaints begins to fall but poor pain management continues to form the highest percentage of those complaints, then the overall reduction is not necessarily an indicator of a better service. A decrease in the percentage of complaints about pain management would signify a better service.

The first and most important rule with any complaint is to reply as quickly as possible. This is usually within 20 days, although by the time it gets to and from the complaints department, you may be left with as little as ten days over all. Some complaints will take only a couple of hours or so to investigate and write a response. Others may take several days or even weeks. If you delegate the complaint investigation to one of your team of staff, you need to ensure that they can alter their workload over the following ten days or so to be able to donate the appropriate amount of time required.

DEALING WITH VERBAL COMPLAINTS

Wherever possible, verbal complaints should be dealt with immediately. A record of the conversation should include:

- the date and time
- who was present
- what information was given
- any apologies made
- any action that was taken at the time or future action you promised to undertake.

It is often a nice gesture to follow this up with a letter to the complainant to summarise what was said and, if possible, what action has since been taken to ensure it doesn't happen again. This should definitely be done if it is suspected that the complainant may wish to consider taking the matter further, or if it has been specifically requested.

DEALING WITH WRITTEN COMPLAINTS

There are four steps to dealing with a written complaint:

Step 1: Check you understand exactly what the complaint is about and what the complainant expects from you. If not, call them to clarify.
Step 2: Draft an initial response letter.
Step 3: Appoint an investigating officer.
Step 4: Finalise the letter or organise a meeting.

Standard layout for a response letter
The response to a written complaint should always include:

1. A 'thank you' for the letter and bringing the issue to your attention.
2. An apology if an error or omission has occurred and a sympathetic sentence or two if not. (People do not complain lightly. They may be recently bereaved, still unwell, emotionally unstable, etc. The complaint may have no substance, but they believe they have something to complain about. You need to put yourself into their shoes and imagine how they must feel.)
3. A full explanation of what happened.
4. A description of what action you have taken/are going to take if there was an error or omission.
5. An outline of what to do should they still not be satisfied, or have any further queries, i.e. your contact details, details of any other helpful sources such as bereavement services, how to go to the second stage if they are unhappy with the response.

TAKE APPROPRIATE STEPS BEFORE YOU INVESTIGATE

Verbal complaints that require investigation and all written complaints need a written response. This needs to be sent on behalf of the chief executive and therefore must always go through your hospital complaints department. You should never attempt to send a written response yourself without informing the complaints department.

CONTACT THE COMPLAINANT PERSONALLY IF APPROPRIATE

Sometimes it is possible to resolve a written complaint simply by making a phone call. If this has been possible, you will need to follow up with a letter confirming the call and any action you agreed to take. This letter will still have to go through the complaints department and sent with the chief executive's signature.

Before investigating any complaint, it is necessary to clarify the precise issues being raised by the complainant and their expectations. Most complainants want to prevent the same thing happening to another patient, but if they have other expectations it is useful to know. Again this can be done over the phone. A telephone call usually serves to reassure them that their complaint is being taken seriously. Maintaining personal contact in the early stages will help ensure the complainant is confident that something is being done.

WRITE A DRAFT RESPONSE (BEFORE INVESTIGATING THE SITUATION)

It is advisable to set aside one hour as soon as possible to write the reply before investigating the circumstances. This is for the following reasons:

1. It helps you and others focus on what the complainant wants without getting sidetracked by other issues that crop up during the investigation.
2. You can write without prejudice by immediately putting yourself in the other person's shoes and writing a response that you would expect.
3. It stops the temptation of putting those 'tricky' letters to one side to be dealt with later.

The sample letter and response outlined in Box 7.1 and Box 7.2 give you an idea of how you can draft a response before you have the results of the investigation. This helps you to focus only on the issues that matter. You are not weighed down too much with information from the investigation that you feel you have to include in the response.

Another good thing about doing it this way is that when you delegate the investigation to someone else, they are clear about what needs to be done. It should make their job a lot easier and less stressful. It is also a good training technique for future managers to get an idea of what a good response looks like.

BOX 7.1: SAMPLE LETTER OF COMPLAINT

Dear Sir

I have had the most unfortunate experience of being a patient in your hospital. The ward I stayed in was disgusting. For the whole week I was stuck in a side room where I had to stay on my own because they thought I had an infectious disease (it so happened that I did not).

I understand the hospital wanting to protect the other patients but the treatment I received was terrible. Not once did a cleaner enter my room. I stayed for one week and during that time the bin was not emptied, the bathroom was not cleaned and the only way I got my water jug refilled each day was to keep pressing the buzzer and constantly pester the nurses.

Getting food and even a cup of tea each day was a constant chore. My plates were often left in my room for several days before I would finally persuade a nurse to remove them. So much for me having brought an infectious disease to the hospital; I'm surprised I didn't catch one while I was there.

It was as if everyone was afraid they might catch something. Don't you train your cleaners? When I complained to the sister, she always seemed to be busy, promising to do things but never coming back. She said that the cleaning was not her responsibility. If that is the case, who is responsible? I thought matrons were back. Well, I never saw one.

I'm so angry about the way I was treated and want to know what you are going to do about it.

Yours faithfully

INVESTIGATE SENSITIVELY

APPOINT AN INVESTIGATOR

Appoint a member of your team to investigate. There is no reason why your staff nurses (both junior and senior) cannot investigate a complaint. It is good to be exposed to complaints early on in their career. The fact that most complaints are down to poor communication and record keeping will help the staff appreciate the importance of such matters, particularly when their own complaint investigation is hampered by poorly kept records.

Ensure that your staff undergo basic training on investigating and writing responses, and then begin by delegating the simple complaints. By doing this, you will generate a team who will be more highly aware and keen to contribute to improving the service. For each complaint investigation, make sure that they have the time and support required. If necessary, go through their diary with them and

BOX 7.2: SAMPLE OF DRAFT LETTER DEMONSTRATING HOW TO WRITE RESPONSE BEFORE INVESTIGATING

Dear x,

Thank you for your letter of 3 October and for being so frank and honest about the problems you encountered whilst in our care.

I was disturbed to read of the conditions you say you had to endure [*Is it true? Did this happen?*]. I am sorry we have let you down and delivered what appears to be a very substandard level of service.

Following our investigation into the matter, we have found that the cleaner did not enter the room because . . . [*Why did they not enter the room?*]. We do aim to ensure that side rooms are cleaned every day and that . . . [*What else does the policy say?*]. I am concerned that this did not happen and have brought it to the attention of John Smith, our Hotel Services Manager. He has assured me that he will . . . [*What is he going to do?*]. All our cleaners do receive a specific training programme which consists of . . . [*Do they? What does it entail?*].

It is the sisters' role to ensure that the cleaning does get done. I have since spoken to the sister, Sarah Jones . . . [*What did she say?*].

You are right; we do have matrons now and I am disappointed to hear you were not given information about this. The matron for that particular area is Jane Smith and her contact details are [*give details*]. I am sorry you did not have these details earlier. The reason you didn't see or know about the matron is because . . . [*Why?*].

Since your letter, I will ensure that . . . [*What can be done to ensure it doesn't happen again?*]. I hope the proposed action I have outlined will go some way to restoring your faith in us.

I do hope you have now made a full recovery despite your unfortunate experiences with us. I can't put things right for you now but please rest assured that I will do everything I can to ensure it doesn't happen again to future patients who need to be cared for in a side room.

Once again, please accept my sincere apologies. If you would like to discuss anything further, please do not hesitate to contact me on [*telephone number*] or the matron, Jane Smith, on [*telephone number*].

Yours sincerely

help to reprioritise their work to ensure blocks of time can be freed up for them to carry out a thorough investigation. Ensure they let you know if anyone is not cooperating. Do not let them struggle with senior staff who refuse to make time to talk to them, or are being deliberately rude. Support them by intervening if necessary.

COLLATING THE WRITTEN INFORMATION

The investigator should start by collecting the relevant written documentation and speaking to the staff involved. Your initial draft response letter will outline to the investigator what information will be required. This usually includes the following documents:

1. The complainant's medical records.
2. Any trust-wide or local policies/procedures relevant to the complaint.
3. Copies of relevant 'off-duties' or on-call rotas to identify who was on duty at the time.
4. A copy of the original complaint and any other correspondence.

Relevant papers from the medical records may include medical and/or nursing progress sheets, consent forms, test request forms, GP referral letters, etc. Remember that physiotherapists and occupational therapists tend to keep separate case notes stored in their own departments. These may need to be located too.

RESPONSIBILITIES FOR MAINTAINING CONFIDENTIALITY

The complaints department will have informed the complainant that their records may be used and have given them the option of refusing to allow this.

The Data Protection Act (1998) requires all processing of data to be 'fair and lawful' and all 'personal data to be protected against unauthorised or unlawful processing and against accidental loss, destruction or damage'. This means that whilst the investigator has the documents in their possession but is not using them directly, they should be kept in a locked drawer/filing cabinet and the office should be locked at all times when no one is there. They should not take the medical records home with them under any circumstances.

As a health care professional, the investigator should follow their own professional code of confidentiality and the Caldicott principles (Box 7.3). You should also ensure they are aware of the NHS Code of Confidentiality which emphasises that patient information must remain confidential and seen only by those with direct involvement (Department of Health 2003, NHS Scotland 2003, NHS Wales 2004).

GETTING INFORMATION FROM THE STAFF INVOLVED

Once all the documents have been obtained, the next stage is to identify the staff involved and make appointments to see them all. Note the word 'interview' has not been used. This is not a formal process. It is also not a disciplinary process. The meeting is simply trying to ascertain the facts. Statements are therefore not formally required, although it is wise to advise staff to write down for their own record what happened should they need to refer to the details later.

> **BOX 7.3: CALDICOTT PRINCIPLES**
>
> 1. Justify the purpose.
> 2. Don't use patient identifiable information unless it is absolutely necessary.
> 3. Use the minimum necessary patient identifiable information.
> 4. Access to patient identifiable information should be on a strict need to know basis.
> 5. Everyone should be aware of their responsibilities.
> 6. Understand and comply with the law.
>
> (Caldicott Committee 1997)

If you do decide that witness statements are required, you must ensure that the interviewees are informed of their rights to have a union representative, colleague or friend present. You should also ensure they are aware that their statements may be used if the complainant decides to take legal action at a later stage.

When the investigator meets with individual members of staff, they should always ensure that the appropriate records are available to help 'jog' their memory. If any of the staff involved cannot remember the patient or what happened then they should say so; it is far better to admit this. Tell the complainant what you have concluded from the notes, but that the practitioner was unable to recall the details.

If at this stage you feel that the investigator can't get all the information together on time, let the complaints department know immediately. A 'holding letter' can then be written. Explain what the problem is and tell the complaints team when you will be able to give them a full response. Remember: always 'under-promise and over-deliver'. If you think you will get the information and response out within the next two weeks, give them a date for three weeks' time. That way they will be impressed if they get the answer within two weeks and it gives you some extra time to allow for unforeseen circumstances.

KNOW WHEN TO STOP THE COMPLAINT INVESTIGATION

WHEN DISCIPLINARY ACTION MAY BE NECESSARY

The complaints and disciplinary procedures should be kept separate. You must stop the complaints process if you suspect any of the following:

- professional misconduct
- negligence
- a serious untoward incident
- criminal activity.

If you feel disciplinary action may be required then you must alert the complaints manager and your line manager. Your line manager together with human resources (HR) support will help you decide which alternative procedure should be followed. A formal investigation into the matter can then be arranged.

The complaints manager will write a letter to the complainant informing them about what is happening and that you will not be continuing with the complaints process until you have the outcome of the alternative investigation. Never do this on your own. It requires the skill and experience of the complaints manager. If the incident only formed one aspect of the complaint, you will be able to continue to investigate the other aspects of the complaint.

WHEN THE COMPLAINANT STATES AN INTENTION TO TAKE LEGAL ACTION

The complaints process is completely separate from the legal process and does not lead to financial compensation. This is why it is vital to be aware of the complainants' expectations from the outset. If they have stated that they want an apology and/or for the standards to improve you may continue. However, if they state at any time during the process that they intend to take legal action, then you must consult with your complaints manager in order to stop the complaints investigation.

Support any practitioners involved

Working in health care is a vocation. There are few other roles where individuals have so much responsibility for so little financial reward. To give care to others every day sometimes under very difficult circumstances and then be the subject of a complaint can be soul-destroying. It needs to be handled very sensitively. Any health care professional is naturally going to feel upset and perhaps even angry. They may feel that they have given so much yet all they get in return is a written complaint about areas of care that may have been missed.

Individuals who are the subject of complaints need to feel that they are fully supported by their manager. You must ensure that you:

1. Don't take sides with either the complainant or the health care professional.
2. Reassure the individual that you are not interested in blaming anyone and you just want to find out if there is anything that can be done to improve the situation.
3. Do not hesitate to ask for advice if the situation is a particularly difficult one.

Never handle a difficult complaint by yourself. The complaints manager is usually very experienced in most types of complaints and will be able to advise. If you feel you need more professional support contact your director of nursing who, in many organisations, has executive responsibility for clinical governance and complaints. They usually have a lot of experience in handling difficult and complicated complaints.

Keep accurate notes of the investigation process

It's a good idea for the investigator to keep a running log of events and findings. An example of an investigation progress sheet that could be used is outlined in Appendix 7.1.

CONSIDER HOLDING A MEETING WITH THE COMPLAINANT

If you feel a written response may not be enough or too complicated, you can call the complainant and offer them the chance of a meeting instead. It may also be offered as a further option at the end of your written response. Inviting the complainant to meet and discuss the complaint can be a more successful option particularly if they have lots of questions. The complaints manager may or may not be involved, but it would be wise to use their expertise in such situations.

USE MEETINGS WITH COMPLAINANTS AS LEARNING EXPERIENCES

Never delegate the chairing of a meeting like this to someone who has no previous experience. As you get used to undertaking such meetings, start bringing one of your staff along to expose them to the experience and get them used to the process. Some health professionals go to great lengths to avoid meeting with complainants fearing that they break some rule or regulation or that they may do something wrong. The more you experience such meetings the more you will be willing to offer them to future complainants without feeling threatened.

PREPARING FOR THE MEETING

Arrange an appropriate venue

The meeting should be as informal as possible. It is preferable to use a nonclinical area, which is more familiar for the complainant. The complainant may bring other people with them for support so it is wise to book a good sized meeting room that can accommodate several people. Make sure there are chairs available in a waiting area outside. If there is more than one staff member involved in the complaint and they need to be present, it is best to call them in one at a time when needed. To be in the same room with a group of health professionals can be quite intimidating for most people not used to the clinical environment.

Prepare a draft agenda with a timetable

This does not need to be formal but you will need some sort of structure to adhere to, otherwise you may end up going around in circles on the same subject with no conclusion. A list of the complaints may be all that is needed so that you can go through each one in turn. It is advisable to start by asking the complainant what they want from the meeting.

Plan on the meeting lasting 1–1.5 hours at the most

If it goes over the hour, make sure the complainant is happy to go on and offer regular refreshments. Do not go over 1.5 hours unless absolutely necessary. By then everyone will be getting tired. Also they will probably have paid for the minimum two hours' parking time, which will cause added anxiety.

Make sure that all documents are available

Include case notes and copies of all correspondence pertaining to the complaint. You may need to refer to these during your discussions. You may also wish to share the contents with the complainant so it's a good idea to familiarise yourself with the contents and be prepared to explain any words or phrases which they may not understand.

Ensure there is someone else present to take notes

These will be used to form the basis of the follow-up letter, so will need to be detailed. If a nurse explained a procedure she undertook, for example, the notes would need to include that explanation. It would not be good enough for the complainant to read that 'the nurse explained the procedure'.

The follow-up letter should confirm the outcome of the discussion. The meeting notes may or may not be included depending on the circumstances. Whatever is decided, the final correspondence to be sent to the complainant must be agreed by all present that it represents a true reflection of what was said. The complaints manager will ensure a cover note is provided signed by the chief executive.

FOLLOW SIX KEY STEPS DURING THE MEETING

STEP 1: LISTEN ATTENTIVELY

Make sure the complainant(s) know they have your full attention. Turn the phone off and put up a 'Do not disturb' notice outside the door. Make brief notes as you go and let them see what you are writing. Don't write too much. You have a note-taker to do that for you. The reason you write notes is to reassure the complainant that you are taking them seriously.

Show them that you are listening through body language and regular prompts. Summarise and reflect back what they are telling you on a regular basis. This not only shows them that you hear what they are saying, it also ensures that you are clear about it in your mind. For example:

- 'Just to clarify my understanding . . .'
- 'Would you mind just going over that bit again with me?'
- 'I have the impression that you feel . . . Is that right?'

STEP 2: EMPATHISE

Let them know you understand what they are feeling or what they must have gone through. For example:

- 'I can see why you must be upset'
- 'It must have been difficult for you'
- 'I can understand why you felt so angry at the time'.

Don't suggest that what they are saying cannot be true or insinuate that they must be exaggerating, with phrases like:

- 'I can't believe she said it quite like that'
- 'Are you sure that's what happened?'

This will only serve to aggravate the situation. It is advisable to neither agree nor disagree but remain neutral. Stick to empathising rather than sympathising. It will help focus the meeting on finding a solution rather than going through the problem over and over again.

STEP 3: EXPLAIN AND APOLOGISE IF APPROPRIATE

Explain why things have apparently gone wrong. If there are nursing records pertaining to the situation, let them see what has been written and explain any technical terms that they may not understand. Be open. If it is clear that a mistake has been made, then apologise and be sincere in that apology. They will want to know that you regret what happened and will take steps to ensure it does not happen again.

If there was no mistake and their complaint is unjustified then say so. Saying that, it is usually the case that poor communication somewhere along the way led them to this meeting. More often than not, you will probably need at least to apologise that they were not better informed.

Make sure you have answered all their questions. Give them time to make sure they have no more questions they would like to ask. Don't be afraid of silences. Good use of silence gives them time to think and feel that they are still in control.

STEP 4: AGREE A COURSE OF ACTION

Once you have listened, empathised and/or apologised and answered all their questions, you need to agree a course of action:

- 'What would you like me to do now?'
- 'How would you like me to take this forward?'
- 'I suggest that from now on, we take the following steps to ensure it does not happen again . . . would you be happy with this?'

If the complainant is satisfied, ensure the course of action agreed is achievable. If what the complainant is asking for is not realistic, then say so. It would be unrealistic, for example, if they want a member of staff sacked for speaking to them in a cursory manner. In this case you might say 'I cannot authorise what you are asking for. This member of staff has been formally spoken to. I do not condone her actions but am prepared to give her a second chance with close monitoring'.

Wrap up the meeting with a promise that you will look into things further if:

● what they are asking for is outside your remit
● they begin asking for too much
● they become angry and abusive
● further issues arise at the meeting that you were not previously aware of.

A few well-chosen words are called for, for example, 'It appears that there are further matters that need looking into, so you will need to give me some more time to look into this properly'.

STEP 5: CLOSE THE MEETING

Close the meeting by summarising what has taken place and what you have agreed. Always explain what will happen next. Tell them they will receive a letter confirming what has been discussed and the changes that you have agreed to implement. Give a timetable; don't say they will receive a letter by the end of the week unless you are absolutely certain that you can get it done by then. Remember to under-promise and over-deliver.

STEP 6: FOLLOW UP

Always do what you agreed to do. If you have promised to call them the next day once you have made further enquires, then do so. Even if you do not have the information, call them and say so, then arrange to call again when you have the information. Follow up is the most important stage in the complaints process. Too many complaints reach the health service ombudsman because complainants do not receive that call/letter which they were promised. Failing to follow up agreed actions only serves to make a bad situation worse.

WRITE A GOOD FINAL RESPONSE LETTER

Get the structure right

Where possible, use the structure outlined on page 127. Thank them, apologise and/or sympathise, explain, outline the action you are going to take and finish up with your contact details plus what they can do next if not satisfied.

If there are several subjects of complaint within one letter, prioritise the main complaint and address the minor points afterwards. Using subheadings for complaints about more than one aspect of care helps to keep it structured.

Represent your organisation

Always keep in mind that your reply is representing your organisation and the overall health care system. Saying negative things about the way they are managed is very unprofessional. It will result in the complainant losing their confidence in you. Don't hide behind the system or processes that are beyond your own control. If the issue is beyond your direct control, say what your organisation is doing about it or who is trying to rectify the 'system problem'.

You are speaking on behalf of your organisation. Complainants do not want to hear about any internal problems you may have with getting things done or poor communication between different departments. They are not interested if the broken toilet has not been mended because the facilities department have not responded to your numerous requests. If this is the case then you are simply showing them that you are not a good enough manager to be able to make things happen.

Write in 'the first person'

Don't try to present an anonymous face. Refer to yourself as 'I' and the complainant as 'you'. For example:

1. *Anonymous response*: 'It is concerning to hear that the standard of care was not satisfactory.'
2. *Personal response*: 'I am concerned to hear that you were not happy with the standard of care.'

Addressing the complainant as 'you' signifies to them that you are treating them as a real person and not just another complainant.

Try not to use the term 'we' unless you are explaining organisational policy or decisions. The complainant is much more likely to believe and trust a single person. An anonymised 'we' represents a faceless organisation.

Add the personal touch

It is always best to put yourself in the complainant's shoes and think how you would feel if you went through a similar situation. Strike a personal note with them. Treat them as you would if you were speaking to a colleague. It helps to write as you speak, so they can almost hear the words. It's not just what you say, it's the way that you say it that makes the difference. The explanation and facts may be right but if they come across as formal and business-like, the complainant will not be satisfied.

Ensure your personality, professionalism and above all, empathy shines through in the letter. The complainant will then feel safe and comfortable that everything that could be done is being done and that it's not just a standard bureaucratic response.

Another way to give your letter the personal touch is to write in the 'active' tense as opposed to the 'passive' tense. Consider the following:

1. *Passive tense*: 'Please rest assured that action has been taken to rectify the situation.'
2. *Active tense*: 'I can assure you that we are taking action to rectify the situation.'

The first sentence distances the writer and absolves any responsibility for the situation whereas in the second example the complainant can be reassured that someone is making sure something is being done. Taking a passive and distant tone is more 'business-like' but not appropriate when writing to a complainant.

Avoid using jargon

Keep it simple or explain technical terms. Most patients still do not know the rank structure for doctors and nurses. Health care assistant, physician, consultant, registrar and staff nurse are all words that should be avoided (or include an explanation about what they are). Try to stick to just using the terms 'doctor' or 'nurse'.

Use the same phrases you would use if you were speaking to the complainant, not the official terms. Use:

- 'about . . .' rather than 'with reference to . . .'
- 'I now know . . .' rather than 'I have been informed . . .'
- 'because . . .' rather than 'due to the fact that . . .'
- 'sorry' rather than 'please accept my apologies'.

IF YOU ARE STUCK FOR WORDS IN STARTING YOUR LETTER

The opening sentence

First impressions count, so the way the letter starts is crucial. It sets the tone. This is why it is usually best to thank the complainant for the letter and for bringing the issue to your attention, followed by either an apology or a note of sympathy for their predicament. The opening paragraph should be kept short. Try not to use latin abbreviations such as 're:'. It depersonalises your reply immediately.

Below are some examples of openings to stimulate your thoughts:

'Thank you for your letter expressing concern about the care and treatment you received . . .'
'Thank you for your letter and for being so frank and open about the problems you encountered whilst . . .'
'Thank for your letter and for bringing this issue to my attention.'
'Thank you for your letter concerning the problems you have had with . . .'

THE APOLOGY OR WORDS OF SYMPATHY

Follow your opening lines with an apology or a few words of sympathy. Remember that an apology is not an admission of liability within the complaints process. Sympathising with the complainant does not equate to apologising. It shows that you are genuinely interested, supportive and understanding. Put yourself in their shoes and imagine how you would feel in the circumstances they describe. Show that you are making an effort to understand their point of view. If you have nothing to apologise for, then don't. You can say you understand without apologising.

Below are some examples of sympathy and/or empathy:

'I am sorry to hear you were not told of your husband's diagnosis at an earlier stage. I can understand how upsetting that would be.'
'I'm concerned to hear that your wound became infected. I can appreciate your anxiety.'
'I was concerned to hear that . . .'
'I know how frustrating it is to be kept in the dark.'
'I can imagine this must have been very distressing for you.'

If you are sorry, say so, even if it is just because the letter is late:

'I am sorry for the delay in replying.'
'First, I would like to say how sorry I am that you feel this way.'
'I am sorry to hear that you are still in pain six weeks after the operation.'
'I am sorry to hear of your recent loss.'
'I am very sorry that you were not satisfied with the care you received.'
'I am sorry to hear that your wound is not healing as well as expected.'
'I am extremely sorry this has happened.'

EXPLANATION OF THE FACTS

Always give a full explanation of the facts but again make it personal. To say that 'this is what happened . . .' or 'these are the facts . . .' is too formal. Try the following examples:

'I'd like to explain what happened so you can see the exceptional and unexpected events which occurred on the ward that day.'
'I have made enquiries and it appears that there has been a major breakdown in communication in your case.'
'We aim to offer good quality food at all times, but unfortunately we cannot cook individual meals to order. We use an external catering firm who bring the ready cooked meals into the wards.'
'Unfortunately, there appears to have been a failure to communicate in this case. The doctor forgot to tell the nurse he had prescribed the tablets to be given that night. The nurse had already given your father his tablets

for the evening and so did not look at his chart again until the morning by which time it was too late.'

THE PLAN OF ACTION

Outlining what you are going to do about the situation is the main part of the letter. The complainant needs to be reassured that something is going to be done as a result of their complaint. They need to know that their letter is being taken seriously. Below are some examples of how to begin this section:

'This unfortunate event has highlighted a gap in our system, so what I've decided to do is . . .'

'This is a very rare occurrence and there is little we can do to prevent it happening again. However, what we will do is . . .'

'Following your letter, we instigated the following system . . .'

'As a direct result of your complaint, we have/will . . .'

'I can assure you that in order to prevent this happening again, I have decided to . . .'

'Since you brought the matter to our attention, we have put in place a process of . . .'

IF YOU ARE STUCK FOR WORDS IN FINISHING YOUR LETTER

Always finish by giving contact details, preferably your own. A few extra words at this stage can help to make it feel more genuine. Here are some examples to stimulate your thoughts (and again to save you time):

'I hope that this will go some way to restoring your faith in us.'

'I am confident that this will not happen again to any of our future patients.'

'Thank you again for bringing this to our attention.'

'Again, I am sorry for the inconvenience caused.'

'I am sorry that we cannot be more helpful on this occasion, but hope you have been reassured that . . .'

'I hope this explains the position, but if you have any other queries, feel free to contact me.'

'I hope this information helps you.'

'Once again, thank you for taking the trouble to write and let me know your situation.'

These are all examples just to stimulate your thinking, especially if you are going through a particularly busy period and do not have the time to spend thinking of the right words.

Remember it doesn't take much to add the personal touch. Rather than write the usual 'please do not hesitate to contact me', the following will have a far better effect: 'I do hope this answers your questions, but should there be anything else you need to know I'll be happy to discuss further if you call me on 01208 1212112. Alternatively, our bereavement service will give you any information you need if you ring them on 02309 5040541'.

Giving them your direct contact details will hopefully ensure that any further issues can be solved through a telephone call. It is far better to do this than end up receiving another letter to which you have to compile yet another response.

CHECK THE LAYOUT IS EASY TO READ

Once you have written the response letter, spend some time on making it look good and easier to read. Ensure the following:

- all paragraphs should be wider than they are long
- use bullet points where you can to break up the text
- use subheadings if more than one complaint is incorporated
- have one idea per paragraph and keep sentences short.

Both examples in Box 7.4 contain exactly the same words, but different layouts. Note how much easier it is to read the second extract as opposed to the first.

CONFIRM THE FINAL LETTER WITH ALL STAFF INVOLVED IN THE ISSUE

The final letter must be checked and agreed by ALL staff involved in the complaint investigation to ensure it is factually correct. Confirm that all points raised in the initial letter have been answered, and the main one is answered first. If you are at all concerned about the wording of the letter, seek advice from the complaints manager.

Once all the staff involved agree that it is a fair and accurate account of what actually happened, return your final response to the complaints department. Never send a response letter straight to the complainant. Most complaints procedures require that either the chief executive signs all response letters or a cover letter by the chief executive is included. The complaints team will ensure that this is done.

FOLLOW UP THE COMPLAINT WITH ACTION

Complaints are a good way of showing where improvements can be made in practice. They often highlight areas that matter more to patients and families than previously thought. Unfortunately, more often than not, the time that is spent on investigating and compiling responses can exceed that which is spent on making the actual improvements.

A two-year UK-wide review of complaints (Department of Health 2001) showed that most complainants simply want:

BOX 7.4: EXAMPLE WHICH DEMONSTRATES HOW TO MAKE YOUR FINAL LETTER EASIER TO READ

First extract:

Thank you for your letter of 5 May, expressing your concerns about the lack of information you received whilst your husband was in hospital. I am very sorry that this happened and can understand your frustrations at not knowing what was going on. I have since talked to the team of nurses who cared for your husband and it appears they were not aware that you were housebound. They assumed that you were not concerned because you rarely called or visited.

I am sorry that your needs were completely overlooked. It seems that on admission, the receiving nurse mistook your daughter to be your next of kin. As you and your husband are divorced, the nurse assumed that you were not living together and little was done to assess your home situation until the decision was made to discharge your husband.

Amended extract:

Thank you for your letter of 5 May, expressing your concerns about the lack of information you received whilst your husband was in hospital.

I am very sorry that this happened and can understand your frustrations at not knowing what was going on. I have since talked to the team of nurses who cared for your husband and it appears they were not aware that you were housebound. They assumed that you were not concerned because you rarely called or visited. I am sorry that your needs were completely overlooked. It seems that:

- On admission, the receiving nurse mistook your daughter to be your next of kin.
- As you and your husband are divorced, the nurses assumed that you were not living together.
- Little was done to assess your home situation until the decision was made to discharge your husband.

- better communication, information and support during the process
- their complaints to be dealt with more quickly
- to ensure that lessons are learned and improvements are made to services as a result.

A complaint that is well handled helps to create a good relationship with the complainant. Complainants will probably tell most people they know about their experience. A poorly handled complaint only serves to create anger and frustration and will cloud their view of their experience. Some complainants may even contact the local press out of sheer frustration. Dealing with complaints requires you to:

- be understanding and appreciate the complainant's point of view
- fully investigate
- respond fully using the right language
- learn lessons and implement changes as a result.

Complaints provide you with important information and feedback about the experiences of patients on your ward. You must ensure that lessons are learned from those who raise their concerns.

SHARE ALL COMPLAINTS WITH YOUR TEAM

Share the issues with your whole team, not just those who were directly involved with the complaint. Make complaints a regular item on your team agenda. Follow up all the actions at each meeting to ensure the issues raised in previous complaints are not overshadowed by those raised in new complaints.

A continuous plan of action from complaints should be maintained and updated regularly. This will ensure your staff view complaints as an opportunity to improve the services and make changes, rather than a hassle. There is nothing worse than managers who continually procrastinate about the number of complaint letters they have to deal with.

COMMENT CARDS/INFORMATION BOARD

Getting no complaints at all does not mean you have a better service; it probably means the patients either don't know how to complain or are worried that you might take offence and their future care may be affected. It is important that you state in your ward leaflet or information board that you welcome comments as a way of finding out what your patients really think.

Having a comment card system on your ward with a board displaying examples of responses is the practice of a progressive ward manager (see p. 94). It helps reduce the number of complaints but enables you to continue getting feedback. Without continuous comments and complaints, you can never be sure that the service you provide is truly meeting the patients' needs.

Make sure your comment notice board is up-to-date with extracts of complaint letters (maintaining patient confidentiality) and their responses so that other patients and users of the service can see that you listen to their concerns and are actually doing something.

ACTION POINTS

- As soon as the complaint arrives on your desk, ensure that you write a draft response; preferably on the day you receive it.
- Appoint a member of staff to investigate the complaint using your draft response as a guide (and with your full support).
- Ensure that you and your staff receive appropriate training and support in handling complaints.
- If there is anything you are unsure about, get help early on from your organisation's complaints department.
- Make sure the complaints process is halted if you suspect an untoward incident, negligence, misconduct, a crime has been committed or anything that you feel requires a formal investigation.
- If you don't have one already, put up an information board in your ward with comment cards and extracts of complaint letters with responses.
- Inform and involve your team in all complaints and resulting action plans, preferably by having it on the agenda of all regular team meetings.

References

Caldicott Committee 1997 Report on the review of patient-identifiable information. Department of Health, London.

Data Protection Act 1998 HMSO, London. Online. Available: http://www.opsi.gov.uk/acts/acts1998/19980029.htm 1 Oct 2005

Department of Health 2001 NHS complaints procedure national evaluation. DH Publications, London. Online. Available: http://www.dh.gov.uk/assetRoot/04/05/89/33/04058933.pdf 1 Oct 2005

Department of Health 2003 Confidentiality: NHS code of practice. DH Publications, London. Online. Available: htttp://www.dh.gov.uk/assetRoot/04/06/92/54/04069254.pdf 1 Oct 2005

NHS Scotland 2003 NHS code of practice on protecting patient confidentiality. Scottish Executive. Online. Available: http://www.show.scot.nhs.uk/confidentiality/publications/6074NHSCode.pdf 1 Oct 2005

NHS Wales, Social Services Inspectorate for Wales and Welsh Assembly Government 2004 Confidentiality: code of practice for health and social care in Wales. Online. Available: http://www.wales.gov.uk/subisocialpolicysocialservices/content/consultations/confid-code-e.pdf 30 Oct 2005

EXAMPLE OF PROGRESS SHEET FOR A COMPLAINT INVESTIGATION

Action	Date completed and any comments
1. Complaint letter received	
2. Contact complainant to clarify their expectations or any unclear issues	
3. Draft initial response	
4. Appoint appropriate investigator	
5. Meet with investigator – Give copy of draft response and agree issues to be investigated – Agree time out in diary to devote to investigation	
6. Investigator: – Locate case notes – Find further relevant documents – Identify and arrange to see staff involved	
7. Investigator: – Meet staff involved – Find out what happened and why	
8. Finalise response letter	
9. Check final response with all staff involved	
10. Send final response to complaints department	
11. Lock away the file in a safe and secure place	

CHAPTER 8

INSTIGATE A ROLLING RECRUITMENT PROGRAMME

Review the post with the person who is leaving   148

Establish why they are leaving   148

Establish if the job description is still appropriate   149

Review the job description and person specification   150

Write good adverts and application packages   150

Put in extra effort   150

Writing the advert   150

Application packages   151

Shortlist and arrange interviews properly   151

Tips for shortlisting   151

Prepare for the interviews   152

Prepare your team for the interviews   153

Get the best out of the interview process   153

Preparing the questions   153

Assessment of practical skills   154

Prepare the environment and interviewers   154

The role of the chairperson in interviews   155

Follow up all candidates personally   155

Calling unsuccessful candidates   156

Follow up promising but unsuccessful candidates   156

Take risks   157

Arrange a good induction programme   157

Before they commence   157

Two-week supernumerary period   157

Allocate a mentor   158

Continually explore all other avenues to get staff   158

Student nurses   159

Bank and agency staff   159

Returning nurses   159

Liaise closely with your recruitment lead   160

Don't discriminate   160

Part time does not mean part skilled   160

Don't waste the skills of enrolled nurses   161

Overseas nurses are not all the same   161

Succession plan   162

Is your staffing establishment conducive to good succession planning?   162

Staff nurse level (band 5)   162

Deputy manager/sister/charge nurse level (band 6)   163

Health care assistants   163

Fully involve your team in all aspects of recruitment 163

Develop their interviewing skills early on   164

Get the team involved with the new staff member early on   164

If you could have all your vacancies filled at all times with the right staff with the right skills, wouldn't life be so much easier? Unfortunately this does not happen in real life, but you can go some way toward making things a lot easier for yourself if you concentrate on the recruitment process all the time, even when all your vacancies are filled. Nurses rarely stay in one post throughout their career. You will always have a fairly high turnover of staff.

It's good for staff to regularly have new people join the team with different skills to offer. It prevents them from becoming too comfortable and set in their ways. It also helps you to continue to review and change your staffing establishment according to the needs of your unit. Make sure you are always one step ahead so that when a person resigns you will be able to replace them quickly without causing too much disruption.

REVIEW THE POST WITH THE PERSON WHO IS LEAVING

Before you even begin thoughts of advertising and filling a forthcoming vacancy, you should first review the role with the person who is leaving.

ESTABLISH WHY THEY ARE LEAVING

Staff may leave your team for promotion or to gain further experience. It could also be for personal reasons such as moving house or wanting to spend more time with children. You should be concerned if any members of staff are leaving for better working conditions, better hours or because of any problems at work. Take note of why they are leaving, and do something to ensure the next candidate will not feel the same way.

Don't leave exit interviews to the human resources (HR) department. Staff have a right to fill in an anonymous exit questionnaire but you need feedback too. You don't need a particular form; just ask them. Remember though that employees have the right to refuse an exit interview. They should always be voluntary.

When you ask why they are leaving, aim to ensure the person talks a lot more than you do. Spend most of the time listening and taking note (even if you do not agree). Ask open questions such as:

1. Are there any other reasons for leaving?
2. What could we do/have done to persuade you to stay?
3. What have you enjoyed or found satisfying about working here?
4. What aspects of work didn't you like or found difficult or frustrating?
5. Is there any more training and development you would have benefitted from?
6. Is there anything that could be improved in the ward which would make things better from your point of view?
7. What is it about your next job that makes it more attractive than this one?

ESTABLISH IF THE JOB DESCRIPTION IS STILL APPROPRIATE

Review the job description with them. Has it changed in any way? If the remit has grown to include other responsibilities such as a vital link nurse role, first ask any of your other staff if they would like to take it on. If not, consider adding it to the job description. If, for example, the person is a link nurse for diabetes and it is a much needed role on the ward, then think about recruiting someone who has, or is willing to develop, those skills. Add it to the job description before you advertise.

The job could have changed so much that the person leaving may say it needs someone more senior with specialist experience or perhaps even someone who does not need the skills of a registered nurse any more. If this is the case, review this idea with the rest of the team. You may all come to the decision that it would be beneficial to replace this person with someone requiring entirely different skills from another pay band. It is advisable in such cases to meet with your finance manager and line manager to go through what you would need to do to change the post and pay band but remain within budget.

Changing the job and associated pay band

You cannot change your budgeted establishment immediately because it has to be done through the business planning process. However, you do not have to match the budgeted establishment exactly. You can recruit a band 5 nurse into a health care assistant (HCA) post, for example; but only if you consult with your finance advisor and line manager first, to make sure that at the end of the year you will not go over budget in order to do so. The finance advisor will work it out for you, taking other issues into consideration such as :

- part-time staff in full-time posts
- staff who are on maternity leave
- staff off on long-term sick leave
- current use of agency and bank staff.

Be daring. There is no reason why you cannot redesign the job into one that suits your ward. You may, for example, like to devise a new role such as an HCA who can also take on ward receptionist duties. This could help enormously at times when your current ward receptionist is on annual leave or off sick.

REVIEW THE JOB DESCRIPTION AND PERSON SPECIFICATION

The job description may need completely rewriting or just a few minor changes. Do this together with the person who is leaving the job. Your HR advisor will advise you on what you can and cannot do with the job description according to your organisation's policies and procedures.

Redesigning roles when staff leave helps replace outdated jobs and allows your remaining staff to progress by taking on different responsibilities. You can design jobs around the patient and changing workloads rather than the other way around. It is not a difficult thing to do. The key is to ensure you involve the right people, i.e. your finance advisor, your HR advisor and your line manager. Guidelines were produced by the Department of Health in 2005 to help guide health care managers with the process of redesigning roles (Department of Health 2005).

WRITE GOOD ADVERTS AND APPLICATION PACKAGES

Don't leave the writing of your job adverts and application packages to your HR department. State exactly what you want in the advert and give them the material for your application packages. List what you want to be sent out to each prospective candidate.

PUT IN EXTRA EFFORT

Don't leave anything to chance. The recruitment teams in HR departments have a huge remit. They have to oversee the recruitment for all personnel within your organisation. Don't expect them to give you special treatment. They will send out standard application packages and do not usually have the capacity to make up specific ones for your ward. So send them additional information to add to your application packages. Don't approach it with the attitude 'it's not my job'. That will get you nowhere. If you really want to recruit the right staff, then you have to put in the effort, whether it's your job or not.

WRITING THE ADVERT

Involve your whole team in devising what to put in the job advert. Include the person who is leaving. They are the ones who browse through the job adverts regularly. Ask them which adverts are the ones which catch their attention. Ask them which parts of the job would be the most attractive for new staff. Getting that advert right is crucial.

Make the closing date for three to four weeks' time. If you give only two weeks, you are ruling out all potential candidates who are on annual leave at the time of the advert. Put the interview date on the advert too. It quickens up the process. The interview date could then be around two weeks after the closing date.

Having the interview date on the advert gives the candidate plenty of time to prepare.

Waiting until you shortlist candidates before you decide on an interview date only serves to delay the process unnecessarily. You will also have a number of candidates who will not be able to attend, thus prolonging the process even further by having to set a second date. Make things easier and straightforward for you and the candidate by putting both the closing date and interview date on the advert in the first place.

Remember to attach the revised job description and person specification when you give the final advert to your HR recruitment department.

APPLICATION PACKAGES

When the HR team receive enquiries, all they are required to do is send out a copy of the job description and person specification. Some send out information about your organisation too. If you really want to interest potential candidates, give your HR department further information about your ward. Make sure it is typed up and ready to send, so that all they need to do is photocopy further ones if needed.

Again, ask your team what they think would be good to include in the application package. A group of people are a lot more creative than one or two on their own. Possible options include:

- a photograph of your team, happy and smiling
- a copy of your team's annual plan of goals/objectives
- some quotes from your staff saying what is good about working on your ward
- an explanation of your method of working, e.g. team or primary nursing, and perhaps even a sample of your 'off-duty' showing how you organise yourselves and to prove that you do not expect them to work awful shift patterns.

Be careful not to give the impression that the ward is better than it is. The last thing you need is to recruit people under false pretences; they won't stay long. Disillusioned newcomers will disillusion your team.

SHORTLIST AND ARRANGE INTERVIEWS PROPERLY

Most health care organisations now have a database of professionals who have been removed from the register or any former employees or agency staff who should not be employed with you again. Before you shortlist the candidates, make sure that all the names have been checked against this database.

TIPS FOR SHORTLISTING

1. *Shortlist within five days of the closing date.* Make sure you block out some time for this in your diary when you put in the advert.

2. *Shortlist with another senior person from your team.* Don't shortlist on your own. At least one of the people involved in the shortlisting needs to be on the interview panel.

3. *Base the shortlisting on the person specification.* Check that the candidates meet all the 'essential' criteria. The 'desirable' criteria need only be used when a particularly large number of candidates meet the 'essential' criteria.

4. *Keep a note of the reasons for selection and rejection of all candidates* which confirms that the same criteria were used for all candidates. Send a copy to the HR department, so that they can deal with any follow-up requests for information from rejected candidates. It will also help should there be any complaints or allegations of discrimination.

5. *Get the results of the shortlisting over to your recruitment department as soon as possible.* Do not rely on the internal post system. You want to ensure that the process goes smoothly and without any hitches. It is in your interests to show prospective candidates that this is a good place to work. Receiving an interview letter with only a few days to spare does not create a good impression.

6. *Try to ensure that requests for references are sent out at the shortlisting stage.* This will prevent any delays in offering the post to the successful candidate. Most application forms give the individual the option to not have references taken up until after the interview, so you need to make sure that you do not breach the individual's stated wishes.

PREPARE FOR THE INTERVIEWS

You will already have your interview date set from the advertising stage. You need a minimum of two people, but it is advisable to have your HR advisor as a third person. They will also help ensure that the process is fair, that you abide by legislation and are not discriminatory in any way.

At least one of the interviewers should have had formal training in recruitment and selection which includes information on the equal opportunity aspects of recruitment and the relevant legislation. Avoid having any more than three people on the interview panel as it can be intimidating to candidates at this level.

Holding interviews in your ward or department office is a good idea so long as you have the space and can guarantee there will be no interruptions. Make sure there is an allocated area outside the room where candidates can wait. The candidates will feel at ease because it is an environment they are used to. It can be daunting for clinical staff to enter formal office environments. They are unfamiliar places for health care professionals, particularly the more junior ones, and may serve to make them more nervous.

Remember also that there are obligations under the Disability Discrimination Act to ensure that disabled applicants are not discriminated against or disadvantaged in any way (Directgov 2005). The HR team should have asked in the interview offer letter if individuals require any special assistance on that day. You should check before the interview if anyone has requested such assistance.

PREPARE YOUR TEAM FOR THE INTERVIEWS

Check the 'off-duty' to ensure you have good 'numbers' on at the time of interviews and ensure all your staff are aware to be prepared for the arrival of prospective candidates. Agree with your team what they should do to greet them when they arrive. Everyone needs to create a good impression. Your staff on that shift should:

- keep a look out for the interviewees arriving
- greet them warmly with a welcoming smile
- show them where they can wait
- inform them where the nearest toilets are
- offer them a drink
- offer to show them around the ward while they are waiting.

All this serves to confirm that your ward is a good one to work where all the staff are nice and friendly. Even if you do not offer the candidate a post, they will go away thinking what a nice place it is and tell all their friends and colleagues, who will tell their friends and colleagues. Word spreads quickly among health care staff. You don't want a disgruntled candidate telling everyone they wouldn't have taken the job anyway because it didn't look like a good place to work.

GET THE BEST OUT OF THE INTERVIEW PROCESS

Each candidate should leave feeling they have been welcomed, treated fairly and given every opportunity to demonstrate their suitability for the job.

PREPARING THE QUESTIONS

Prepare the interview questions in advance. Questions should be tailored to the person specification. In other words, you want to find out how the candidate meets the desirable criteria. You have already determined the essential criteria from the application form. Questions should also be included to find out :

- why they have applied for this job
- what qualities they can bring to the team
- what their plans are for further career development.

You can also ask questions to get them to expand on what they have written on the application form. What you must not include are any questions about the candidates' personal circumstances such as how they organise their childcare or whether they are married or in a relationship, etc.

Be consistent

You should ask the same set of questions to each candidate. This is to ensure they all have the same opportunities to present the best of themselves. It does not mean you have to keep rigidly to the wording of each question. You can vary them according to the answers given. There is also nothing wrong with asking further probing questions to expand on the answer(s) given.

Try and stick to open-ended questions to encourage the candidate to talk freely. The aim is to ensure the candidate does most of the talking. Avoid leading questions; encourage them to give their own answer, not the answer that you would like them to give.

ASSESSMENT OF PRACTICAL SKILLS

It is very difficult to assess a candidate's practical competence in an interview. Presentations serve mainly to assess their presentation skills. One of the ways you can assess their practical skills is to include a set of questions based on scenarios:

- 'What action would you take if . . . ?'
- 'How would you deal with a situation where . . . ?'
- 'If x happened, what would you do?'

Another good way of eliciting information from candidates is to get them to quantify their experience, using questions like:

- 'How many times have you . . . ?'
- 'What is your experience to date regarding . . . ?'

The use of some sort of written test can help you to assess the practical aspects too. Present them with a couple of scenarios and ask them to write down what they would do. You could give them a situation where they have to prioritise as they would if they were in charge of a shift. Ask them to write down their rationale for each action.

If you decide to include a written assessment, you must:

1. Let the HR department know at the shortlisting stage, so they can inform the candidates in the letter inviting them for interview.
2. Allow for the extra time required in the interview timetable.
3. Organise a separate quiet room where candidates can undertake the exercise undisturbed.
4. Make sure that the questions relate specifically to criteria outlined in the person specification.

Whatever method you use for assessment and interviewing, it is essential to set up a scoring system such as marks out of five for each question. Each interviewer will then score the person separately. These can assist with the final decision.

PREPARE THE ENVIRONMENT AND INTERVIEWERS

Tidy up the room if needed. Set out the chairs, preferably so that you can see the clock on the wall behind the interviewee. Continuously looking at your wristwatch during the interview is disconcerting for the candidate. Sit in the candidate's chair to see if it is a comfortable distance away from the interviewers' chairs and there are no diversions such as glaring sunlight from the window.

Divert the phones and any pagers, and ensure everyone turns off their mobile phones. Put a very big notice on the door saying 'Interviews in Progress' with the date and time. Include the time when you will be finishing.

THE ROLE OF THE CHAIRPERSON IN INTERVIEWS

Before you begin the interviews, identify which one of you will chair the process. Normally it would be you, but your junior staff have to gain the experience some time and it's best they do it at a time when they can receive support and guidance from a more experienced interviewer. The role of the chair is to:

1. Introduce yourself and the other interviewers.
2. Settle the candidate by using small talk such as 'Did you find your way alright?'.
3. Explain the interview plan and that you will be taking notes throughout the process.
4. Give some background information about your ward.
5. Facilitate the flow of questions.
6. Allow silences to ensure the candidate gets a chance to consider their thoughts before answering.
7. Ensure that the candidate does most of the speaking.
8. Keep to the timeframe.
9. Ask if the candidate has any questions at the end.
10. Ensure they give you the appropriate documents, e.g. occupational health form, ID such as passport, etc. (HR will advise you beforehand as to what is required).
11. Thank the candidate for attending.
12. Inform the candidate what will happen next, and when you will be making the decision.

FOLLOW UP ALL CANDIDATES PERSONALLY

Make your choice and write up your notes immediately after interview. Keep all your notes and scoring results from the interviews. They help when feeding back to candidates especially if you are required to feedback a few weeks or even months after the interview. Make sure the records are accurate and objective with no reference to personal opinions. Under data protection laws candidates may have a right to see these notes after the interview if they so wish.

Most people prefer to call the candidates personally. Don't promise to call them that evening. Remember: 'under-promise and over-deliver'. It will cause you undue hassle if you say you will call them that evening then find that you are unable to make a final decision for some reason. Give yourself at least a day's grace, in case of any problems. Always caveat any verbal offers with them being subject to satisfactory checks (e.g. Criminal Records Bureau clearance).

Don't offer the job before receiving the references. It will cause you immense problems if you receive unsatisfactory references after offering the job. The references usually just confirm that you have made a good decision, but if they do not you will need to follow them up. That takes time. You can telephone the referees if you have not received a written reference. You can ask them to send you a fax or email. A detailed record of the call including the date, time and the person you spoke to may suffice.

CALLING UNSUCCESSFUL CANDIDATES

Nobody likes to be the bearer of bad news. However, it is a nice gesture to call the unsuccessful candidates as soon as possible after the interviews, rather than let them wait for the official letter. Handle the situation by turning it into a positive experience :

1. Begin by telling the candidate they were unsuccessful.
2. Follow this immediately by telling them what they did well and which parts impressed you.
3. Then, tell them the reason why they did not get the job. Be precise but do not dwell on this part. Stick to one or two comments then follow it up by offering further feedback at a later date should they want it.

Once the candidate is told that they have been unsuccessful they are not usually in the mood to have a discussion about what they did wrong. However, they may want further feedback at a later date. Offer this service and make sure you are genuine in your offer. Tell them you have made lots of notes and are more than willing to spend time giving them further information about what they can do to improve next time. Your aim is to make sure that everyone sees your ward in a positive light, even unsuccessful job applicants.

FOLLOW UP PROMISING BUT UNSUCCESSFUL CANDIDATES

If you only have one vacancy but two or three really good candidates, don't just take one and say goodbye to the rest. Speak to your colleagues. Do they have any vacancies? Do your HR team know of any other vacancies which you think the candidates may like to consider? Make a point of finding out this information before you call them. It's far better to let them know you think they have such good potential that you have talked to your colleagues and found another position they might like to apply for. Even if they are not interested, they will remain positive about themselves and have positive memories of the whole process.

TAKE RISKS

If you know you have a further similiar vacancy coming up in other couple of months, take the risk and employ one of the other good candidates as well. The turnover in nursing is so high that you would be foolish not to. Obviously you must get your finance advisor to work out all the costings and ensure you obtain your line manager's approval. It is usually a cost-effective way of dealing with things by the time you take into account the cost of further adverts and interviews.

ARRANGE A GOOD INDUCTION PROGRAMME

As soon as the candidate has confirmed their starting date, prepare their induction period together with your team. This is a crucial part of their employment. A good induction period makes the candidates feel welcome and reinforces their positive feelings about your ward. If you do not ensure this is done properly and then have problems later on with poor performance or incompetence, you could be found at fault because you failed to ensure an adequate induction period.

BEFORE THEY COMMENCE

You can start the induction before the candidate even commences the job by sending them any information that may be of interest together with a personal welcome letter from you. Include any forms that need signing to ensure they receive things in good time and save them unnecessary hassle, such as:

- car parking pass
- email address and IT password
- ID badge and security pass
- uniform measurements.

  Other items you might like to send them are:

- a copy of their two-week initial induction programme
- a copy of their first 'off-duty' with details of shift times
- a list of staff names in your team and any particular responsibilities, e.g. link nurse
- minutes from the last team meeting
- the name and details of their allocated mentor.

TWO-WEEK SUPERNUMERARY PERIOD

It is advisable that the new recruit is supernumerary for the initial two-week induction period, making sure that they are not shown on the 'off-duty' at all. If they are, there is the possibility that they may be used to cover in times of short staffing. You cannot afford to let this happen in those first few weeks. Their initial induction should include:

1. *A warm welcome on their first day.* Make sure you or a senior member of your staff are there to greet them and can spend some time going through things with them.
2. *An induction checklist.* Most organisations have an induction checklist to be completed. Encourage them to complete this over the first couple of months, not the first two weeks. Don't overload them with information.
3. *Mandatory training.* Try and fit all their annual mandatory study requirements within the two-week supernumerary period. If you get the statutory sessions such as manual handling awareness, health and safety and cardiopulmonary resuscitation (CPR) out the way in the induction period, it will not impinge on the study time available for the rest of your team in that financial year.
4. *Clinical work.* Allocate time for working full- or half-shifts during the induction period. They need to get the practical experience working alongside members of your team. Don't allocate them patients to look after on their own. That is not induction, it is using them as a pair of hands.
5. *Attendance at meetings.* Take them along to any meetings you have. Let them observe the sisters' meeting and perhaps even meet the director of nursing if present. Give them an insight into your role, vision and values right at the beginning no matter how junior their grade. It would be good to do this with all new HCAs too.
6. *Attendance to individual needs.* Tailor each induction programme to each individual. If someone has just returned to work after some time out, their needs will be very different from someone who has transferred from another department within the same organisation.

   It's a good idea to develop the induction programme with someone in your team of the same grade as the new recruit. They will be more understanding of the individual's needs.

ALLOCATE A MENTOR

Allocate them a mentor for the first three months and ensure this person works with them regularly on the 'off-duty'. After three months, the individual will be settled enough to choose their own mentor. Most areas will have some sort of competency package for new members of staff to guide their skills development during the first few months. Following this, they should have their first appraisal at around three to six months to agree objectives and a personal development plan for the coming year. Don't neglect this part; it is very important.

CONTINUALLY EXPLORE ALL OTHER AVENUES TO GET STAFF

Even if you are 'up to establishment', you can't afford to become complacent. Always be on the lookout for new staff. Create such a warm and welcoming environment for anyone visiting your ward that you'll end up with a queue of people wanting to work there.

STUDENT NURSES

Word spreads around student nurses like wildfire about which wards are the best to work on, so make sure that all students allocated to your area are:

- warmly welcomed
- rostered to work with their mentor at least twice per week
- given lots of feedback about their progress
- invited to any staff social gatherings.

If you do not receive students to your area because of your specialism you will be losing out on a major source of future staff. Contact your local university and offer day- or week-long placements where students can shadow an experienced member of staff. Even spending a short time with you can make a huge impression.

BANK AND AGENCY STAFF

Some choose to work for the bank or agency on a permanent basis so that they can have more flexiblity around their home life. However, they may change their minds and apply for a post on your ward if they see that they would have some choice over their shift patterns. Team self-rostering is a good way of letting your staff have flexibility around their home life (see p. 80). Implementing this may help with your recruitment of these people. In the meantime, make sure that your staff treat all bank and agency staff well by:

1. Greeting them each time with a warm welcome and full introductions.
2. Taking time to find out the person's name, qualifications and experience.
3. Taking time to show them around the ward and going through their patients' needs with them.
4. Continually checking on how they are doing throughout the shift.
5. Giving feedback on how they are doing (temporary staff rarely receive this unless they have done something wrong).
6. Giving thanks at the end of the shift for anything specific that they have achieved or done well, not just a general thankyou for turning up.

RETURNING NURSES

Around 20 000 nurses leave the register each year (Nursing & Midwifery Council 2004). Surveys of nonpractising nurses show that they would consider returning if:

- they received support in their decision to return
- refresher training was available
- part-time and family-friendly employment practices were available

- they could spend more time with patients and have a less stressful working environment.

(Select Committee on Health 1999)

On a national level, nurses are actively being encouraged to return, and 'return to practice' courses are now being run by many organisations. On a local level, all that you need to do now is provide part-time and family-friendly practices and an environment where your nurses can spend more time with the patients and be less stressed.

When you advertise for further staff, make sure you also advertise in the local paper for those who are not practising. Adapt your advert accordingly; advertise for nurses who wish to return stating the benefits such as flexitime, child care or nursery availability, and offer sponsorship through your organisation's 'return to practice' course. There may be a large untapped resource of potential staff in your local community who are currently not working.

LIAISE CLOSELY WITH YOUR RECRUITMENT LEAD

Most health care organisations employ someone who deals solely with nursing recruitment. Their job is to make sure everything is being done to attract staff to your organisation. They will have knowledge of all current recruitment initiatives such as the cadet nursing programmes, return to practice courses and various job fairs. They will have a good idea of what vacancies are where, plus who is interviewing for what and when. If you keep in close contact with your recruitment lead they can let you know of promising candidates from elsewhere. They will also keep you informed about when the next batch of students are due to finish and start looking for jobs.

The recruitment lead soon gets to know which wards are popular and which are not. They will deter promising students from the worst wards where it is known they will receive little support and attention. They do not want to put all that effort into recruiting staff who would leave within a few months due to unsatisfactory working conditions.

You cannot blame the national shortage of nurses for all your vacancies. Nurses are out there and to find them you have to put more time and effort into:

1. Making your ward one of the most popular wards to work on within your organisation.
2. Finding the right places and right times to recruit.

DON'T DISCRIMINATE

PART TIME DOES NOT MEAN PART SKILLED

Nursing remains a female-dominated profession and, as a result, there will always be a high percentage of part-time workers. Health care professionals usually start off their careers working on a full-time basis, but many will reduce to part time at some time during their careers in order to balance family and work commitments. This does not mean that they should be demoted or passed over for promotion. Don't assume that because a person does not want to work full time they are not as highly committed and motivated as those who do. If you do, you are being discriminatory.

In addition to this, some part-time workers will not apply for promotion because they have the impression that a higher grade means working more hours. Try not to condone this culture; a higher grade means that higher skills are needed, not a higher number of hours.

If you do need to cover a certain number of shifts with a certain level of skill then consider employing two people to share one job. Two people sharing one job will give you far more than one person in terms of experience. (You have to be careful that they are truly job sharing, i.e. not working the same shifts.) The key to this working successfully is to ensure they jointly take responsibility for the one role. In other words, they can't blame the other for not getting things done.

DON'T WASTE THE SKILLS OF ENROLLED NURSES

Enrolled nurses have been discriminated against for many years, particularly since grading was first introduced. Many have been kept at junior staff nurse level for most of their careers. Few have been able to attain promotion above staff nurse level. Enrolled nurses have much to offer; often as much, if not more than, some of their first level registered colleagues. Fortunately, many have now had the opportunity to convert from enrolled to registered nurse but there are still some who either choose not to or have not had the opportunity.

If you feel that a more senior level position requires the person to be at diploma level academically then advertise the position as diploma level. However, don't waste the potential opportunity for a good enrolled nurse internally or externally who could be an asset to your team.

Add an extra part to the advert (and job specification) that if enrolled nurse candidates can demonstrate the relevant experience and competency for the role, they should be prepared to undertake the diploma as a condition on which the offer of a job is made. You will increase your choice of candidates.

OVERSEAS NURSES ARE NOT ALL THE SAME

You may be familiar with the following expressions from nurses within organisations who have recruited from another country:

'They are all so hard-working.'
'They don't understand that nursing is different here.'
'Where they come from, they do what the doctors tell them to.'
'They are quick to learn our ways.'
'They demand so much of our time.'

We would not dream of talking about all UK nurses in such a manner, because we accept that they are all individuals. Yet people will often take the attitude that nurses who train in another country are all the same. Be careful not to condone this attitude. Accept that all these nurses are individuals, with their own unique blend of strengths and weaknesses. Work on their strengths as you would any other new member of staff.

Overseas recruitment is a fantastic opportunity to bring in new ideas and different experiences to your team. Yes, it will be a hassle to ensure they have the appropriate competencies and skills for the role but no more than any other staff nurse you recruit to your team. If you have a new recruit who is struggling in the role, look to improving your own systems of support and methods of staff development before blaming the individual nurse. If you undervalue individuals in any way, you will undermine their confidence and self-esteem. It will not help them work well. If you value each individual for the unique qualities that they bring to the team, they will feel good about themselves and consequently be motivated to work well.

SUCCESSION PLAN

IS YOUR STAFFING ESTABLISHMENT CONDUCIVE TO GOOD SUCCESSION PLANNING?

Think carefully about posts your staff can fulfil once they have reached the appropriate standard. If you only have one deputy, for example, you could be limiting promotion prospects for your staff. Having two deputy managers rather than one may be more helpful in terms of succession planning. If you have ten staff nurses and only one deputy, you will be putting yourself at risk of losing good staff who will look elsewhere to get in the next pay band. It reflects poorly on you if one of your senior staff leaves and you have nobody in your team who is ready to replace them. If this does happen, review and improve on what you are doing to develop the skills of your team.

STAFF NURSE LEVEL (BAND 5)

Since the advent of pay bands, the perpetual headache of having two grades of staff nurse has finally been removed. It became quite ridiculous having to interview D grades for E grade jobs, which only served to hinder rather than help staff retention. Things are a lot easier now that all staff nurses are in band 5. However, having one staff nurse grade does not mean you can forgo any thoughts of succession planning. You still need to ensure they are competent enough to get through that gateway halfway through the pay band. You also need some system in place so they have the opportunity to get to deputy manager standard (band 6) over a certain time span.

Good succession planning means that when senior people leave you will have at least one person who is up to the standard of taking on that role. Make sure you have a system in place so that each junior nurse who joins your team has a detailed personal development plan linked to the knowledge and skills framework (KSF). This should give them every opportunity to be able to get through the first gateway. Do the same for your senior staff nurses to get to the level where they can apply for the next pay band.

Your recruitment plan for registered nurses should continually aim for the newly qualified or junior staff nurse level, however don't always promote internally. It is good to regularly employ nurses higher up the pay band scale from external sources. They will bring valuable experience, new ideas and, more importantly, they will challenge your ways of working.

DEPUTY MANAGER/SISTER/CHARGE NURSE LEVEL (BAND 6)

Be on the constant lookout for your next deputy. If any of your staff nurses have particularly good management and organisational skills, you will want to develop those skills and get them ready for when your current deputy decides to leave. Don't wait until people resign before looking around to replace them. Be proactive and ensure you have staff ready to take on the post should the opportunity arise.

HEALTH CARE ASSISTANTS

You should also provide a system of career progression within your staffing establishment for HCAs. They should be able to access NVQ level 2, then NVQ level 3 followed by the opportunity to access nurse training. They may not wish to progress any further than their current level but the opportunity to do so should always be there. Some may prefer to specialise into areas such as taking on a link role or diversifying into taking on some ward administrative duties. As with the registered nurses, when a senior HCA leaves, you should have at least one other HCA ready to take their place.

FULLY INVOLVE YOUR TEAM IN ALL ASPECTS OF RECRUITMENT

People sometimes get the words 'inform' and 'involve' confused. Involving your team in the recruitment process entails more than just ensuring they are fully informed at each stage of the process. Keeping them fully informed is better than nothing but it will be far more beneficial to go one step further and actually involve them all in the process.

As soon as any team member resigns, meet your team to review the role and discuss whether it should remain the same or whether a different role would further enhance the team. Involve them in redesigning the job description if that is needed.

When you are ready to write the advert, get your team together to discuss and agree how to word the advert to make it more attractive to potential candidates. If you do not have time to meet with all your team, use other means of communication. Add it to the agenda of your regular team meetings rather than set up a special meeting.

DEVELOP THEIR INTERVIEWING SKILLS EARLY ON

Include at least one of your team in the interviewing process. Guidelines usually recommend that at least one of the interviewers should be a higher grade than the candidate. There is no reason why you cannot include someone from your team who is the same or even a lower grade than that of the candidate; they have to start somewhere. Don't wait until staff become a senior grade before inviting them to sit in on interviews. The experience is extremely valuable. If they are only observing, give them one of the questions to ask. Everyone remembers their first interview when they had to ask questions and were too nervous to listen to the candidate's reply. It's something that should be done at an early stage in people's careers and not left until they are deputy or ward manager level (as is so often the case).

Take time after the interviews not only to discuss and agree the successful candidate but also to discuss the process. If you have a team member with you who is new to the process, ask what they have learned. Discuss the process with the whole panel. Was there anything you felt you could have done better?

GET THE TEAM INVOLVED WITH THE NEW STAFF MEMBER EARLY ON

Once you have offered the post, let your team know who the new team member is and a bit about their background, then immediately appoint someone to take the lead in planning their induction. Make sure your culture of involving all the team also applies to team members. In other words, encourage the person planning the induction to ask the rest of the team for their ideas on what should be included.

If you can, get someone of the same grade as the new team member to sort out the induction programme. They will understand the new person's needs better than anyone else. That includes HCAs; you do not need to be a registered nurse to be able to organise an induction programme.

The key to having a strong and healthy recruitment process is to ensure you show that you value the input from all your team members. It's the fundamental difference between leading your team and managing your team. Lead them well and you will have a far stronger and healthier team than if you simply administer and maintain the team using a transactional (solely managerial) approach.

ACTION POINTS

- Each time a member of your staff leaves, review the post and job description with the 'leaver' and the rest of your team.
- Involve your team in writing job adverts and customising the application packages for your ward.
- Include the interview date on all adverts and shortlist within five days of the closing date.
- Include your team in the whole process. Ensure at least one team member is included in the interview process and ensure all prospective candidates are given a warm welcome by your team when visiting the ward.
- Make sure all new team members receive a two-week supernumerary induction programme devised by your staff and including mandatory updates.
- Network widely to ensure that you and your team are continually aware of new recruitment opportunities.
- Review your staffing establishment and systems of developing your staff to ensure they have every opportunity to develop the skills for the next post and are ready within two to three years of commencement in their current role.
- If you do not already do so, start involving your team in the whole process of recruitment rather than just keeping them informed.

References

Department of Health 2005 Improvement leaders guide: redesigning roles: personal and organisational development. DH Publications, London. Online. Available: http://www.wise.nhs.uk/cmsWISE/Tools+and+techniques/ILG/ILG.htm 30 Sep 2005

Directgov 2005 Disabled people: your rights. Online. Available: http://www.direct.gov.uk/DisabledPeople/RightsandObligations/YourRights/fs/en 30 Sep 2005

Nursing & Midwifery Council 2004 Statistical analysis of the register, 1 April 2003 to 31 March 2004. NMC, London. Online. Available: http://www.nmc-uk.org Search: 'Annual statistics 2003-2004' 30 Sep 2005

Select Committee on Health 1999 Minutes of evidence: supplementary memorandum, medical and nursing staff in the NHS (SR 56A), 3 March 1999. The Stationery Office, London.

CHAPTER 9

BE POLITICALLY AWARE

Understand how health care is managed nationally 168

The NHS in England 168

The NHS in Wales 169

The NHS in Scotland 169

The NHS in Northern Ireland 170

Private health care 170

Be aware of the wider organisation 170

Know your board of directors and their priorities 171

Getting to know your board of directors 172

Choose your meetings carefully 173

Board meetings 173

Sisters' meetings 173

Directorate meetings 174

Sending staff to meetings on your behalf 174

Impromptu meetings 174

Network – get to know the right people 174

Other ward managers 175

Senior managers and directors 175

Be alert to opportunities 175

Building up your networks 175

Be diplomatic 176

Guard your opinions 176

Try not to be too critical 176

Don't take sides 177

Control your temper 177

Talk of 'we' rather than 'I' 177

Think as a manager 177

Service users 178

Voicing your disagreements 178

Work with your director of nursing 178

The professional development team 179

Shadowing 179

Mentoring 179

Get recognition for your work 180

Hospital newsletter 180

Conferences and study days 180

Compare your ward with others 180

Choose your mentor and mentees with care 181

The mentor role 181

Choosing your mentees 181

Plan ahead for your own needs 182

Identify your special interests 182

Keep a box file for your CV 183

Writing your CV 183

Tailor your CV to the job 184

Sending a cover letter 184

Being politically aware means knowing how your organisation ticks, who's who and how to use this knowledge to get things done. Without this knowledge, you can become cocooned in your own small environment. You may be taken advantage of because of your ignorance. You also run the risk of missing out on opportunities to improve your working environment, your staff and patient care. To be a good manager, it is essential that you know:

• how your organisation and others within health care operate
• the health strategy and policy at a national and local level and be able to include them when planning your goals with your team
• who the key people are to make things happen (both internally and externally to your organisation) and how to access them.

A good manager should learn how to network and build strong alliances in order to become more powerful and effective in the role.

UNDERSTAND HOW HEALTH CARE IS MANAGED NATIONALLY

It is advisable that you find out what the key strategies and policies are, where they come from and how they influence your day-to-day practice.

THE NHS IN ENGLAND

All health care work in England is influenced by the Department of Health. The Department of Health sets the national standards and shapes the direction of the NHS (Department of Health 2005a).

The NHS is currently managed through strategic health authorities (SHAs) across England. The role of the SHAs is to make sure that the hospitals and primary care facilities in their area are performing well. Both community and hospital services are managed locally and referred to as NHS trusts. Foundation trusts are the only trusts not accountable to the SHAs. They are accountable to a local body of elected governors. Primary care trusts (PCTs) are currently at the centre of the NHS in England and receive 75% of the budget from their SHAs. Contracts, called service level agreements (SLAs), are set up between the PCTs and their local hospitals.

The main strategy that influences the NHS is the 'NHS Plan' (Department of Health 2000). It is a ten-year plan and is where all the current targets originate. In addition to the NHS Plan, there is a national rolling programme of national service frameworks (NSFs) which was started in 1998. These are long-term strategies for improving specific areas of care such as coronary heart disease, cancer and the care of older people.

The Healthcare Commission is a separate independent body, which inspects the performance of health care organisations. Their role includes the publication of performance rating for trusts (Healthcare Commission 2005).

The Department of Health employs the Chief Nursing Officer (CNO) who is the most senior nurse advisor to the government. Accessing the monthly CNO bulletin on the website is a wise move for all sisters and charge nurses (Department of Health 2005b). It gives updated information about relevant issues in the NHS which are of specific interest to all nurses. It also enables you to access link websites to obtain further information about issues of particular interest.

THE NHS IN WALES

The NHS in Wales is managed through 22 local health boards (LHBs), which assess what health services their populations need and then pay hospital trusts, family doctors and dentists, etc. to provide those services. They receive 75% of the Welsh NHS budget. The Welsh Assembly Government is responsible for policy direction and for allocating funds to the NHS in Wales (NHS Wales 2005). It has three regional offices based in mid, north and southeast Wales. These offices coordinate and manage the performance of LHBs and NHS trusts.

Wales also has an NHS plan, 'Improving Health in Wales' (NHS Wales 2001). It is the source of the targets that influence the planning, organisation and delivery of health care services in Wales. NSFs have also been developed to ensure the NHS plan is implemented effectively.

The Healthcare Inspectorate Wales (HIW), a department of the National Assembly for Wales, is responsible for inspecting and investigating the provision of health care by and for Welsh NHS bodies (HIW 2005). The CNO for Wales provides professional advice to the Welsh Assembly Government and direction in the development of specialist health and community services.

THE NHS IN SCOTLAND

The Scottish Executive Health Department is responsible for producing health policies and administering the NHS in Scotland (Scotland's Health on the Web 2005). It is managed through 15 NHS boards. These NHS boards are responsible for developing local health plans with local hospitals, GPs and other NHS bodies. The NHS trust system was abolished in 2004.

The Scottish NHS plan, 'Our National Health', was published in 2000 (Scottish Executive 2000). Like the NHS plans for England and Wales, it has the same emphasis on tough targets such as waiting times, but through a different management structure, i.e. unified NHS health boards rather than separate NHS trusts.

NHS Quality Improvement Scotland set clinical standards and targets for continuous service improvement (NHS Quality Improvement Scotland 2005). They review and monitor performance against set targets. A performance assessment framework is used, similar to the star rating assessment in England and Wales.

Scotland also has a CNO, who is the most senior nursing advisor to the Scottish Executive.

THE NHS IN NORTHERN IRELAND

The Northern Ireland Office (NIO) administers the NHS through a dedicated minister who deals with health, social services and public safety in Northern Ireland. The Department of Health, Social Services and Public Safety (DHSSPS) creates the policy and legislation (DHSSPS 2005a). The NHS is managed locally through four health and social services (HSS) covering northern, southern, eastern and western areas and their associated HSS trusts. Like England and Wales, the HSS trusts manage staff and services on the ground and they control their own budgets.

The NHS plan for Northern Ireland: 'Investing for Health' was published in 2002. The content differs from those in England, Wales and Scotland, because the HSS have been integrated as one system since 1972. The CNO contributes to the development and implementation of health and social care policy on behalf of the profession (DHSSPS 2005b). The Regulation and Improvement Authority regulate and monitor the quality of the health services in Northern Ireland.

PRIVATE HEALTH CARE

There are many private hospital companies in the UK, the biggest being BMI Healthcare which has 49 hospitals, closely followed by Nuffield Hospitals with 43 hospitals, BUPA with 25 hospitals and Capio Healthcare with 21 hospitals. Many consultants who undertake private practice are also employed by the NHS and private hospitals tend to base their standards along the relevant NHS regulations and guidelines.

BE AWARE OF THE WIDER ORGANISATION

This is basic information about how health care is run in the UK. If you did not know much of it before, do rest assured that you are not alone. Nurses are often so focused on managing their day-to-day pressures that being aware of the wider organisation has never been a priority. However, once you become a nurse manager, you will find it helpful to become more aware of the 'bigger picture'. Without developing an awareness of the wider structure, you will be unable to build up appropriate networks needed to achieve your goals. Don't fall into the trap of cocooning yourself in the safe environment of your unit, with the attitude that 'what happens out there does not concern me' or 'I haven't got time for that'. If you do not know how the system works, you cannot influence it.

Make it a personal goal from now on to regularly look up the appropriate websites and keep yourself abreast of the ongoing changes both nationally and within your own organisation. All this information is now freely available on the internet. Because it is for the general public, it is easy to understand and most of the jargon has been removed.

KNOW YOUR BOARD OF DIRECTORS AND THEIR PRIORITIES

Services within NHS hospitals tend to be divided into directorates, each managed by a directorate team. This team usually consists of a clinical director, general manager and a lead, senior or head nurse. They report directly to the board of directors. All NHS trusts are managed by a board of directors, led by a chief executive and overseen by a chairman.

The trust board of directors comprises the following members:

- chairman × 1
- chief executive × 1
- executive directors × 5 (including the chief executive)
- nonexecutive directors × 5.

(In Scotland, the system differs; hospitals are no longer run as separate NHS trusts. They still contain a similar management system with a chairman and chief executive but there are fewer directors. In addition, the chairman and chief executive sit on the NHS board which oversees all aspects of health care in their area, not just their own hospital.)

Nonexecutive directors

The chairman is a nonexecutive role. The chairman and nonexecutive directors are lay people whose role is to act as advocates for the community. Some might have business or financial skills whereas others may have experience as a carer or even as a patient. The chairman and nonexecutive directors are not responsible for the operational management of the trust. The idea is that they bring in extra skills to help the trust board to ensure a high quality service. They are expected to draw from their experiences in the local communities to make sure that the patients' interests are paramount.

Both the chairman and nonexecutive directors are employed on a part-time basis. The chairman works three days per week and the nonexecutive directors work two to five days per month.

The chairman

The chairman's role is to lead the trust board and ensure it fulfils all its responsibilities. They chair all the board meetings and ensure the smooth running of the board by supporting, constructively challenging and setting the appropriate managerial style. The chairman's other main role is to communicate effectively both internally and externally to gain the views and commitment from the trust staff and the local community. This is why you'll often see the chairman walking around the trust talking with staff and attending trust events.

The chairman and nonexecutive directors interview and appoint the chief executive and executive directors.

Executive directors

Of the five executive director members, the following are a statutory requirement:

- the chief executive
- the director of finance
- the medical director
- the director of nursing.

The fifth executive director appointment to the board is at the discretion of the trust. Some appoint an executive director for human resources. Others may decide on having an executive director for operations or planning. In addition to the five executive directors, there may be a small number of further directors who are not in an executive role. This means that they attend board meetings but do not have voting rights.

Executive directors are responsible for a particular function within the organisation such as nursing or finance, but as board members they are required to contribute to other trust-wide issues and policy outside their particular brief. All directors of the trust have a corporate responsibility for:

- setting the strategic direction
- ensuring effective financial planning and control
- promoting quality and clinical governance
- agreeing annual business plans.

The chief executive

The chief executive has personal responsibility for the overall operational management of the trust and reports to the chairman. The chief executive is accountable for the performance of the trust both in terms of meeting statutory requirements such as financial stability and health and safety legislation, and also quality targets.

GETTING TO KNOW YOUR BOARD OF DIRECTORS

The trust board is a very powerful body. In order to be politically astute, it is wise to build the appropriate alliances and networks in order to access this power. The trust board usually holds a meeting in public every month. Anyone can attend to listen and ask questions. Going along to these board meetings is an easy way of getting to know and understand what is going on. Take staff along for the experience and to help develop their political awareness.

Many chief executives also hold regular 'open forums'. They book a couple of hours in their diary where they will be available at a certain venue for anyone to come along and ask questions. These are not information-giving meetings; they are there for the staff to bring up issues only.

Another easy way of finding out what your trust board's priorities and plans are is via the intranet or in the annual business plan. This plan is open to the public and therefore written in an easily readable style. You need to know what the trust board's priorities are. If the priorities of your unit are different to those of the trust board, you will not get very far with them.

For those working in private health care, the system is different, but it is necessary that you make yourself aware of what your company's priorities are, if you have not already done so.

CHOOSE YOUR MEETINGS CAREFULLY

Select your meetings carefully; this is not only for time management reasons. There are certain meetings that you should attend and contribute to, to ensure you are part of the organisation's important network and remain up-to-date with what is going on. As a general rule, if the person chairing the meeting is not particularly influential within your organisation and does not have the authority to make decisions, then think twice before going; your time could be better spent.

BOARD MEETINGS

The monthly meetings of the trust board are extremely useful. It is worth putting the dates down in your diary to remind you to organise yourself or one of your team to attend that day. Add it to the top of the 'off-duty' to remind your team about it. It will also make them realise the importance of the role of the trust board (and perhaps even to keep them aware that there is one).

Consider adding an attendance at a trust board meeting to your staff induction programme. It will stimulate their thinking about the wider organisation. In addition, the directors will probably note the continual attendance of members of your team. It can do you no harm to be seen as a forward-thinking manager within the organisation.

SISTERS' MEETINGS

Many nursing directors hold regular sisters' meetings in order to:

- find out what is going on on the 'shop floor'
- gain your views and opinions (which will influence decision making at board level)
- discuss any issues that are currently affecting your practice
- keep you informed about any changes in policies or guidance
- get you involved in specific projects for improving patient care.

Add the dates of sisters' meetings to your 'off-duty' too. They are very important and often your only access to the director of nursing. You will not be able to attend every time, so always make sure that at least two of your senior staff are familiar with the meeting structure. They will then be able to attend in your absence with confidence.

DIRECTORATE MEETINGS

Your directorate meetings are just as important for you to attend. If you do not, decisions will be made without your input but may affect your work. Prepare for these meetings; look at the agenda beforehand. Think about anything you need to know or ask about. Do not go to meetings just with the intention of getting information. That is a waste of your time. It will be quicker to read the minutes. Go to meetings prepared in order to contribute and influence decisions.

SENDING STAFF TO MEETINGS ON YOUR BEHALF

Try not to send any of your staff to meetings without prior experience. The main reason for sending a substitute to a meeting is to contribute to the decision-making processes. Putting a member of staff in a room full of senior colleagues for the first time and expecting them to speak confidently on your behalf is expecting too much. It could be quite a damaging experience. Whenever you can, take a member of your staff along with you to meetings to gain the appropriate experience. Once they are familiar with the process, you will be able to send them along as your representative when you cannot attend in person.

Try and ensure you are always represented at every board, directorate and sisters' meeting. Never be concerned about missing out on important information. You will get all the information you need from the minutes. The main reason for attending meetings is to contribute, on behalf of your staff, to future changes and development within your organisation. It is important that you are part of the nursing agenda in your trust. Staff on induction would also benefit by coming along with you to observe.

IMPROMPTU MEETINGS

Prepare for impromptu meetings with influential people. The chairman is often wandering around the hospital meeting people to get a feel for what is going on. That's their job. Don't just say hello and generally pass the time of day. Prepare in advance something that you would want to say or ask, in the event that you may pass them one day in the corridor. You may even have a politician or the media visit your trust. These visits are often booked with very little notice. It is a good idea to always have three questions in your mind should such a situation arise, to avoid these chance meetings becoming wasted opportunities.

NETWORK – GET TO KNOW THE RIGHT PEOPLE

The right people to know are not necessarily the most senior people. Often they are the secretaries or teams who work for senior people. Medical secretaries, for example, have a wealth of information about what is going on. The personal assistant who works for the chief executive or director of nursing is also a very useful person to know. They know how their boss thinks and are usually full of very helpful advice.

Always smile and say hello when you walk in through your hospital reception. Stop every now and then to pass the time of day. Do the same with the porters, the people who serve you in the canteen and the person who mops the corridor outside your ward each day. The more people you know, the more you will get to know about what is happening in your organisation.

OTHER WARD MANAGERS

You should also cultivate a good friendship with your peers. Working in isolation from the managers of other wards and departments will weaken your influence in the organisation. Get together with the others as a group and you will strengthen your position and voice. Try and ensure you support and help each other in times of pressure.

SENIOR MANAGERS AND DIRECTORS

Get to know the senior managers. Don't shy away from them. One way to do this is to hang back after meetings where senior managers are involved. Usually after such a meeting, the clinical staff dash back to their familiar clinical environment, but it's worth staying behind for a short while. Tidy up the coffee cups or put the chairs back in order to stop you feeling awkward. You may find you are drawn into a conversation with a senior manager asking you for your opinion about something from a clinical perspective. The more you do this, the more you will become confident in speaking with them.

Sometimes you will notice a senior manager or director sitting on their own at a lunch occasion or a presentation meeting. Go up and introduce yourself. Be genuine. Don't try and use the occasion to influence any changes. You need to build up a trusting relationship first.

BE ALERT TO OPPORTUNITIES

Take your time to develop your alliances. It will not happen overnight. Just be alert to opportunities for getting to know the right people. They will not come to you; you have to go out and find them. Having the appropriate networks can mean the difference between success or failure in your role.

BUILDING UP YOUR NETWORKS

Networking is about building a two-way alliance. You should be prepared to give more than you receive. Tips for increasing your networks include:

1. *Helping others out.* Offer to send some information about something you have talked about and ensure you follow it up. Nobody forgets a simple, friendly gesture like this. Make sure you add your contact details on your cover note.
2. *Saying thank you.* If you hear an interesting speaker at a meeting or teaching session, go up afterwards and thank the speaker. People rarely do this but speakers do appreciate some feedback. This may or may not spark up a short conversation, which you could follow up afterwards. Whatever the outcome, they will remember your face.
3. *Giving out business cards.* This is not pretentious. You are a senior manager and business cards are a good way of getting people to remember you. Give them out at external meetings and conferences.

Remember that the junior staff you come across such as medical and nursing students may well get to be in more senior and influential positions than you one day. Try to ensure that they always remember you in a positive light.

BE DIPLOMATIC

GUARD YOUR OPINIONS

Know when to keep your opinions to yourself. Don't express your point of view unless you have been requested to do so. People who offer opinions without being asked can be irritating. They tend to do so because:

- they have an audience
- they want to make people think they are clever
- they want to get attention
- they think it will make a difference.

Learn when to say something and when to keep quiet. Opinions don't usually make a difference unless they have been asked for. When you are asked for your thoughts or judgements, try to avoid using phrases such as 'in my opinion'. It would be better to present your opinion as a solution. For example:

Question: 'What do you think about the changes in the admission procedure?'
Answer 1: 'Well, in my opinion, the paperwork takes too long to complete.'
Answer 2: 'The paperwork needs to be reviewed. It takes too long to complete.'

The second answer sounds like a well-considered answer. The person is confident and appears to know what they are talking about. Opinions are more likely to be accepted if presented as a fact rather than as an opinion, if they are presented in a confident and adept manner.

TRY NOT TO BE TOO CRITICAL

If you have problems with a colleague or a senior manager, don't criticise them personally. If you think a senior manager is lazy or incompetent, never say so.

Getting personal is not professional. On the other hand, you cannot ignore a senior manager's behaviour if it is affecting others. You just need to be diplomatic about it. Focus on the behaviour, not the person. You could say, for example, that perhaps they need to increase their motivation or update their clinical skills.

DON'T TAKE SIDES

Don't take sides in times of conflict between others. As soon as you do this, you become part of the dispute. Stay objective, remain calm and don't be drawn in. You will come across as more confident and self-assured. Calming down situations of conflict also gets you noticed in a positive light. In the same way, getting into heated arguments is totally unprofessional. You will be seen in a negative way, no matter how right you are.

CONTROL YOUR TEMPER

If a major decision has been made without your consultation, do not create an argument and never become aggressive. Always think very carefully before you act. There are times when you need a mentor or clinical supervisor to help you find an alternative way of dealing with the situation.

Usually there is nothing you can do but accept a bad decision but take action to ensure something similar never happens again. Always learn from your experiences. It is usually best to let the individual(s) know how you feel about the decision but then leave it at that. Don't let these things fester. After all, it is only a job!

TALK OF 'WE' RATHER THAN 'I'

Having the right attitude makes all the difference. You may find some of your colleagues develop a 'them and us' attitude. They like to side with their staff and moan about 'the management'. Try not to become one of them; your staff will not respect you, nor will the management. Besides, you are now part of the management. Even if you do not agree with some managerial decisions, try to keep your adverse feelings away from your staff. Just stick to the facts when explaining the situation to your team. If you talk of 'we' rather than 'I', you automatically assume a position of greater authority when talking to others.

THINK AS A MANAGER

When problems occur, it is easy to see things from your own point of view, but it's the manager's role to regard things from the staff and organisation's perspective.

Don't waste time thinking:

'Will this mean I will have to work more weekends?'
'Will this mean I won't get Christmas off this year?'
'What do I get if I put us forward to be part of the pilot project?'
'Will this make me look good?'

Consider things from as a managerial point of view:

'How can I ensure adequate senior cover at weekends?'
'How can I make sure the Christmas 'off-duty' is fair to all members of staff?'
'Will this pilot project improve patient care?'
'How will this benefit the staff?'

SERVICE USERS

There are some ward managers who have not grasped the concept of being part of an organisation. This often becomes apparent when something goes wrong. Phrases such as 'it's not our fault. It was the admissions department who cancelled your appointment, not us' or 'sorry, there are no pillows, the linen service here is terrible' may reflect the true facts of a situation but this is not the stance a manager should take.

Always remember that you are representing your organisation as one of their managers. If patients complain about services that have nothing to do with your department, empathise and reassure them that you will relay their concerns to the appropriate people to ensure that services will improve. Don't be defensive.

VOICING YOUR DISAGREEMENTS

If you do disagree with something, be careful how you do it. You may wish to say, for example, 'if we are going to open up four more beds, we need to consider how it will affect the staff' instead of 'I think you're mad to even suggest it'. There will always be disagreements with others within your organisation; just be careful about how you deal with them.

WORK WITH YOUR DIRECTOR OF NURSING

The director of nursing is an executive director. This is a very powerful position. They have far greater authority than your line manager and even your general manager. The director of nursing is the professional lead for nurses throughout the organisation. They work closely with the chief executive and other board directors in making decisions about what happens in the organisation over all.

The majority of nursing directors do not directly manage the nursing workforce, so some nurses get the impression that their role is not important; they could not be more wrong. You should make it your goal to build a strong alliance with your director of nursing.

THE PROFESSIONAL DEVELOPMENT TEAM

The director of nursing is responsible for the professional development of the nursing workforce and will usually have a small team of senior nurses to assist them in this role. This includes one or more deputy directors and various practice development nurses. It is a wise move to develop close working relationships with the professional development team. Their role is to help you develop practice, so you should make maximum use of this resource. Much of their work is currently dictated by national and local policy so close liaison will help keep you abreast of new policies and procedures.

SHADOWING

Try and arrange to spend a day shadowing your nursing director to give you an insight into their role and responsibilities. If you feel too awkward approaching them out of the blue, introduce the idea via an email. Make it short and succinct. Point out that you would like to learn more about their role and to pick up tips about how you can manage your ward more effectively. Many directors welcome this approach as it also gives them a chance to get to know more about what is happening at a clinical level in your area. They will let you know what dates they have available which will be appropriate for your learning.

MENTORING

Following the shadowing experience, it may be an idea to follow it up with a request for mentoring for the next six months. Having a director of nursing as a mentor for a while would be an invaluable experience. You do not have to be the ambitious type to do this. You will benefit from lots of hints and tips to help you in your current role.

You may have the added benefit of increasing your networks as they introduce you to other senior members in your organisation. The greater your network the more influential you will become.

Your nursing director will also get to know you. They will see that you run a good ward, that you are forward thinking and that you have leadership potential. When opportunities arise, they may think of you first of all as the person who may benefit. They may have access to some funding, for example, to assist with a project. If you had mentioned that it is something you are currently working on, you may find that you are nominated for the funding. Keeping your director informed of your work can bring all sorts of benefits.

Being closely associated with your director of nursing will give you the opportunity to influence the wider agenda and contribute to any major decisions affecting your organisation. But it will not just happen; you have to make it happen.

GET RECOGNITION FOR YOUR WORK

If you don't get to know the right people, your work and that of your team will have less chance of being recognised and appreciated. Celebrate your successes and let the rest of the organisation know how good your team are.

HOSPITAL NEWSLETTER

Write something regularly for your hospital newsletter. You do not have to be an accomplished journalist. The communications team are there to help you. Try not to just use the newsletter as a way of keeping people up-to-date with matters such as 'Nurse Jones just had a baby' or 'Nurse Smith has been promoted'. Talk about any innovations or changes that have made an improvement to patient care. Put forward ideas that other wards may benefit from. It could be something like a successful change in your handover system or how a new system of restricted visiting times helped your patients get a much-needed rest.

Aim to get an article in every six to twelve months. One of the board directors usually has to read through and approve the newsletter before it is finally published and distributed. Your team's contributions will not go unnoticed.

CONFERENCES AND STUDY DAYS

Encourage your staff to speak about their successes at local workshops and conferences. You can find out about these through your organisation's practice development team. Keep them informed and involved in all new initiatives on your ward. They will hopefully tell others of your good work and help promote it to others too.

COMPARE YOUR WARD WITH OTHERS

There is nothing more soul-destroying than to read an article or see people being praised for implementing a new way of working that you've been doing for years. The problem is being able to recognise the things you do that are better than other areas. One of the best ways of doing this is to invite others to shadow you. Having a student nurse work closely with you for a day is a great way of finding out what people do on other wards and to point out what things you do well on your ward.

The benchmarking process is another good way of finding out what you do well compared with other areas. Promoting the work of your team is not a selfish thing to do. It is recognising their hard work and rewarding them for a job well done. This is one of the five fundamental behaviours of a good leader (see p. 5).

CHOOSE YOUR MENTOR AND MENTEES WITH CARE

THE MENTOR ROLE

When you become a manager, it is wise to have a mentor who is a lot more senior than yourself. The role of a mentor is to provide advice, guidance, information and contacts to help you in your work. A good mentor can be invaluable because:

- they have far more experience than you
- they have often 'been there and done it' before
- they will help you benefit from the knowledge they have in their current position
- they can introduce you to their wider networks.

Aim high

Try not to settle for someone who is just one or two grades above you; aim higher. The more senior your mentor is within your organisation, the more they can help you become influential in your role. A member of the board is ideal. A nonexecutive director in particular can give you the benefits of their skills from outside the NHS. They are usually keen to take on the mentor role because they want to understand your role better. Having a mentee at clinical level gives them a valuable insight into the complexities of running a ward.

Having a board director as a mentor can open doors for you. They will explain how to get things done. If you feel you need extra staff for your unit and are getting nowhere, having a finance director as your mentor can be extremely advantageous. Don't expect them to do things for you; it's not that easy. However, you can get them to explain the system clearly to you and point out where you are going wrong.

Don't choose a mentor who has little or no influence in your organisation. It will be a waste of time. If they have no influence, how can they help you to gain those skills? How will they help increase your networks? Managers within the NHS who are not politically aware do not make good mentors.

Change your mentor as necessary

You don't have to keep the same mentor all the time. Once you have achieved your objectives, you can move on. Set a limited time span such as six to eight months to start with. By this time you will have got to know them well and can choose to either stay with them or move on to another mentor more suitable for your current needs.

CHOOSING YOUR MENTEES

It is advisable not to have more than a maximum of three people to mentor. Your time is precious. Don't waste your time on people who are only looking for your help to improve their career prospects. Watch for staff who have good potential. You'll know them when you see them. They are usually committed, hard working and produce high standards of work. Often they don't know they are good. Their work may go unnoticed. Only you are experienced enough to know that with a bit of extra guidance and support, this person could go a long way and really make a difference.

Being a mentor to someone with potential can be a very rewarding experience through watching them become more confident in themselves with your guidance and support. They may well become more senior than you one day. It can give a huge sense of satisfaction knowing that you were part of the process. And what's more, they'll never forget you.

Steer clear of your own junior team members

Try not to mentor a junior member of your own team unless it is your deputy. It may cause resentment among the rest of the team. If you do have someone in your team that you feel would flourish with good mentoring, ask one of your colleagues (fellow ward managers) to become their mentor.

Mentoring new ward managers

It's a good idea to get together with your peers and set up a system whereby the more experienced ward managers mentor the newer and less experienced ones. No ward manager should start their new role without being assigned a more experienced manager to mentor them. Show them the ropes. Introduce them to the essential people and systems they need to know to get things done. Don't let them struggle like you probably did. A good internal mentoring system will build a stronger team of ward managers within your organisation.

PLAN AHEAD FOR YOUR OWN NEEDS

Don't neglect your own needs. Being politically aware can also help you with where you want to go. Have you thought about where are you heading? You may wish to go into management, education or a more senior specialist clinical role (e.g. nurse consultant). Even if you want to stay where you are until retirement, it is still wise to plan ahead to ensure you get the best out of your job.

IDENTIFY YOUR SPECIAL INTERESTS

If your ultimate aim is to become a nurse consultant, start specialising in your subject now. Become a member of the appropriate specialist association and ask the appropriate nurse specialist or medical consultant to become your mentor.

If your aim is to go into senior management or teaching you would benefit by developing your skills in a particular area. Make sure that your name is linked with the specialist interest throughout the organisation. You could join the appropriate project group or perhaps even write an article for your hospital's newsletter such as '10 Tips For Managing Your Budget'. Get yourself recognised.

Don't leave it to chance. That ideal job won't just fall in your lap; you have to make it happen.

It is easy to allow your own needs to get overlooked when your time is taken up with meeting the needs of your patients and staff. Boosting your individual status is something nurses find hard to do. You have to make your mark so you stand out and your potential is noticed. Having a specific area of interest will enable you to do this. Although your job requires you to have a general knowledge of all issues, becoming an expert in one or two specific areas can help your future career prospects.

KEEP A BOX FILE FOR YOUR CV

It is doubtful if anyone has the time or inclination to keep their CV up-to-date at all times, but it is helpful to keep a box file labelled CV and each time you attend a course, workshop or study session, add any relevant papers, certificates or reflective notes. You'll find it easier when you come to writing or updating your CV to have everything together in one place rather than having to search through papers and diaries trying to remember what you did.

WRITING YOUR CV

The basic outline of a CV (see Appendix 9.1 for a sample CV) should contain the following:

- your name
- your address
- your contact details
- a summary of your current role.

Write a brief couple of paragraphs outlining your current role. This is one of the most important parts of your CV. Don't use the job description. Everyone knows the responsibilities of a ward manager. Promote what is special about you.

A summary of your educational achievements
List in date order, starting with the most recent courses. Don't include your school education; you are too senior for that to matter now. Your registered nurse qualification should be the last one on the list.

A summary of your work experience
List where you have worked since registering as a nurse. Put it in date order starting with the most recent experience. Don't repeat your current role here. You have already outlined this at the beginning of the document. Write in any key achievements. Try not to just list what your responsibilities were. You need to convince your new employer that you are a person who achieves things, rather than just does the job.

References

Two references are required, one from your current employer and one from your previous employer. If you have been in your current post for many years, you could use someone else like a link lecturer or course tutor. (Remember always to ask your referees first. Never just assume that they will provide one. It is inconsiderate to put down someone's name as a reference without asking.)

TAILOR YOUR CV TO THE JOB

Each CV should be tailored to the job you are applying for. Don't be tempted to include everything. No matter how senior or experienced you are, your CV should be no more than two pages long. Your potential employers need to see that you have the relevant skills for the job. They do not want to wade through everything you have done and have to try to decipher for themselves which bits are relevant.

SENDING A COVER LETTER

If you are asked for your CV only, send a cover letter. Outline in it why you want the job and why you feel you are the right person for it.

If you are required to send an application form as well, don't write 'see CV' on the application form. Pick out the pertinent parts from your CV and add them to your application form. The application form usually asks you why you want the job and why you feel you are the right person for it. This information is not specifically outlined on the CV, so you will need to add it to the form. A cover letter is not normally required when submitting an application form.

ACTION POINTS

- Access the NHS website each month to keep yourself up-to-date with what's going on nationally.
- Find out the membership of your hospital board and what their priorities are.
- Aim to attend or send a representative to all the board meetings, sisters' meetings and local directorate meetings.
- Aim to add at least one new contact to your network each month.
- Concentrate on presenting facts when asked your opinion and never criticise others.
- Never use the phrase 'the management'.
- Make a date to shadow your director of nursing.
- Write a short article for your hospital's newsletter about a recent achievement.
- Get yourself a senior mentor.
- Consider whether your current mentees are relevant.
- Start up a box file for your CV.

References

Department of Health 2000 The NHS plan: a plan for investment, a plan for reform. HMSO, London. Online. Available: http://www.dh.gov.uk/assetRoot/04/05/57/83/04055783.pdf 29 Sep 2005

Department of Health 2005a Welcome to the Department of Health. Online. Available: http://www.dh.gov.uk 29 Sep 2005

Department of Health 2005b Chief Nursing Officer. Online. Available: http://www.dh.gov.uk/cno 29 Sep 2005

Department of Health, Social Services and Public Safety 2002 Investing for health. DHSSPS, Northern Ireland. Online. Available: http://www.dhsspsni.gov.uk/publications/2002/investforhealth.asp 29 Sep 2005

Department of Health, Social Services and Public Safety 2005a DHSSPS, Northern Ireland. Online. Available: http://www.dhsspsni.gov.uk 29 Sep 2005

Department of Health, Social Services and Public Safety 2005b Chief Nursing Officer. DHSSPS, Northern Ireland. Online. Available: http://www.dhsspsni.gov.uk/pgroups/nursing 29 Sep 2005

Healthcare Commission 2005 Healthcare Commission: inspecting, informing, improving. Online. Available: http://www.healthcarecommission.org.uk 29 Sep 2005

Healthcare Inspectorate Wales 2005 Healthcare Inspectorate Wales. Online. Available: http://www.hiw.wales.gov.uk 29 Sep 2005

NHS Quality Improvement Scotland 2005 Raising healthcare standards. Online. Available: http://www.nhshealthquality.org 29 Sep 2005

NHS Wales 2001 Improving health in Wales. National Assembly for Wales, Cardiff. Online. Available: http://www.wales.nhs.uk/publications/NHSStrategydoc.pdf 29 Sep 2005

NHS Wales 2005 Health of Wales Information Service. Online. Available: http://www.wales.nhs.uk 29 Sep 2005

Scotland's Health on the Web 2005 Scotland's Health on the Web. Online. Available: http://www.show.scot.nhs.uk 29 Sep 2005

Scottish Executive 2000 Our national health: a plan for action, a plan for change. Scottish Executive, Edinburgh. Online. Available: http://www.show.scot.nhs.uk/sehd/onh/onh-00.htm 29 Sep 2005

SAMPLE CV

Jane Smith
21 St James Street, Newbury, Gloucestershire GN23 4FN
Tel: 08900 400300
Email: *jane.smith@internet.com*

Current role:

Ward manager, Flower Ward, Tree NHS Trust from 2004 to present.
I manage a 28-bed medical ward, using a primary nursing model, which I successfully implemented two years ago. I have a special interest in integrated care pathways and led the development of two ICPs for patients admitted with CVA and MI, which are currently in use on the ward.
I manage a team of 24 staff with a budget of £500 000. I use a transformational leadership approach in all aspects of my work by ensuring that I involve my team in all decisions and encouraging them to consistently challenge the status quo.

Educational achievements:

Dec 2005 Diploma in Health Service Management
Aug 2005 Advanced Life Support Update
Jan 2003 BSc Professional Nursing Studies
Feb 2000 RN (PIN 123456 Exp 05/10)

Career history:

2002–2004 Junior Sister, Stroke Unit, Another Trust, London
Key achievements:

* Successful implementation of team nursing
* Instrumental in reducing staff vacancies from 50% on commencement of role to no vacancies within one year

2000–2002 Staff Nurse, Medical Ward, Another Trust, London
Developed an in-house one year training programme to develop the skills of newly qualified nurses in caring for medical patients.

References:

Current employer
Mrs A Smith
Medical Unit
Tree NHS Trust
08900 000000
jdeq@internet.com

Senior Lecturer
Mr B Jones
Management Dept
Tree University
08900 333333
jq@university.com

CHAPTER 10

LOOK AFTER YOURSELF

Recognise symptoms of stress 188

Positive and negative stress 189

Consider taking a break 189

Options for reducing the pressure 190

Recognise and deal with any staff stress 190

Recognising the signs 191

Dealing with stress in others 191

Get yourself a mentor 192

How to approach prospective mentors 193

People to avoid as mentors 194

Set up a peer support group or action learning set 194

What is action learning? 194

Support and challenge 195

Train up your deputy ward manager 196

'Acting up' in your absence 196

Delegate to improve their skills 196

Ensure they get appropriate support 197

Don't feel threatened 197

Work on their strengths 197

Delegate with care 197

Get a union representative or steward on your team 198

Union stewards 198

Union representatives 198

Reap the benefits 199

Choose carefully whom you talk to and what you say 199

Members of your team 199

Your line manager 200

Be wary of the informal network or grapevine 200

Get to know influential people 200

Be careful what you say 200

Get over mistakes and move on 201

Be wary of perfectionism 201

Be confident 201

Dealing with mistakes – changing the culture 202

Drink plenty of water and eat regularly 202

Drink at least 8–10 glasses of water per day 203

Cut down to 3–4 cups of coffee/tea per day 203

Cut out fizzy drinks 203

Don't forget to eat regularly 204

Night shifts 204

Remember it's only a job 204

Taking on the role of a manager gives you greater power and authority. However, this power and authority comes at a price; your staff will have greater expectations. They will require you to:

1. Support them through difficult times.
2. Take over in difficult situations when they don't know what to do.
3. Provide the appropriate resources and environment to enable them to do their job properly.
4. Know everything.
5. Be confident.
6. Always make the right decisions.
7. Never be off sick.
8. Never have any problems of your own.
9. Never make mistakes.

When you were a staff nurse, you were safe in the knowledge that there was often someone more knowledgeable and experienced to turn to. When you become a ward manager, you are that more knowledgeable and experienced person on every shift you work.

You have more pressure than many nonclinical managers. You are responsible for ensuring that sick and vulnerable people get appropriate care and treatment 24 hours a day, seven days a week. Everyone, including your team, the patients and their relatives, have very high expectations of you. It's an incredibly responsible job and there are few who would not buckle under the pressure at times. The key is to look after yourself and set up your own support system.

RECOGNISE SYMPTOMS OF STRESS

Stress is a word used very liberally nowadays. Everyone seems stressed. People talk of suffering from the stress of exams, interviews, giving presentations, holding dinner parties, starting a new job, etc. Stress is not something that happens to you. Stress is your *reaction* to something that happens to you. It's 'the adverse reaction people have to excessive pressure or other types of demand placed on them' (Health and Safety Executive 2005a). In other words, how you react to the *'excessive pressure'* or *'other types of demand'* in your job determines the amount of stress you feel.

You will always have pressure of some sort or other in your work. A certain amount of pressure is needed to keep you motivated, but if you allow it to spiral out of control, it can lead to stress, which in turn can make you ill. So the answer is to stop the pressure spiralling out of control. This sounds easy but when you are in the midst of dealing with continual excessive day-to-day demands it can be difficult to recognise the signs.

POSITIVE AND NEGATIVE STRESS

We all need a certain amount of pressure. Our bodies respond to it by producing a positive stress response. This positive stress response allows us to meet deadlines and generate new ideas by giving us energy and motivation. However, when we feel out of control with the pressure of work, we experience a negative stress response. If the pressure continues day after day, we may experience the physical, emotional or mental symptoms brought on by negative stress. It is important to recognise the signs. Ask yourself:

1. Do people easily irritate you at work?
2. Have you lost your ability to have fun and enjoy yourself at work?
3. Do you find yourself becoming more cynical, critical and sarcastic particularly when talking about the future?
4. Do you suffer with continual aches and pains, a tight stomach or indigestion?
5. Do you suffer with frequent colds and infections?
6. Do you get in a panic after handover when you actually have to get up and take charge?
7. Do you often think at the beginning of the shift 'here we go again'?
8. Do you feel that you cannot get things done; that the barriers are too big?
9. Do you feel that you simply do not have the energy to do the job any more?
10. Are you fed up with people asking if you are alright?
11. Are you taking comfort in food, i.e. putting on weight, or alcohol, i.e. drinking every evening after work?
12. Does thinking about work keep you awake at night?
13. Do you constantly think about work on your days off?
14. Do you feel out of control?

It is important to recognise the symptoms of negative stress. If you allow them to persist, you are risking serious health problems. At the end of the day, is your job really worth risking your health for?

CONSIDER TAKING A BREAK

Continuously feeling stressed is an indication that your work is controlling you. Your only option is to reduce the pressure. One way to do this is to take a break. A holiday may not be sufficient. The job of a ward manager is not highly paid. You can earn similar money working in a far less demanding job. There are plenty of alternative jobs you can undertake on a temporary basis. Do a spot of agency work for a while or even work in an office or the local supermarket. It doesn't mean you have failed. Call it a sabbatical.

Sometimes a three to six month break can do you the power of good. With the current national emphasis on flexible working policies you could take a six month break and have the option of returning to the same job. If you are really feeling the pressure, think about it.

OPTIONS FOR REDUCING THE PRESSURE

There are many less drastic options you can take to reduce the pressure other than taking a long break. These include:

1. Going to see your manager to identify and agree areas where your workload can be reduced (see Ch. 2).
2. Identifying areas for further training and development to enable you to deal with certain pressures.
3. Getting a mentor to help you deal with difficult situations and learn from them.
4. Setting up a group with your peers to support and learn from each other's experiences.

You may also need to look at yourself and identify any personal traits that need attention. These include:

● poor health habits, e.g. smoking, consuming too much processed food and fizzy drinks
● negative attitudes and feelings, e.g. thinking that everyone else is right and you must be wrong
● unrealistic expectations, e.g. expecting all staff to know everything and work as hard as you do
● perfectionism, e.g. expecting to complete work to the same standard even when adequate staffing or resources are not available.

RECOGNISE AND DEAL WITH ANY STAFF STRESS

If your staff are stressed at work, it will only serve to increase your problems. Stress in the workplace is a health and safety issue. Organisations are required by law to look at what the risks are and take sensible measures to tackle them (Health and Safety Executive 1999). You have certain responsibilities for the health, safety and welfare of your staff. It is important for you to ensure systems are in place to respond to individual concerns. Guidelines are available to help managers meet their legal duties (Health and Safety Executive 2005b). These guidelines outline standards that should be met. Your staff should be able to say that:

● they are able to cope with the demands of their job
● they have a say about the way they work
● they receive adequate information from you and their colleagues
● they are not subject to any unacceptable behaviours at work such as bullying
● they understand their roles and responsibilities
● they are engaged frequently when undergoing any organisational change.

Some people are more vulnerable to stress than others particularly if there are recent changes in their personal circumstances. If allowed to continue, it can affect their health and their performance. It can also affect other staff who have to continually cover when their stressed colleagues ring in sick. Ultimately, patient care will suffer.

RECOGNISING THE SIGNS

Be alert to changes in a person's mood or behaviour. They may become quiet and withdrawn, bossy and aggressive or irritable. Their performance at work may be affected. Their standard of work may gradually deteriorate. One obvious sign is increased sickness levels or lateness. Other symptoms often missed are becoming too involved at work, staying behind to make sure things are done or expecting higher and higher standards from self and others.

Look out for the physical symptoms too. These include frequent coughs and colds, headaches, perpetual tiredness and an inability to smile or join in with any banter. The symptoms of stress vary and if you don't know a person well it can be difficult to determine. It is therefore imperative that as their manager you make it your business to know all the individuals in your team. You should be familiar with how they think, how they organise themselves and how they work together with the others as a team. A noticeable change in someone's behaviour is the main symptom to be alert to. If you do not know how they behave normally then spotting the changes will be a lot more difficult.

DEALING WITH STRESS IN OTHERS

Once you have spotted the symptoms of stress, you need to do something about it. The first step is to find out the cause. The only way to find out is to ask, and listen closely to what they have to say. Some common causes of stress in nursing are:

● feeling overloaded
● feeling out of depth
● feeling undervalued
● feeling alone and unsupported
● lack of confidence
● uncertainty about the future of role or work environment
● pressures from home such as childcare or money worries
● being bullied or harassed.

If any of your staff say they feel overloaded, out of their depth, undervalued or alone, then they need extra support. You can do this yourself or it may be more appropriate to assign one of the more senior and experienced people in your team to do this.

Giving support is more than just spending time listening and giving advice. On its own, this solves little. Support involves taking practical action too. If the problem is work overload or feeling out of depth, try working closely with them for a few shifts, observing how they manage their time and helping them to improve any skills deficit. If the problem is feeling undervalued or a lack of confidence, try increasing feedback (both positive and negative) on their day-to-day performance. Consistent feedback helps by showing them what they do right and what they need to do to improve. It helps individuals to take control of their work and feel that they are making progress.

If members of your staff are stressed due to uncertainty about changes at work, this may indicate that you have not involved them enough in the process of change. You may have kept them informed, but there is a huge difference between informing and involving staff. Make sure they feel their opinions are heard and acted upon.

If someone has pressures at home causing undue stress at work, you are not obliged to sort out their home circumstances but consider what you can do to help at work. Possible solutions may include allowing them a short period of leave or a change in working hours.

If any members of your staff are being bullied or harassed, take action to stop it now. Give them some time out from the situation or move staff if necessary. Involve human resources (HR) straight away for advice and support on the best approach to follow. Never leave a situation like this to solve itself (see p. 251).

GET YOURSELF A MENTOR

Having a mentor will help you develop the knowledge and skills to achieve not only the objectives in your personal development plan but they will also help in your day-to-day practice by giving you support and guidance or pointing you in the direction of someone who can help. Having a mentor is the key in helping you develop your leadership skills. You need to find someone with the right position and experience to enable you to build your confidence in the role. If you are ambitious, a good mentor will also help you further your career.

Don't confuse a managerial mentor with the role of the mentor in nurse education. Nurses are familiar with the term 'mentor' used in the context of supervising and assessing student nurses and for postregistration nurses undertaking formal courses of study. However, the role of the mentor in the world of management is totally different from the role of the mentor as advocated by the universities.

Mentoring in nurse education

In nursing, the term mentor is used to denote the role of the nurse, midwife or specialist community public health nurse who facilitates learning, supervises and assesses students in the practice setting (Nursing & Midwifery Council 2004). A mentor is allocated to preregistration nurses to help them achieve their learning outcomes through assessment, planning, clinical support and role modelling. Postregistration nurses undertaking further modules or courses of study are also encouraged to have a mentor for similar reasons. There is usually some sort of formal assessment and paperwork associated with the role.

Mentoring in management

Mentors for managers should be more experienced managers but not the individual's line manager. They usually meet regularly but do not work together in the same department. The relationship is more informal and no formal records are required. The mentor assists the individual not only in their current position but also helps them develop for future roles. The most significant difference for managerial mentors is their role in introducing you to their networks so that you can broaden your horizons and become more politically aware.

Most senior managers within health care are familiar with the latter definition of the mentor role. Mentoring at managerial level is seen as a two-way process. It enables the senior managers to become aware of new talent as well as giving them an insight into what is really happening at the clinical level. The role of the mentor in management is to:

1. Offer a different and objective view of the issues you wish to discuss.
2. Offer a nonjudgemental relationship.
3. Develop your skills of reflection to enable you to continually learn from your experiences.
4. Advise, guide, support and help you to solve problems.
5. Widen your network to give yourself more of an insight into the politics of the wider organisation.

What a mentor in management won't do is:

● carry out any form of formal assessment
● sort out all your problems for you
● tell you what to do
● offer clinical advice.

Don't choose a mentor because they are 'nice' or you happen to know them. Find someone who can help you reach the goals in your personal development plan. If, for example, you wish to develop your skills in dealing with patient complaints and writing response letters, the complaints manager or one of the nonexecutive directors who is involved with the complaints department would make an appropriate mentor. As mentioned previously (see p. 181) nonexecutive directors make ideal mentors.

HOW TO APPROACH PROSPECTIVE MENTORS

It is not easy to go up to someone you don't know and ask them to be your mentor. What if you do not like them or feel uncomfortable in their presence? In order to find out, one option is to shadow them first. Shadowing a senior experienced manager is becoming the 'in' thing to do for managers. Call or email the person you have chosen, asking if you could shadow them for a day to find out more about their role and to develop your skills in a certain area. If the day turns out well and you feel it would be beneficial, you can then ask them to be your mentor. Otherwise, thank them for their time and find someone else.

PEOPLE TO AVOID AS MENTORS

Be careful about who you choose to be your mentor. There is no point in wasting your time having someone who cannot devote the time and effort to the role. This includes managers who:

● are new to their own job and therefore finding their feet
● are not respected within the organisation
● have little influence within your organisation
● are always busy
● have achieved little in their role.

And one last tip is to ensure your line manager knows who your mentor is. It can be quite disconcerting to learn that you have formed a professional relationship with someone who is senior to them. Some managers will need reassuring that the liaison is to improve your skills, not to 'tell tales' about them.

SET UP A PEER SUPPORT GROUP OR ACTION LEARNING SET

The ward manager's job is a lonely one but it needn't be. It never ceases to amaze me why ward managers within organisations rarely get together apart from at formal sisters' meetings. The biggest source of support is from others who do the same job and therefore have similar problems.

There is no reason why you cannot set up a small support group of like-minded individuals. It's usually advisable to start off with a small number of around six people. Make sure you focus on solutions. Some nurse managers are adept at having lengthy discussions about a problem without ever considering what the solution could be. *Action learning* is a solution-orientated method of learning from each other's problems.

WHAT IS ACTION LEARNING?

Action learning is a process that involves looking at problems from a different perspective, taking action and learning from the result of that action taken. The idea is that the whole group learns from the actions that the person takes rather than just one person alone. It involves a number of stages:

Stage 1: A member of the group presents their problem and the rest of the group listen without interruption.

Stage 2: The group questions the individual further, encouraging further reflection and discussion.

Stage 3: Following further discussion, the individual together with the group focuses on possible solutions. This enables the individual to devise a plan of action to tackle the problem.

Stage 4: After the meeting, the individual goes back to their workplace and follows through the agreed actions.

Stage 5: At the following meeting, the individual feeds back to the others what happened as a result of their actions. Together they discuss whether the action worked and what they learned from the process, i.e. if it happened again, what would they do next time?

Stage 6: If the action was not successful, another plan can be devised. The group learn as much from unsuccessful approaches as they do from successful ones.

Action learning has become popular in the UK since Reginald Revans founded the idea over 50 years ago (Revans 1983). Revans was a nuclear physicist working in Cambridge who found that whenever he came up against complex problems there was no-one else working in his field to advise him. He decided to get together with his colleagues to question each other to stimulate reflection and sharing of each other's problems. Together they came to workable solutions for their own and each other's problems.

When Revans began working for the coal industry in 1945 he managed to increase productivity by 30% by getting the pit managers to meet regularly in small groups to share and learn from each other's experiences.

SUPPORT AND CHALLENGE

Action learning is a simple but very effective method of learning and supporting each other. To get the most out of an action learning group, it's a good idea to get someone external to the group to facilitate the process to start off with, but not essential. If there is nobody available within your organisation with the right skills and you do not have the funding for an external facilitator, don't let it stop you setting up some sort of 'support and challenge group' yourself. As long as you meet regularly, you will be able to help each other learn from your experiences and the actions you take.

The key to the success of your group depends on:

● ensuring all discussions are solution-orientated, as opposed to problem-orientated
● meeting regularly, at least every month
● ensuring that all discussions remain confidential within the confines of the group
● sticking with the same group members as far as possible to enable you to build up trust in each other
● each member being voluntary, i.e. wanting to take part and actively contribute.

The group members need to be able to build up trust and confidence together to be able to challenge each other to think differently about things. Joint reflection with other ward managers is an ideal way of helping you become more effective in your role. It offers the chance to give and receive feedback, which you may not get in such an isolated position. The team you manage will give you a certain amount of feedback but they do not fully understand your issues, having never been in the role themselves. Your line manager's feedback is also limited in that they are working at a distance and in an entirely different role.

TRAIN UP YOUR DEPUTY WARD MANAGER

Your deputy ward manager is your greatest asset. Your aim should be to enable them to develop the skills and ability to do your job within two years of being in the post.

'ACTING UP' IN YOUR ABSENCE

When you take annual leave, you should be able to rest in the knowledge that your ward is in safe hands. You need to be confident that any crises will be dealt with, all your emails will be sorted and you do not have to return to a 'shed load' of work that accumulated while you were away. The only way to do this is to prepare your deputy. Help them to develop the skills to 'act up' in your absence.

To prepare your deputy for this role, make sure that you share everything with them. They should be familiar with all aspects of your job. Take them along to meetings so that they are knowledgeable about the groups to which you belong and will be able to represent you in your absence. Don't ask them to replace you at a regular meeting when you have not familiarised them with the process beforehand; it would be unfair. They need to feel confident to speak up on your behalf. If you are just interested in getting the information, send your apologies. There is no need to waste your deputy's time. Read the minutes instead on your return.

DELEGATE TO IMPROVE THEIR SKILLS

Make sure your deputy has some responsibility for aspects of your role such as parts of the budget, investigating complaints or writing reports on your behalf. Delegate early and support them through the process. Don't just show them how to do it. Help them to learn by doing it themselves.

When you are on days off, assign your deputy to deal with your emails. You can do this by giving them 'proxy access' using their own password. It serves to give them an insight into your responsibilities. Ensure they have the authority to deal with them as they see fit. Give feedback (not criticism) on your return so they can identify what they are doing right and wrong and learn a better way of doing things if appropriate.

ENSURE THEY GET APPROPRIATE SUPPORT

Make sure your deputy has access to a good senior mentor from elsewhere in the hospital. You can be one of their mentors, but it's advisable to encourage them to have someone who is not working in your ward. This will enable them to gain an external and thus more objective view on issues at work. A more experienced ward manager from another ward would make a good mentor for them. Your way is not always the only way, so having an external mentor will encourage them to challenge your ways of working.

Encourage your deputy to join or set up a peer support group or action learning set. They also need an outlet in which to be able to discuss issues and learn from their experiences and mistakes in a safe environment with others who are in similar roles.

DON'T FEEL THREATENED

Don't feel threatened if your deputy picks things up quickly and you feel they are becoming better at the job than you. Your job is not at risk. Use the situation to your advantage. Their success is a reflection of your efforts. Your own job is made easier. Having a good deputy takes a huge weight off your own shoulders. It helps you to have peace of mind when you are away from the ward for any length of time.

WORK ON THEIR STRENGTHS

Your deputy will probably have strengths that differ from yours. Use this to your advantage. If you are not good at presentations, for example, but your deputy excels at them, ensure it is your deputy who gives presentations at important events.

When you undertake a managerial task in the presence of your deputy, such as dealing with aggressive relatives, discuss your performance afterwards. Identify together which aspects went well and which aspects did not go well. By doing this, you are enabling them to learn from your strengths.

DELEGATE WITH CARE

Don't 'dump' tasks you don't like. Your deputy will come to resent this and it does not help their learning. Only delegate tasks that will assist in their learning and development. Don't delegate tasks you don't know how to do yourself. On the other hand, don't feel that you must learn something first before your deputy can take it on. If you do not know how to do something, then learn together with your deputy.

Don't be put out when you find that members of your team prefer to approach your deputy with issues rather than you. It usually has nothing to do with your management style or approachability. People tend to abide by the old hierarchical rules, i.e. go to the person of the next grade, not two grades up. They are just respecting your authority.

GET A UNION REPRESENTATIVE OR STEWARD ON YOUR TEAM

It is advisable to encourage and support one of your team members to become a union representative. Don't be discouraged by the fact that you have to give them time off to represent staff outside of your ward because the advantages far outweigh the disadvantages. It's something you could put in as a business case for extra funding if necessary (see Ch. 6). Both the Royal College of Nursing (RCN) and Unison provide full training for these roles.

UNION STEWARDS

Union stewards have to undergo specific training which provides knowledge of employment law, terms and conditions, and disciplinary and grievance procedures. Through this training and their representative work, they learn the skills of:

- communicating
- negotiating
- how to work with management
- leadership
- networking.

They also attend regular seminars to keep them up-to-date with issues such as bullying and harassment legislation and diversity. A union steward will bring enormous benefits to your team through the knowledge and experience they gain in the role. If you have any serious HR issues at work, your union steward will be an invaluable resource for you and the other members of your team, simply because they are so easily accessible.

As part of their role, they also meet regularly with your organisation's senior management team (including board directors and the chief executive) to ensure that the employment rights of workers are promoted and poor practice and decisions are challenged.

UNION REPRESENTATIVES

Members of your staff could also be encouraged to become a union representative or workplace contact, with the option of specialising in subjects such as health and safety or learning. This role demands less time and commitment but is still advantageous in terms of the knowledge and experience they bring to your team.

Union health and safety representatives work to ensure the environment is safe and healthy for the workers. Their work includes:

● raising awareness about health and safety issues
● alerting their work colleagues to risks and their obligations
● carrying out regular investigations into unsafe conditions at work.

They need paid time off to receive training and to regularly update their skills, but the investment is worth the end result. They will be knowledgeable about important issues such as health and safety legislation, accident investigation and audits/risk assessment.

Union learning representatives offer education and advice particularly in relation to changes such as in the use of the knowledge and skills framework (KSF). They help their colleagues know what they need to know to meet the criteria and help with their career progression.

REAP THE BENEFITS

Be prepared to invest to reap the benefits. Remember that the role and responsibilities of union stewards and representatives have a far wider remit than their immediate work environment. You have to be willing to invest time to enable them to represent members and issues outside your ward or department. It costs you money but is well worth the extra expense to have all that extra knowledge and experience within your team. In addition, becoming a union representative or steward helps members of your staff to develop their confidence and skills in negotiating. They will gain invaluable insight into the work of committees and develop extensive networks, which can benefit your whole team.

CHOOSE CAREFULLY WHOM YOU TALK TO AND WHAT YOU SAY

MEMBERS OF YOUR TEAM

Try not to turn to members of your staff for emotional support of any kind. Although you will work together as a team and hopefully have some fun times together, it is not wise to use them as a sounding board for any problems you face. If you do, it may make things difficult for you in the future. It could result in:

● your future judgement of that person being affected
● difficulties in dealing with any future inappropriate behaviour
● resentment among those who see their colleagues as 'teacher's pet'.

If you are frustrated, angry or upset because of a situation either at work or at home, talk to your mentor, clinical supervisor, your spouse, etc. – just not anyone from your team.

YOUR LINE MANAGER

Be careful when talking to your line manager about your problems and frustrations. Always keep in the back of your mind that this person undertakes your appraisals and they or their colleagues may even interview you for future posts. Whether you like it or not, your line manager will talk about you with their colleagues so you want to ensure you create the right impression.

Although you may always be honest, reliable and never talk about people behind their backs, not everyone else is the same. Be wary of others and try not to convey anything negative about you for them to discuss with their colleagues.

BE WARY OF THE INFORMAL NETWORK OR GRAPEVINE

You can never be sure who knows who, who is related to whom and what sort of relationships people had before you joined the organisation. The director of nursing could have trained with your line manager and still meet socially. Your ward receptionist may happen to be a good friend and neighbour of the chief executive. The only safe bet is to ensure you never talk negatively about anyone.

GET TO KNOW INFLUENTIAL PEOPLE

When you attend a work gathering such as a meeting, presentation or conference, choose carefully who you talk to. Make sure you talk to people who are influential. Don't just stick with your peers where you feel safe and comfortable; you will get nowhere. You already know them and see them regularly. See if there is anyone there that could be quite handy to know. Make a point of talking to someone that you don't already know at every meeting you attend.

BE CAREFUL WHAT YOU SAY

If you speak in negative tones, the people you talk to will return those negative tones. If you use positive language, people will be positive in return. If you criticise others, you will be criticised. If you bitch or gossip about others, they will bitch and gossip about you. What you give out is what you will get back. Always think before you speak.

Be careful also of those who try to manipulate you into divulging information, using statements such as 'I hear your line manager has been having problems with the team in ward x'. Never agree with a statement such as this. Reply with something like 'I know nothing of it' or 'have you talked to her about what you've heard?'. Never be drawn into such conversations even if you agree and do not like the way your manager is handling things. Let your manager know how you feel by all means, but never let it be known to others. Disloyalty earns disrespect.

GET OVER MISTAKES AND MOVE ON

'Success is the result of good judgement.
Good judgement is the result of experience.
Experience is often the result of bad judgement.'
(Robbins 2001; p. 34)

Don't dwell on things. In any job you will make mistakes; it's all part of the learning process. It is so easy to feel pressured when you have made a mistake, particularly in the clinical environment where patient care has been, or could have been, compromised. The worry over a poor clinical decision, the distress from having upset people or the anguish of feeling you have let the side down can be overwhelming, that is if you allow it to be.

All mistakes should be dealt with in the following three stages:

Stage 1: Take corrective action and/or ask for help as appropriate.
Stage 2: Talk it through with someone (individual or group) and learn from it.
Stage 3: Take action to reduce the risk of you making the same mistake again.

The key is to be open and honest. Never cover up, always talk it through with someone and learn from it. If you allow yourself to continually worry about your mistakes, it will increase your stress levels and gradually affect your health and self-esteem.

BE WARY OF PERFECTIONISM

Are you a perfectionist? Perfectionists tend to get more upset and are more likely to cover up mistakes than others. They are also less likely to ask for help. Excessive worry over mistakes puts perfectionists at risk of developing mood disorders and even phobias (Kawamura & Frost 2004). If you have tendencies towards perfectionism or are a perpetual worrier, you need to work on changing your mindset. Even if you have compromised patient care, don't let the worry take over your life. Learn from the experience.

Discuss your mistake with your peer support group and let others learn from the experience too. Experience is built on mistakes. If you allow your mistake to make you think and feel negatively, you will become reluctant to try new things. Treat mistakes as learning opportunities.

BE CONFIDENT

Don't feel sorry for yourself and make statements like 'it's all my fault' or 'if only I hadn't done this or that'. You are a manager and need to set an example to others. Talking about yourself like this will not only erode your own self-esteem, it will reduce respect from others. Be honest and say something like 'Sorry about that. It was my decision and I accept it was not appropriate. I guess the best thing to do now is . . .'

DEALING WITH MISTAKES – CHANGING THE CULTURE

Over the past few years, a more open system is being encouraged where people can learn from their mistakes out in the open. In the past (and to some extent, even now) some health care managers have been guilty of perpetuating a 'blame culture' where people are punished for making mistakes. Things have gradually been changing since the publication of an important document in 2000 entitled 'An organisation with a memory' (Department of Health 2000). It looked into how the NHS learns from errors and adverse events. Since this report, a national reporting system was set up to record mistakes, adverse incidents and near misses in the NHS and make sure lessons are learnt. The aim was to promote a blame-free culture, which encouraged people in the health service to report mistakes without fear of reprimand. For the first time in its 50-year history, the NHS had a structured universal system to learn from mistakes.

However, changing the structure of the system is the easy part; changing the culture takes a lot longer. Changing the mindset of people working in the NHS after 50 years of punishing people for mistakes is no easy task. Nurses today still do not feel entirely comfortable with sharing information when they have made a drug error, for example.

You can help by being a role model. Show your staff that you learn from your mistakes. Create an environment where they can admit and learn from their mistakes without being under threat of punishment or blame. 'Learning through mistakes can often be a very effective way of improving competence and understanding. But to acknowledge errors and shortcomings, professionals must feel safe to do so. Employers, therefore, must create an environment which enables this to happen' (Bristol Royal Infirmary Inquiry 2001; Ch. 25, No. 7).

DRINK PLENTY OF WATER AND EAT REGULARLY

Do you get home from work feeling completely shattered? Are you often starving when you get in? Do your legs ache? Do your eyes feel tired and dry? Do you find you can't concentrate on what your kids are saying when you pick them up from school? Do you get frequent headaches? All these symptoms may not just be the result of having been through a busy shift; they can be the result of not drinking enough water or eating regularly throughout your shift. If you tend to do this often, you may find that you have enough energy to get you through the shift but it's all used up by the time you get home.

You need to be in the best of health to be alert enough to make the right decisions and support your staff. If you do not drink water regularly throughout your shift you will suffer from symptoms of dehydration. These include lack of concentration, irritability and headaches and not necessarily just a feeling of thirst. If you do not find the time to eat properly at work, you may find yourself compensating when you get home. It's not a healthy habit to get into.

If you make time at work to eat and drink sufficiently you will not only be more productive at work, you may also have some energy left for when you get home.

DRINK AT LEAST 8–10 GLASSES OF WATER PER DAY

Hospitals are hot, humid places and you are on your feet all day. It doesn't take an expert to tell you that you need to drink more water to compensate. But so many nurses rarely drink enough water during their shift to sustain their body's needs. If you arrive home tired after each shift with aching legs and dry eyes, you are not drinking enough. If you feel thirsty, you have allowed yourself to become very dehydrated.

The UK Food Standards Agency (2005) recommends that in normal circumstances you should be drinking six to eight glasses of water each day. Being on your feet all day in a hot, stuffy environment is not normal circumstances, so you should be drinking even more. Try and aim for eight to ten glasses of water per day, drinking at least six of these during your shift. You will feel a lot more alert at the end of the shift and have more energy to devote to your home life. It's easy to fit drinking water into your working day if you plan it:

1. Drink a glass of water just before handover.
2. Have one at the beginning of your first break and another just before you return to the ward.
3. Drink two glasses with your meal at your lunch or supper break.
4. And one just before you go home.

CUT DOWN TO 3–4 CUPS OF COFFEE/TEA PER DAY

Don't rely on tea and coffee to meet your fluid requirements. The caffeine acts as a mild diuretic and simply adds to problems of dehydration. Tea and coffee also affect the body's absorption of iron from food and women are at particular risk of anaemia from drinking too much tea and coffee. The iron-deficiency symptoms of tiredness, lethargy, difficulty in concentrating and a short attention span are often ignored and put down to being busy at work. It's not always just the work that makes you feel like this. You could be drinking too much caffeine.

However, there are numerous studies now to show that a moderate intake of tea, i.e. three to four cups per day, is good for you over all so the message is to cut down but don't cut out altogether (The Tea Council 2005).

CUT OUT FIZZY DRINKS

These are full of caffeine, laden with E numbers and additives and have few nutrients. There have also been links to cancer of the oesophagus, kidney stones, hyperactivity, weak bones, dental erosion and obesity. Why bother drinking them at all?

DON'T FORGET TO EAT REGULARLY

Ideally you should eat something every two to three hours, but at work getting the chance would be a fine thing! Taking frequent breaks is no easy task. One alternative is to eat food that will give you lasting energy levels. Chocolate, cakes and crisps give you energy for the first hour or so but then your energy and concentration levels will plummet. By the time you get your break, you will feel shattered.

The key is to plan ahead. Before an early shift, eating a substantial breakfast such as porridge or muesli will give you longer lasting energy. If you cannot face breakfast early in the morning, take it to work and eat it on your first break. Taking ready snacks such as nuts and raisins or sandwiches with brown bread will give you longer lasting energy.

Try to eat more slowly to aid your digestion and prevent stomach problems later on in the shift. It takes concentrated effort to do this especially on early shift when you have been 'on the go' all morning.

NIGHT SHIFTS

You have to be particularly attentive to your health on night shifts. As well as drinking plenty of water to keep hydrated and alert, some tips on remaining healthy during night shifts include:

- avoiding caffeine three to four hours prior to sleep
- eating a banana or drinking some warm milk before going to bed, because they contain L-tryptophan, a natural sleep inducer
- avoiding alcohol prior to sleep, because of its diuretic effects
- trying to keep to regular meal times.

(Clayden 2003)

REMEMBER IT'S ONLY A JOB

Don't let yourself succumb to work-related burnout. You are at risk if you regularly:

- work more than 37.5 hours per week
- take work home with you
- come in on your days off for meetings or to catch up with things
- think about work when you are not there
- allow staff to call you at home
- cancel days off or annual leave because of work commitments.

If you are allowing any of the above to happen regularly then you are investing too much in your job and not enough in other areas of your life. Take action now. Don't say 'I can't'. It equates with saying 'I choose not to'. Take stock and think about what you can do and what you will do to ensure that you lead a more balanced and fulfilling life rather than putting all your energies into work.

People who suffer from burnout often blame their jobs, but that isn't necessarily the case. It could be because they have invested too much into their jobs and not enough into other aspects of their lives. The first step is to prioritise your workload to fit into 37.5 hours per week (see Ch. 2). The next step is to review what your priorities are outside of work. These could include getting exercise on a regular basis, seeing more of your family, spending evenings out with friends, taking up or renewing an old hobby. Anything is better than nothing. You have to find that balance.

Plan to take some annual leave every three to four months and book it at the beginning of the financial year. Don't save it up; spread it throughout the year to give yourself regular breaks. Avoid the 'if only' way of thinking:

'If only we had more staff . . .'
'If only I could get on top of all this paperwork . . .'
'If only the 'off-duty' didn't take me so long . . .'

Don't prolong getting your life in balance by waiting for all the 'if only's'. You could be waiting a very long time! Don't let life pass you by. Enjoy the journey not just the destination.

You have a huge responsibility and remit to your role but it's certainly not reflected in your salary. You could earn just as much in a far less stressful job. What's more, you could walk into that job tomorrow. You could even join an agency and earn just as much money with far less responsibility. Always remember that. The reason why you are in your job should hopefully be because you gain job satisfaction. If you are not satisfied in your role, take a break. A break serves to allow you to stand back and take a look at your life, think about what you enjoy and what you really want to do. Put yourself first, not your job.

ACTION POINTS

- If you are under too much pressure at work and feeling stressed, identify possible solutions and take action.
- Make sure all members of your staff displaying any signs of stress are managed appropriately.
- If you do not have a mentor, work out what your personal objectives are and choose one. Shadow them first if necessary before asking them.
- Focus on developing the skills of your deputy so they can fully support you in your role, especially in your absence.
- Find out about what is involved in being a union representative or steward and offer the opportunity to one of your staff.
- Get a group of five or six other ward managers together and set up an action learning group to learn from each other.
- Focus on getting to know more influential people within your organisation.
- Focus on learning from your mistakes rather than worrying about them.
- Ensure you have a competent and confident team behind you by encouraging staff to be open and learn from their own and each other's mistakes.
- Look after your health by drinking a minimum of six glasses of water throughout the shift and eating good food regularly.
- Book some annual leave to take every three to four months. Work to live; don't live to work.

References

Bristol Royal Infirmary Inquiry 2001 Learning from Bristol: the report of the public inquiry into children's heart surgery at the Bristol Royal Infirmary 1984–1995. Chapter 25; Competent healthcare professionals. The Stationery Office Ltd, Norwich. Online. Available: http://www.bristol-inquiry.org.uk/final_report/report 24 Sep 2005

Clayden J 2003 Tips for surviving and enjoying the night shift. Whiteria Nursing Journal, 01/01/03. Online. Available: http://www.findarticles.com Search: 'Clayden' 24 Sep 2005

Department of Health 2000 An organisation with a memory. HMSO, London. Online. Available: http://www.dh.gov.uk/assetRoot/04/08/89/48/04088948.pdf 24 Sep 2005

Health and Safety Executive 1999 Management of health and safety work regulations. HMSO, London

Health and Safety Executive 2005a Stress information. Online. Available: http://www.hse.gov.uk/stress 24 Sep 2005

Health and Safety Executive 2005b Tackling stress: the management standards approach. HMSO, London. Online. Available: http://www.hse.gov.uk/stress/standards 24 Sep 2005

Kawamura K, Frost RO 2004 Self-concealment as a mediator in the relationship between perfectionism and psychological distress. Cognitive Therapy and Research 28:183–191

Nursing & Midwifery Council 2004 Standards for the preparation of teachers of nurses, midwives and specialist community public health nurses. NMC, London

Revans R 1983 The ABC of action learning. Chartwell-Bratt, Kent

Robbins A 2001 Notes from a friend. Pocket Books, London

The Tea Council 2005 Tea and antioxidant properties. Online. Available: http://www.teahealth.co.uk 24 Sep 2005

UK Food Standards Agency 2005 Eat well, be well: helping you make healthier choices. Online. Available: http://www.eatwell.gov.uk/healthydiet/nutritionessentials/drinks/drinkingenough 24 Sep 2005

CHAPTER 11

BE A GOOD ROLE MODEL

Be smart   210

Uniform policy   210

Set the standard with your own uniform   210

Personal grooming   211

Make a good first impression   211

Visitors to the ward   212

New members of staff   212

Centre the spotlight on the other person   212

Always smile and be positive   213

Be eternally optimistic   213

Focus on the solution, not the problem   214

Speak clearly   214

Focus on your pronunciation   214

Your telephone manner   215

Stop apologising   215

Be relaxed and in control   216

Keep your cool   216

Manage conflict with confidence   216

Use of empathy   217

Make your writing distinguishable   218

Handwriting   218

Care plans and evaluations   218

Emails   219

Be aware of how others see you   220

Ask people to point out your key strengths and weaknesses   220

Ask people about their work satisfaction   220

Making use of feedback   221

Set an example with your choice of language   222

Never moan or gossip about others   223

Why do people gossip at work?   223

Moaning about work   224

Stop any moaning and whinging   224

Don't stagnate   224

Sharing your learning and experiences   225

Involvement in the wider organisation   225

Involvement in wider professional issues   225

Having others shadow you   226

A good manager sets standards concerning the way their staff and patients should be treated. A major part of your role is to set an example for your staff to follow by showing them:

- how you can cut through bureaucracy to make things happen
- how you expect them to conduct themselves
- how you expect them to treat the patients
- the high standards you expect them to attain at all times.

Behaviour is highly contagious. Few of us have spent time with a friend in a low mood and not felt a lowering of our own mood as a result. The way you behave has a huge effect on how your staff behave. Always bear that in mind.

BE SMART

Where expression of feelings and attitudes are concerned, it has been found that 55% of the impression we make on others is determined by what they see, 38% by what they hear and 7% by the words we use (Mehrabian 1981). In other words, people are very much influenced by how you look and sound a lot more than by what you say.

Appearance counts; there is no doubt about it. Pleasant looking people get on better than those who take less pride in their appearance. Just because you have a set uniform, it does not mean that you do not have to bother with what you look like. The image you present to others at work will be seen as a reflection of your level of confidence and self-esteem. The way you control your posture and use your body language can persuade others that you are more or less confident.

UNIFORM POLICY

Make a point of adhering strictly to your organisation's uniform policy. If you deviate in any way at all, it gives the green light for others in your team to do so. You may think that wearing nail varnish is fine, for example, but if it flouts the uniform policy it is not fine. If you wear nail varnish, you would not be able to reprimand staff for wearing large earrings or not tying up long hair.

Don't blame the system if you have only been given three uniforms and therefore cannot keep them clean. You are the manager; it's up to you to cut through the bureaucracy and get yourself and your team the required seven uniforms each.

SET THE STANDARD WITH YOUR OWN UNIFORM

1. Make sure your uniform is pressed and stain-free (and fits properly).
2. Make sure your shoes are clean and/or polished. Many people consider scruffy shoes to be a bad reflection on the wearer.

3. Remove all extra jewellery. Wearing items such as a wristwatch instead of a fobwatch will give your team members the opportunity to start wearing extra bits of jewellery too. It's unhygienic, unprofessional and a health and safety hazard. Don't encourage it.

4. Ensure that you have an appropriate name badge where your job title is prominent. Use only the title of ward manager, sister or charge nurse. All other titles are not instantly recognisable by the general public (nor often by other health care professionals).

PERSONAL GROOMING

Personal grooming should also be in tip-top condition:

1. Don't neglect your hands and nails. Hibiscrub, alcohol rubs and the constant use of paper towels can play havoc with your skin. Keep a small tube of hand cream in your pocket. Keep your nails short.

2. Keep your hair neat and tied up if long. Your hairstyle can soften or sharpen your image. You will look less confident if you hide behind your hair or have straggly bits hanging over your face. Be wary that very short hair on men can look aggressive.

3. For women, be sparing with make-up. It's advisable to wear some, particularly for older women, as going without make-up can suggest you don't really bother about yourself.

4. If you have to smoke, camouflage the smell when you return to the ward. Use mints and wash your hands. The smell is very distinctive and off-putting for nonsmokers. (Like any strong odour, it can exacerbate nausea in sick patients.)

Be professional at all times. When you are on nonuniform days such as awaydays, meetings or office days, continue to dress smartly. A manager can take no days off from being smart. Your appearance is the most noticeable thing about you.

Some feel that it is unfair to judge people on their appearance but when you meet many people for a few minutes each day (i.e. patients, relatives, senior managers, other health care professionals) they do not have the time to get to know the 'real' you. Like it or not, they will be influenced largely by how you present yourself.

MAKE A GOOD FIRST IMPRESSION

First impressions are powerful and permanent. You never get a second chance to make a good first impression. People form an opinion within the first few seconds of meeting you so it's important to get your image right with all new acquaintances.

VISITORS TO THE WARD

Show your staff the way you would like all visitors greeted. Everyone in your team should take the initiative in making people feel welcome. Don't allow your staff to continue writing at the main desk while visitors wait to speak. Their reticence to address the visitor may be considered as rude and intimidating. It will leave a lasting first impression that will affect all other future contacts with that visitor and your team.

Ensure all your staff wear proper name badges. The enormous array of uniforms and job titles in health care today make it extremely confusing for people to work out who's who and who does what. While they are not a substitute for a personal introduction, they do help visitors recognise instantly who people are.

NEW MEMBERS OF STAFF

Make it your aim to greet all new members to the team. Starting a new job is such a daunting experience. Having someone pointedly come over, introduce themselves, shake your hand and ask how you are is a very welcoming experience and one that is often not forgotten. New pre-registration house officers (PRHOs) become future consultants and GPs. Student nurses may well go on to become future nurse managers that you will liaise with. Those first impressions of being on your ward will stay with them.

CENTRE THE SPOTLIGHT ON THE OTHER PERSON

The key to making a good first impression is to centre the spotlight on the other person. Demonstrate immediately that they are the centre of the conversation. This is particularly pertinent in the case of patients and their relatives. They are not there to hear about you; they want to feel confident that they have your full attention and that you are in control. Think how you would feel as a relative presented with the following greeting: 'Oh hello. We are a bit busy at the moment. I'm afraid that your father's admission was unexpected. We are a little short staffed but I promise I will come over and see you as soon as I can'.

This greeting is focused on the person who is making it and creates the impression that they are not in control of things. If you focus your greeting on the other person, it creates a far better first impression: 'Hello there. Your father has been admitted to bed ten. If you'd like to take a seat in the dayroom, I'll come and explain everything to you in about ten minutes once we've settled him in'.

Visitors do not need to know all about your problems. They need to be reassured that their relatives are in a safe environment and cared for by competent professionals.

The same applies when you are meeting other health professionals:

Focus on self: 'Hello. I'm the ward sister. I've been here for a good few years and know how the place runs like the back of my hand. If you need anything, let me know.'

Focus on other person: 'Hello Dr Smith. You must be the new SHO. How are you settling in?'

Both the above greetings are perfectly acceptable, but the latter example demonstrates that if you focus your greeting on the other person it can help them to feel a lot more comfortable and relaxed. Using the name of a new acquaintance also makes it more personal.

Focus also on listening to what the other person has to say. You'll make a good initial impression if you demonstrate good listening skills. Give positive verbal cues such as 'that's useful to know' or 'what happened next?'. Try not to take over by giving unsolicited advice or relating a similar experience; this only serves to refocus the conversation on to you. Aim to listen to your new acquaintance, not to make them listen to you. It also helps if you maintain steady eye contact. Don't be constantly looking over their shoulder thinking about what you should be doing next. Try not to interrupt by answering the telephone or busying around doing other things.

Giving a good first impression gets you off to the right start and will save a lot of time and effort later on. The benefits far outweigh the inconvenience of dedicating a few minutes of your time.

ALWAYS SMILE AND BE POSITIVE

Your facial expressions affect the mood of your team. If you look gloomy and depressed, it is not only unattractive, it will make others feel gloomy and depressed too. Yet when you smile at someone, they will feel happier in an instant; few people would not smile back. It makes people warm to you.

Always smile even in the face of adversity. However, do make sure it is genuine. People who put on a smile all the time without being genuinely happy can be irritating. If you are not happy and cannot smile, do something positive about it. Being deliberately positive increases the mood in both you and your team. Smile to yourself now and notice how it increases your mood. Smiling makes you feel happier; feeling happier makes you smile!

Be aware that your facial expressions and body language affect the way the people around you feel and the way they work. It ultimately affects the standard of patient care. A positive attitude produces a good working atmosphere. It not only increases morale, it leads to increased performance and job satisfaction. Search for opportunities to invest in each person who works for you. See each interaction with a member of your team as an opportunity to increase their positivity.

BE ETERNALLY OPTIMISTIC

Being consistently optimistic is a prerequisite for great leaders. You do not have to be a born leader to have this attribute; it can be learned. Start thinking positively and tell yourself that things are going to be good today. Act like things are going well and before long you will start believing it.

When people ask you how you are, don't reply 'oh, not so bad really' or 'can't grumble'. When people ask this question, they are usually only being polite and not asking how you really are. Smile and be positive. Use phrases like, 'I'm good' or 'I'm very well indeed. How are you?'. Be continually upbeat. It's infectious.

FOCUS ON THE SOLUTION, NOT THE PROBLEM

Present solutions. There is always something positive in any situation; you just need to draw it out. If you are greeted with a statement such as 'we are three staff down today and there are no agency available; how on earth are we going to cope?', don't let your facial expression fall with a reply like 'oh no, I don't believe it'. Keep smiling, be positive and say something like 'never mind, we'll just have to decide what the priorities are and leave whatever work is nonessential'.

Associate yourself with people who make you feel good. If your manager is one of those people whose glass is always half empty, listen and learn. Experiences with managers like this help you grow. Watch the effect that they are having. You'll learn how negativity breeds negativity. Strive to ensure you do not emulate such habits.

Luckily, the attributes of great leaders can be developed by anyone who is passionate and committed in their work. Start today by being cheerful, smiling and eternally optimistic, no matter what the situation you are in.

SPEAK CLEARLY

Your speaking style conveys more about you than maybe you would wish. People determine your intelligence, education, even your leadership ability by the words you use and by how you say them. The whole reason for speaking is to impart information clearly and effectively. If you tend to speak too softly or mumble, it could result in:

- others not being able to hear or understand you
- being misheard or misunderstood
- giving the impression that you lack confidence
- giving the impression that you don't really have anything interesting to say and are insignificant. As a result, people will quickly forget you.

If you stand upright with confidence, make eye contact and speak clearly, people will assume that you are knowledgeable and have something specific to say which is relevant to them. They will remember you.

FOCUS ON YOUR PRONUNCIATION

The nature of your role means you have to be able to think fast and make quick decisions throughout your shift. For some health workers, this comes out in their speech. It is a natural tendency to talk quickly when pressured or stressed.

Speaking too quickly means that people cannot keep up with you and there is a tendency to 'fall over' your words. The result is that not all of your message will get through. Some find it happens more often towards the end of the shift. Focusing on your pronunciation is a good way of slowing down your speech. People will be more attentive and more likely to understand what you are saying without having to ask you to repeat it or glazing over and stopping bothering to listen.

Concentrate on how you pronounce your words. Some people get into the habit of dropping the 'g's and 't's from the end of their words. This results in words being slurred together and can make you come across as uneducated. Say the following sentences out loud as if you were talking to one of your colleagues at work:

'Are you going to start the ward round in a minute?'
'Do you want to start taking your breaks now?'
'I'll sort out the discharge arrangements if you just take this phone call?'

Did you articulate each syllable and pronounce all the 'g's and 't's? Be aware that not doing so can inhibit you getting your message across clearly.

Filler phrases such as 'you know', 'actually', or lots of 'um's and 'er's also distract people from listening to what you are saying. People will notice these repetitive phrases more than they notice what you are saying. Lazy, sloppy speech indicates a lack of commitment and energy, and even arrogance. It can be construed that you don't care and you can't be bothered. This is not an image you want to portray, nor one you want others to copy.

YOUR TELEPHONE MANNER

The way you answer the telephone speaks volumes about you. Saying something like 'ward ten?' is really not sufficient. 'Ward ten, Sister speaking' is an improvement, but 'ward 10, Sister speaking. How may I help you?' is more warm and welcoming. It also makes you come across as more confident and professional.

Body language is extremely important. The way you stand and the way you speak affects your total image. If you are constantly fidgeting or looking anywhere but at the person you are speaking to, you will appear ill at ease. This affects your telephone manner too. If you are slouched across the desk talking to someone over the phone, you will come across as less controlled than if you sit upright.

STOP APOLOGISING

Be wary about apologising before you speak and if you do tend to do this, try and break the habit unless you have genuinely done something to be sorry about. It can come across like you are apologising for your presence and people are quick to pick up on that. Take the following examples:

'Sorry to bother you, would you mind taking one of our patients to theatre?'
'Sorry. I can see you are busy but Dr Smith has come to see Mrs Jones.'

If you find yourself using phrases such as those outlined above, try using the following alternative approaches:

'We have a patient ready for theatre. Is anyone available?'
'Excuse me interrupting you. Dr Smith is here to see Mrs Jones.'

These things may seem minor, but the way you convey yourself is so important if you want to be taken seriously.

And one last tip: swearing is not appropriate for someone in a managerial role. It is not only unprofessional but some consider that people who swear are of lower intelligence. It is often seen as a sign that someone's vocabulary is inadequate. When used very sparingly, it can have a powerful effect and make people take notice, but when used regularly, it will lower people's opinion of you and sets a bad example.

BE RELAXED AND IN CONTROL

If you are smart, articulate, always smiling and positive in your outlook, you will come across as warm, friendly and confident. In other words, you are creating the impression that you are in control; your work does not control you. Walk upright (no rounded shoulders) and greet people with a good strong handshake. It's an attractive quality; people are drawn to attractiveness.

KEEP YOUR COOL

Never lose your temper. Loss of temper means loss of control. By all means, say how you feel but ensure you remain cool, calm and collected as you do so. There is nothing wrong with saying 'I know you have a job to do, but I find your attitude quite impossible' and walking away if necessary. Don't get into a heated argument. It is unbecoming of a senior manager and will be talked about for years to come by the other party and any onlookers.

MANAGE CONFLICT WITH CONFIDENCE

It helps in times of conflict if you can identify whether you and the other party are adopting a parent, child or adult state. Eric Berne (a psychoanalyst who wrote the best-selling book called 'Games people play') puts forward the theory that people tend to take on the persona of a parent, adult or child depending on what situation they are in (Berne 1968). In times of conflict, try and decipher what role you are playing:

Parent state: Are you nurturing the other person by trying to give advice or protect them by not giving enough responsibility? Are you being critical perhaps by telling them off for breaking the rules?

Child state: Are you feeling insecure and expecting to be told what to do? Are you trying to rebel against 'the rules'?

Adult state: Are you being sensible, calm and logical? Are you able to keep your emotions from interfering with the situation?

According to Berne, there is no 'best' or 'worst' state. Each can be helpful if used in the right situation. Being in adult mode all the time can make for a very boring person. However, having an awareness of what state you and the other person are in can help you manage relationships more effectively.

Situations of conflict can be resolved by concentrating on bringing both parties into 'adult state'. If, for example, you have some members of your team who decide that they can behave how they like with complete disregard about the effects it has on others, you may be tempted to take on the role of the controlling parent. This can exacerbate the situation, whereas if you take on the adult role, which tends to be more unemotional and detached, it could help diffuse the situation and help produce a matching adult state in others.

USE OF EMPATHY

Use of empathy is often a good way of resolving the situation if someone is being difficult. Being empathic means showing that you understand the other person's point of view by using phrases such as 'I understand what you are saying; I get frustrated with the system too sometimes'. Self-disclosure also helps. Tell them how their behaviour makes you feel such as 'your tone is making me feel uncomfortable'.

When you are in a situation of conflict, try and match the other person's parent or child state by empathising with them, then move them into more of an adult state by suggesting a joint solution. Using 'we' rather that 'you' or 'I' also helps in diffusing heated situations. This is illustrated in the following example:

Manager: 'I'm not happy about the way you run the ward. You should not allow staff to be drinking coffee at the main reception desk.' *(Angry critical parent mode.)*

Sister: 'I can understand why you think like that. I feel the same myself at times.' *(Use of empathy and self-disclosure.)* 'The problem is when we are short staffed, the staff are unable to leave the ward for their breaks. Perhaps we could come up with an alternative solution?' *(Sensible adult mode, suggesting joint solution.)*

Whatever you do, always keep your cool. Working in health care, we are all subject to chronic staff shortages, bed pressures, poor resources and relentless government targets. No wonder working relationships are constantly put under strain. Some would say that conflict is inevitable, but if you keep your cool it does not have to be. Further tips that may help in times of adversity include:

1. Always manage difficult people face-to-face. Leaving voicemail, email, fax, notes, etc. will only serve to increase their animosity.

2. Control your own emotions; do not get angry and shout back. If you feel threatened or intimidated, say that you will leave and come back later when you have both calmed down. Put some time and distance between the two of you until you have calmed down. Never walk out in a huff.
3. Notice those in your team who are not being difficult, those who work hard and without complaint. Reward them. Just a simple thank you may be all that is needed. Don't allow the difficult ones to claim most of your attention.

MAKE YOUR WRITING DISTINGUISHABLE

How you write is very important. You will be judged not only on what you write but also on how your writing looks. If your staff see that you write scruffily on patient documentation, they will not bother to be neat and tidy either. If you don't bother to refer to the care plan when writing your evaluations, your staff will not bother either. You set the standard in everything you do, so don't let your writing let you down.

HANDWRITING

Using a distinctive pen, a black fountain pen, for example, will show out on documentation. Take the time to ensure that everything you write is:

- neat and legible
- large and noticeable
- joined up with complete rounded letters
- consistent.

Make sure that your staff notice your handwriting. When they recognise it, they will notice the content. Your aim is for them see your high standards of documentation.

In law, the clinical record portrays the standard of care. You should role model a high standard of care at all times. Remember that patients' records are also reviewed by an array of health professionals – anaesthetists, surgeons, physiotherapists, complaints managers and even solicitors. They will all judge the standard of care based on the standard of your records.

CARE PLANS AND EVALUATIONS

Unfortunately, the task of writing care plans and evaluations is still often relegated to the end of the shift. This is a time when people are tired and rushing to get everything done so that they can get off home. It's not the best time to write such an important document. Demonstrate to your staff that they can make entries throughout the shift. Each time you complete an episode of care or if there is a change in the patient's condition, write an entry in the evaluation section (in your distinguishable writing). Obviously it is not possible for you to do this each and every time but try and get into the habit of writing your evaluations and any care plan updates throughout the shift rather than saving them all until the end. Make a particular point of doing this when you have a member of staff or student to shadow you for a shift.

EMAILS

Emails are another area where it is wise to role model how you would like others to email you. People will also judge your intellect through the way you write your emails. As a general rule:

1. Go through your emails on a daily basis. Answer them quickly, preferably within 24 hours.
2. Keep all emails short; never more than one screenfull or three paragraphs.
3. Always make the best use of the subject heading such as 'Re: Impending staffing shortage across medical unit next week' or 'Benchmarking meeting on Monday cancelled'. Subject headings like these means your emails are more likely to be opened and noted.
4. Make your emails easier to read by writing the most important information in the first paragraph and the background/supporting information in the rest of the email. If you need to send more than one screen of information, send it as an attachment.
5. Never use your work email account for private or personal emails. All your emails should come as no surprise if another member of your team gains access to them. It is good development for a deputy or someone who is shadowing you for the day to go through your emails with you. It helps them to gain an excellent insight into your role and responsibilities.
6. Bear in mind that no email is confidential. If you wish to send a message that is confidential or controversial in any way, use the phone or use face-to-face contact.
7. Don't send blind copies (bc) casually. They imply that you are going behind someone's back.
8. Don't ask for a receipt unless absolutely necessary. It implies that you do not trust the recipient to read or respond promptly to your emails.
9. Use the urgent icon sparingly. If not, future really urgent emails will be ignored.
10. Don't use CAPITAL LETTERS. In email language, this is construed as SHOUTING!
11. Never send jokes via email. If you receive them just delete; do not forward them.
12. Always use a positive tone and be aware that the tone of emails can be misconstrued.
13. Never leave your computer unattended. You don't want your staff or any others sending emails to people in your name.

Everything you write, whether by hand or computer, speaks volumes about you. Make sure you are conveying the right image and encourage others to have the same high standards.

BE AWARE OF HOW OTHERS SEE YOU

To be a good role model, you have to know yourself. Hopefully you know your strengths and weaknesses from your own point of view, but are you sure that others see you in the same light as you see yourself? How realistic is your image of yourself?

You may, for example, see one of your strengths as being assertive and getting things done, but others may regard you as aggressive and loud and as a result may shy away from you. You may feel that you are weak at organising your team, whereas your team may see it as a strength that you allow your team to organise their own work and make their own decisions.

ASK PEOPLE TO POINT OUT YOUR KEY STRENGTHS AND WEAKNESSES

A simple way to find out what others think of you is to ask. Ask each of your peers, members of your team and your line manager to write down what they think your three key strengths are and identify one area that could be improved. This can be quite a humbling exercise and some would have difficulty asking their colleagues what they think about them.

ASK PEOPLE ABOUT THEIR WORK SATISFACTION

Another way to find out how you are perceived is to ask people about your leadership skills but to put it to your team in a way that makes it seem like you are asking about their work. One way to do this would be to devise a questionnaire based on leadership behaviours. Kouzes & Posner (2002) outlined five behaviours of a good leader:

1. Challenging the process.
2. Inspiring a shared vision.
3. Encouraging the heart.
4. Enabling others to act.
5. Modelling the way.

Think of some questions that would enable you to find out how your behaviour affects your team. Here are some examples.

Challenging the process

'Do you feel we should spend more time and effort on finding different ways of doing things at work?'

'Do you feel that the work of the team could be improved if we looked outside the organisation for more ideas?'

'Do you feel we take the time to learn from our mistakes?'

Inspiring a shared vision

'Do you feel that you are fully aware and involved with what's going on in the ward?'

'Are you excited about working in this ward over the coming year?'

'Do you feel enthusiastic about the future of the ward?'

Encouraging the heart

'Do you feel your work is valued within the team?'

'Do you feel that your work is noticed and appreciated?'

'Are you usually thanked when a job has been done well?'

Enabling others to act

'Do you feel your views are listened to seriously?'

'Do you feel that you have sufficient opportunities to learn new skills in your role?'

'Do you feel that you have enough autonomy in deciding how to go about your work?'

Modelling the way

'Are you comfortable with what the expectations are of you in your job?'

'Do you feel that the team have a good plan with achievable goals about where you are all going?'

'Do you feel well led as a team?'

Make it simple. Don't get them to start grading the answers. You do not have time to collate lots of different answers. Ask members of your team to answer a simple yes or no to each of the questions. The sections that have two or more 'no' answers suggest that you could perhaps improve in that particular behaviour. This is a less threatening way of achieving personal feedback than if you were to ask individuals to identify your strengths and weaknesses.

MAKING USE OF FEEDBACK

If, for example, you have consistent 'no' answers in the section for 'Encouraging the heart', perhaps you need to work on your feedback skills (see p. 51). If you received consistent 'no' answers in the section for 'Inspiring a shared vision', you may want to look at establishing shared goals for your team (see p. 48) and perhaps shadowing someone senior within your organisation for a time to pick up on the skills required to inspire a team.

Make sure you get feedback from as many team members as you can. Don't just pick the 'nice' ones. You may get a biased view or they may complete it in a certain way to try and please you. Try and get the views from a good cross section of staff within your team. Once you get more confidence, asking individuals what they think your strengths and weaknesses are will give you more specific and individual feedback with which you can work on. To be a good leader it is advisable to be aware of what others think of you.

SET AN EXAMPLE WITH YOUR CHOICE OF LANGUAGE

Don't let negative people set the tone. There is always at least one person in a team who will consistently use language such as:

'We can't do that.'
'They'll never allow us to do that.'
'We've tried it all before, it won't work.'
'We've got enough to do.'
'We haven't got enough staff.'
'They don't know what it's like for us.'
'There's nothing we can do.'

These people have the attitude that someone else is always in control. They are not choosing what they do; other people rule their lives. They have a tendency to absolve responsibility for any choices they make.

Think about the language you use:

'I have to go to the sisters' meeting this afternoon.'
'We have to do it this way because . . .'
'I've tried but it makes no difference.'
'If only we could recruit one more member of staff.'

Using language like this will give the impression you are not in control. Not only that; others will adopt this negative tone. Blaming outside forces for your situation makes you a victim and is hardly the quality required of a leader. Think carefully about the language you use. Make sure others see you as someone who is in control of the situation. Do you have to go to that meeting or do you choose to go? Surely no one is standing there with a gun to your head making you attend that meeting.

Managers will often use negative phrases to cover up their guilt at leaving staff extra work in their absence. Instead, just explain why you have chosen to go to the meeting: 'I shall be leaving you this afternoon for a couple of hours to attend a meeting about the future changes within the directorate'. This is just as acceptable but shows that you are in charge of what you are doing.

Use positive language such as:

'What is the alternative?'
'I will . . .'
'I choose to . . .'
'I prefer to . . .'
'I shall . . .'
'OK, so that didn't work, what shall we try instead?'
'I have decided to . . .'
'I am going to . . .'

It's all in the mind. If you think you are powerless, you will be powerless and others will see you as such. You will start producing every excuse you can to justify why you have to do something or why you cannot do something. It becomes a self-fulfilling prophecy. Change your way of thinking and you change your way of seeing things and the way others see you.

NEVER MOAN OR GOSSIP ABOUT OTHERS

Keep your opinions to yourself. Don't allow yourself to get pulled into a situation where a group of staff sit around talking about individuals who are not present to defend themselves. Retrain yourself to look for the good in each person and in each situation. Change the conversation around by pointing out the positive things about the individual or change the subject completely. If you gossip, your staff will gossip. As their role model, think about what behaviour you are portraying to them.

Moaning and gossiping about others is contagious and achieves nothing. Once one person starts whinging, others join in and it creates an overall negative atmosphere. Your job is to maintain a continual positive atmosphere. In addition to this, if you do moan and whinge about others, your staff may well think 'if they say this about others, what do they say about me when my back is turned?'.

People are wary when in the company of gossips and will not talk freely. As a manager, you need to be seen as someone that people can be open and honest with. Being heard gossiping will only hinder you. Never let your guard down, even on ward nights out. Socialising with your staff is part of your role but be careful. Don't get involved in negative conversations about other people at work.

WHY DO PEOPLE GOSSIP AT WORK?

People who spend a lot of time gossiping at work are usually either bored with their jobs or haven't got enough work to do. If it is happening on your ward, perhaps you need to look at how their work is being organised. Staff who spend their time completing a set list of tasks (e.g. washes by 11:00, observations at 12:00) find their work neither challenging nor inspiring. Make sure your staff are not delegating tasks like this to their juniors. Show them how they can empower staff to take on responsibility for the whole patient rather than just tasks. If you encourage your senior staff to take on more responsibilities, they should hopefully take note and encourage their juniors in the same way.

MOANING ABOUT WORK

If you find yourself moaning about work, make yourself think of a solution to the issue instead. If there isn't one, then stop moaning; it only serves to waste time. If there is a solution, put your efforts into solving the issue instead of wasting your valuable time moaning about it. People tend to moan or procrastinate when faced with:

● a large workload
● unrealistic time commitments
● too many interruptions
● work requiring skills they do not have.

If this is happening to your team regularly, perhaps you need to take a step back and look at what you and your team can do to control your workload rather than allowing it to control you (see Ch. 2).

STOP ANY MOANING AND WHINGING

If you are one of those people whose glass is more half empty than half full, try and make a conscious effort to look on the bright side. People are much more likely to warm to you if you're talking positively rather than negatively. Get into the habit of it and you'll not only give yourself a lift, but others too.

Make the staff room a nice place to be in by adding things that lift people's spirits. Put photos on the wall from ward nights out. Ensure there are nice mugs for tea rather than drab paper cups. Make sure there is always a plentiful supply of coffee, tea, sugar and milk. Perhaps even get the staff to add an extra £1 to the kitty and when things are particularly challenging, buy some cream cakes for the team. These may seem small gestures but together they will help to prevent a climate of moaning and gossiping and general dissatisfaction.

DON'T STAGNATE

Demonstrate a personal commitment to improving yourself and others by showing that you are continually willing to learn and develop professionally. Methods you can use to role model that commitment are through:

● sharing your learning and experiences
● involvement in the wider organisation
● involvement in wider professional issues
● having others shadow you.

SHARING YOUR LEARNING AND EXPERIENCES

If you personally attend any courses, teaching sessions or conferences, make a point of sharing what you have learned with the rest of your team. If you have a patient with a condition rarely seen by the team, find out about it and share the knowledge with your team. Don't just encourage others to do this. Show them the way and how it should be done. Your staff will be more willing to share what they have learned with the team if they observe you doing it all the time.

Always practice what you preach. Most nurses remember being told to share their learning as a student or junior staff nurse. It can cause a lot of unnecessary anxiety for them if they are the only ones required to do this. If you and your senior staff put on sessions regularly where you share your learning, it will become common practice and junior staff will be more willing to take part.

INVOLVEMENT IN THE WIDER ORGANISATION

Becoming involved in hospital committees not only widens your networks, it can help your staff to broaden their horizons too. Take one of them along with you to the meetings every now and then to introduce them to the higher 'workings' of the organisation. Show them just how important your meetings are and how they influence clinical practice.

Demonstrating to your staff how influential you are at a higher level gives them an insight as to how influential they can be in their future careers. Give them firsthand knowledge of any decisions made and how and why they will affect future practice. Seeing you have wider influence will increase their respect in your skills and abilities too.

INVOLVEMENT IN WIDER PROFESSIONAL ISSUES

Make sure you are a member or are involved in the professional association linked with your role. If you do not have a specialist association, try other professional bodies. The Royal College of Nursing (RCN) holds various management and leadership forums with which you could become involved. Another option is to join a community group or a group run by one of your local primary care trusts (PCTs).

Don't become involved in any more than two groups. It would not be appropriate to allow outside commitments to interfere with your day-to-day managerial responsibilities. Make sure also that this commitment is in your work time and recognised as a core responsibility. Some nurses regard work for hospital-wide or professional associations as an extra task that should be done in their own time. That could not be further from the truth. You are furthering the knowledge and expertise of your team. If you elect to do this in your own time you are conveying the message to your team that you expect them to do that too.

HAVING OTHERS SHADOW YOU

Encourage members of your staff (registered and unregistered) to shadow you regularly, at least once per month. Having someone to shadow you keeps you on your toes. They will ask questions and make you think about the way you work. Having to explain why you make decisions makes you think again about why you do things. It's hard work and can be quite challenging but is an enormous benefit to your learning. You can also learn new ideas from those that shadow you. They will be fresh with ideas from other wards where they have worked or new techniques and knowledge from various courses or study they have undertaken.

Never think you know everything. No matter how long you have been in your job or specialty, there is always more to learn. It is advisable to adopt this attitude at all times. If you still have lots to learn, then your staff will too. If you allow yourself to stagnate, your staff will follow suit.

ACTION POINTS

- Check your uniform policy and make sure you strictly adhere to it as an example to others.
- Make a point of warmly greeting all visitors to your ward and focus the conversation on them.
- Start smiling more and focusing on the positive aspects in all situations.
- Speak slowly, clearly and focus on pronouncing your 'g's and 't's particularly if you have a tendency to talk quickly.
- In times of conflict, try and identify what state you and the other person are in – parent, child or adult. Use empathy and self-disclosure to bring both into an adult state.
- Buy a pen that will distinguish your writing from others and ensure that everything you write is neat and legible with large, rounded letters.
- Think of ways you can get feedback from your team (in a nonthreatening manner) to identify areas you can improve upon.
- Stop yourself each time you say 'I can't' or 'I have to' and change it to 'I will' or 'I choose to'.
- If you have a tendency to gossip or moan about things at work, think about why you do this and what you can do to stop this habit.
- Consider ways in which you can demonstrate to others that you are continually learning by sharing your experiences.

References

Berne E 1968 Games people play. Penguin, London

Kouzes J, Posner B 2002 The leadership challenge, 3rd edn. Jossey Bass, San Francisco

Mehrabian A 1981 Silent messages: implicit communication of emotions and attitudes, 2nd edn. Wadsworth, California

CHAPTER 12

MANAGE YOUR MANAGER

Clarify expectations   228
Be clear about what you expect from your manager   228
Be clear about what your manager expects from you   229

Work with, not against, your manager   230
Meet regularly   230
Remain loyal   230
Put a stop to any interference in clinical issues   230
Assist in decision making   231
What if your manager is always too busy?   231

Act, if an important decision has been made without your consultation   231
Take immediate action   232
Prevent it happening again   232
Organisation-wide decisions   232
Is it bullying?   233

Act, if a change in another department has a knock-on effect in yours   233
Coping is not taking action   234

Don't be pressurised into taking on extra work without funding   235
Emergency situations   235
Nonemergency situations   235
Opening up extra beds   236

Project work   236
Work with your manager   237
If you are doing extra work without funding, take action   237
Keep the communication channels open   238
Why some managers 'micromanage'   238
Keep in constant contact   239
Give feedback   239
Write good and timely reports   239
Stage 1: Write a basic outline   240
Stage 2: The introduction   240
Stage 3: Background description   240
Stage 4: Results/implementation   240
Stage 5: Conclusion   241
Stage 6: Recommendations   241
Actively manage incidents, mistakes and accidents   241
Serious untoward incidents   242
Know how to conduct a good investigation   243
Make a provisional plan of action   243
Review all the documentary evidence   244
Interviews   244
Prepare a written report   245

A very important, but much neglected, part of being a good manager is building up a good working relationship with your own manager. This may not seem your foremost concern because you are focusing so much on building your own team. But if you make time for your manager, you will ensure that you:

● are involved in important decision making that affects your team
● have greater access to appropriate help to achieve your team's goals
● gain their respect and be taken seriously
● learn from their experiences (including their mistakes)
● keep well informed
● have more freedom and authority to act.

If you do not put time and effort into managing your manager, you will become low on their priority list. This means you could end up having any concerns you raise falling on deaf ears. You may find that they forget to give you information which your colleagues already know. They may not be interested in listening to you. You could even find that you end up arguing regularly and get labelled as the 'difficult' one.

Having a poor relationship with your manager does you no favours at all. It will hinder your progress. It doesn't matter whether you like them or not, they have access to knowledge and information that you don't. You should find the right ways of working with them to help achieve your goals.

CLARIFY EXPECTATIONS

Problems tend to arise if there is a lack of clarity about your tasks and responsibilities.

BE CLEAR ABOUT WHAT YOU EXPECT FROM YOUR MANAGER

You do not have to become great friends with your manager, but you must understand their role and the demands placed on them. If you know what the organisation expects from your manager, then you will understand more readily why they work the way they do, why they make the decisions they do and perhaps why you disagree about some things.

Your manager may have a different leadership style to you. They may not be as transformational as you. They may be used to giving out orders, rewarding those who do well and punishing those who don't do so well. This may not sit well with you. If that is the case, then say so. Be clear about your expectations in that you want to be involved, not just informed. Ask them for regular feedback, both positive and negative, so that you can continuously improve in your work, rather than wait for your appraisal to find out how you are progressing.

Make sure you get your appraisal each year. Don't wait for your manager to initiate the process. Write down what you want to discuss:

1. The objectives you feel are the priorities for your ward.
2. Your personal development needs in order to achieve those objectives.

Forward this information to your manager in preparation for your appraisal. Take control of the process, as you would hope your own staff would do for you. If the meeting is cancelled more than twice, point out what is happening and how it makes you feel. Unfortunately, there are still some senior managers who will regularly cancel appraisals with their staff (usually because they are disorganised) without realising the damage it can cause to staff morale.

You need to understand what your manager's own objectives are too. A good manager will ensure that your objectives reflect their own. In that way, you will know that you are both heading in the same direction. It would be detrimental if your objectives were totally different from your manager's own objectives. That would only serve to create tension in your working relationship, not to mention the effect on practice.

Remember that your manager is only human. Sometimes people are labelled as 'poor' managers because they do not conform to our expectations. Your manager may have become out of touch clinically, for example, but they may be particularly good at helping you to write complaint letters or getting more resources for your ward. Make sure you get the most from what they do well and try not to focus on their weaknesses.

BE CLEAR ABOUT WHAT YOUR MANAGER EXPECTS FROM YOU

Your manager will probably have run a ward or department before taking promotion. Problems sometimes occur when they expect you to run your ward in the same way that they did. The only way you can ensure that you have full control without interference is to keep your manager fully informed about what you are doing. Let them see what you are doing well. Be clear about the skills you have and those you want to improve upon. Your manager needs to believe in your abilities before they will trust you.

If your manager does not communicate their expectations clearly, then it is your responsibility to to ask them what they need or want from you. Your manager may not have good management or support from their own manager; this may affect their own ability to manage you. You need to appreciate their position and accept that perhaps they need prompting to articulate their expectations. Make sure you have what your manager expects in terms of organisational objectives written down clearly during your appraisal. Always refer to these in anything that you do. If your manager comes to you with further projects, ask yourself if it relates to your original objectives. If it does not, question your manager's expectations. Are they perhaps too high?

Don't get into the habit of propping up a failing or struggling manager. Encourage them to get help and support from elsewhere. You cannot provide your manager with the same support that you give your team. It is not fair on you and you must let them know that.

WORK WITH, NOT AGAINST, YOUR MANAGER

Just because someone is your manager it does not mean that they are perfect and know everything. Like you they will also be learning from their experiences and mistakes. Treat them as you would your staff. Don't focus on their weaknesses; nobody is perfect. Focus on their strengths; they would not be in the job if they didn't do something right.

MEET REGULARLY

Have regular review meetings, every two to three months, where you review your objectives. Take the intiative and set up these meetings if your manager does not already do so. The constant changes in health care, including government targets, may result in a need to change your priorities. Make sure any changes to priorities are discussed and objectives changed and agreed accordingly. Without keeping a check on them throughout the year, you could find you are going in a different direction to your manager.

REMAIN LOYAL

If you do not like the way your manager works, do something about it. Don't complain to others about their way of working. Tell your manager how you feel and suggest ways of changing their behaviour or approach. You must be seen to be working on the side of your manager at all times. Disloyal people can never be trusted by both their managers and employees alike. A reputation for disloyalty can be hard to dispel.

PUT A STOP TO ANY INTERFERENCE IN CLINICAL ISSUES

If you feel your manager is interfering too much in clinical issues, it can indicate that they do not have enough confidence in your abilities. You need to ask yourself why. Are you showing them what a good job you do or are you leaving it up to them to find out? Managers do not have time to constantly observe their employees. Take the initiative; keep them abreast of what you do well and any achievements regularly. They will appreciate more of what you do, rather than what you don't do.

Some managers are unable to let go of the clinical side if they have been promoted internally. Sometimes this means they do not have confidence in their more senior role and are taking refuge in what they do know. The key in this situation is to give consistent positive feedback in what they are doing well at in their managerial role. Then intersperse this with small amounts of feedback about how their additional involvement on the clinical side is affecting you and your team in a nonproductive way.

ASSIST IN DECISION MAKING

Some managers find it difficult to decide what to do when confronted with any situation that arises outside the norm. The best thing you can do in this situation is to help them by outlining the possible solutions, making it clear to them which one you feel is the most suited at that time. You may need to follow this up with clear directions on the steps that need to be taken. Remember to always support them in any decision they make including the 'fall-out' should it be the wrong decision. Nobody ever wants to hear the phrase 'I told you so' or 'it was the manager's decision, not mine'.

WHAT IF YOUR MANAGER IS ALWAYS TOO BUSY?

Being permanently busy does not mean that more work is getting done. It means the person is not in control of their workload. If your manager is busy and not in control, it will affect your work too. Meeting with your manager to confirm what you have defined as your workload (as outlined in Ch. 2) may help them to see that it would be a good idea for them to do the same exercise.

Every time your manager comes to you saying 'we have to do this . . .' ask two important questions:

1. 'Do we have to do this, or do we choose to do this?' (if you do not choose to do it, you are not in control).
2. 'If we choose not to do this, what will the consequences be?'

If you do choose to do the extra task, identify the time and resources it will take, then decide which of your current tasks you will discontinue in order to make time for the new more important task.

ACT, IF AN IMPORTANT DECISION HAS BEEN MADE WITHOUT YOUR CONSULTATION

If any important changes need to be made at work, everyone should be consulted. You should be given the chance to say what you think and your manager should genuinely listen, consider and respond to your views.

TAKE IMMEDIATE ACTION

Don't always blame others if you were left out; you have to shoulder some of the responsibility. Ask yourself why your manager did not include you. Don't get angry, don't procrastinate and don't bottle it up. Go and speak to your manager before you speak to anyone else. Remain calm and ask them why you were not consulted. They may have simply forgotten.

If you have views or alternative solutions, then let them know. If you feel there will be serious consequences which may not have been considered, make these very clear. Follow up your discussion with an email confirming what you discussed. Address the email to any others involved in the decision-making process, so that they may also consider your views. Consider your wording very carefully. You must not, under any circumstances, give the impression that you are being disloyal to your manager. Ultimately you may not be able to change the decision made, but you have a right for your views to be considered.

PREVENT IT HAPPENING AGAIN

Treat this as a learning experience, and take action to reduce the risk of it ever happening again. If you find that your manager genuinely forgot to include you or did not realise the importance of involving you, then it is clear that you have not been making enough effort to communicate with them on a regular basis. Make sure you do so in future.

Don't just contact your manager when you have a problem or when they call a meeting. Make the effort to see your line manager regularly. Meet with them at least once a week to update them on current issues. Keep them informed of everything you are doing. It is also important to keep them up-to-date with any projects or work that they have delegated to you.

Nurses are generally not good at promoting themselves, but if you do not promote your knowledge and abilities, how else are they going to know? It is not sufficient to say that's their job to find out. It's also your job to let them know and get yourself involved in activities, meetings and projects in which your knowledge and expertise are required.

ORGANISATION-WIDE DECISIONS

If senior management (i.e the chief executive or board of directors) within your organisation make a decision which affects you and you were not consulted, you do have the right to make a written request for information and consultation, under the 'Information and consultation of employees regulations' (Department of Trade and Industry 2004). However, 10% of the rest of the workforce must also want this information. These rules came into effect in April 2005. To make use of this or any legislation, you should always consult with human resources (HR) and your union representative in the first instance.

IS IT BULLYING?

If you feel you are doing everything you can to improve communications with your manager but feel that you are being deliberately left out of decision making, this could be construed as bullying. It is advisable in this situation that you keep file notes. Record all incidents where you have not been consulted and note all actions you have taken to try to improve the situation.

Try and speak to your manager first. Tell them how their actions are making you feel. Discuss your concerns with them and agree actions to be taken in the future. If your manager refuses to change or even to listen to you, seek further advice from a senior HR manager. They will guide you through the process outlined in your local policy for bullying and harassment. They will also provide you with support and access to counselling if required.

ACT, IF A CHANGE IN ANOTHER DEPARTMENT HAS A KNOCK-ON EFFECT IN YOURS

Health care is continually changing to meet changing demands and targets. We barely have a chance to settle down after one move, merger or restructuring of services when the next change is being announced. Decisions are often having to be made quickly, and sometimes they are not properly thought through. Certain aspects may be overlooked, particularly the effects on other neighbouring departments.

Mistakes happen. Don't put up with the consequences and just make the best of things. A common example is disruption through building work. The facilities department may be doing building work nearby and you find the noise is intolerable for patients returning from theatre who need optimum rest to recover. Don't just moan about the system and accept it. Nurses are so good at coping with severe disruptions that often they will think nothing of it. But you must not continue to cope if it is affecting the patients. You are their advocate and it is your duty to ensure that patients do not suffer unduly. Waking up from surgery to the sound of very loud drilling and banging is not conducive to a good recovery.

Getting on the phone and shouting at a member of the facilities department will have little effect. You will be a lone voice from one small insignificant department and easily overruled by others. Gather your information or data first. Find out:

- who else is affected?
- are they suffering in silence too?
- what has anyone else tried to do about it?
- who is the senior person in charge of the project?
- was your line manager(s) involved or consulted?

It is sometimes the case where a ward manager's line manager was consulted and gave their permission for the works to go ahead but forgot to inform everyone concerned or did not realise the impact of their decision on the wards. If this is the case, contacting the manager of the facilities department first is not appropriate. Your manager should be the first port of call.

Don't be tempted to complain to your line manager and expect them to resolve the issue (even if they are partly to blame). That is commonly known as 'passing the buck' and is not appropriate. State the problem and work together on possible solutions. It's your ward and your patients, so work together with your line manager to solve the issue. Present your case to the appropriate manager of the building works project, preferably face-to-face, and follow up your discussion and agreed actions with an email. Keep your line manager informed and involved at each stage in the process.

Remember to always keep records; an email will suffice as a good record. Suggest solutions once you have all the facts. These could include: cancelling surgery, closing beds, transferring very sick and vulnerable patients to another ward temporarily. Work with the facilities manager and your own line manager in finding suitable solutions. Don't focus on the fact that you were not consulted in the planning process.

COPING IS NOT TAKING ACTION

Another example concerns bed management decisions. Whilst I was working as a senior sister on a cardiothoracic surgical ward with a team of cardiothoracic trained nurses many years ago, the general manager announced that three of the beds in the high dependency unit (HDU) area were to be designated for major maxillofacial surgical cases. I was given one week's notice. I told my line manager how angry I was, then just got on and coped with the change.

In hindsight, I should have found out all the facts, made a full risk assessment and put my concerns down in writing to both my line manager and general manager; I did none of this. I did not lead my team, I coped with the decision and expected my staff to do the same. The maxillofacial patients did not receive the high standard of care they should have received. I thought I was acting as a good manager and patients' advocate by setting up a good liaison with the ward sister and team from the maxillofacial surgical ward, accessing study days and teaching sessions for the staff and ensuring the staff always had access to specialist advice when needed.

My actions ensured that we coped well with the decision. However, I would have managed the situation far better if I had:

- made a full risk assessment including getting my team to identify all the potential issues and problems
- made an appointment to discuss the issue with my line manager, general manager and the bed manager together, and agreed alternative solutions for the benefit of the patients. This could have included delaying the start date to ensure

staff were appropriately trained through secondments to other wards and specialist courses
● documented the outcomes of the discussion and circulated them to appropriate personnel.

If you find that someone makes a decision that has huge 'knock-on' effects in your department without consulting you, take appropriate action. Coping is not taking action.

DON'T BE PRESSURISED INTO TAKING ON EXTRA WORK WITHOUT FUNDING

Being pressured to take on extra work is a common problem within health care. Because patient care could be compromised, health care professionals often feel they have no choice but to take on the extra work. Unfortunately, nurses are sometimes too willing to work double shifts, stay on in their own time and take work home so that patients will not suffer. It is not a fair situation. Some managers will pressurise you into taking on extra work; others will take on the extra work and expect you to follow suit. You must not be cajoled into accepting more and more work without appropriate funding.

EMERGENCY SITUATIONS

In emergency situations, you have no choice. If you have to take a number of patients who require additional care and need to book extra agency staff, then so be it. But make it clear in such situations that you do not have the funds within your budget to deal with these extra demands. Work out, with the help of your finance advisor, roughly what the cost will be and inform your line manager. Make sure your discussion is documented and a copy sent to your line manager and whoever else is involved in making the decision: that includes members of your hospital board if necessary.

NONEMERGENCY SITUATIONS

If you are asked or 'told' to take on extra work without extra funding, arrange a meeting with both your line manager and finance advisor to clarify and agree how much the extra work will cost. Do this even if your manager has told you not to worry about it and that they will 'sort it'. These situations rarely get 'sorted'. You need to make sure that everyone is clear about how much you will be over-spent at the end of year as a result.

If your line manager informs you that they will or have accessed funding from elsewhere for the extra work, get this in writing first. It does not have to be formal; an email will suffice.

OPENING UP EXTRA BEDS

If you open up extra beds, make sure you have the appropriate staff to provide an acceptable level of patient care. Don't try and cope with your existing staffing establishment. If you do, you are indicating that you do not need extra staff for those beds. How can you prove that this work needs extra funding when you have coped to date without it? It is not unknown for some ward managers, who were asked to open up some extra beds temporarily to deal with a short-term problem, to find themselves a few years down the line with those beds having remained open but with the original funded staffing establishment. Don't let it happen to you.

PROJECT WORK

If you are asked to take on a piece of work on behalf of the directorate or the organisation, such as an audit, clarify how much time and resources it will take (remember that staff time is a resource). If you are required to undertake the work personally, identify and agree with your manager which aspect of your existing workload you will not do, in order to make time to do this extra work. Even a simple piece of work such as writing a report could take a good few hours or days depending on the subject.

If your staff are required to do extra work such as link nurse roles or attending organisation-wide working groups, calculate how many hours' work will be required and work out how much that will cost you in terms of agency cover. Don't expect staff to take the work home or find time during their shift to undertake extra work (unless your staffing levels are regularly above the minimum safe levels per shift).

If your staff need to take on a new link nurse role, for example, work out how much time they will need to fulfil the role. A link nurse role could include:

- a two hour meeting each month
- follow-up actions from each meeting
- keeping the ward team informed and up-to-date on the subject
- teaching sessions.

The above tasks may require the equivalent of a whole day's worth of work per month. How much will this cost in terms of agency cover? Even if you find the link nurse stays on for a short time after each shift to fulfil the duties required and accrues time owed, the time they eventually take will come out of your budget. It costs money to cover a shift or half a shift when the nurse actually takes her time back. There is no allowance to cover time owed within your funded establishment (see Ch. 6).

WORK WITH YOUR MANAGER

If you regularly say yes to more work, your manager will assume you have the time and the resources to do it. Some managers do not realise the impact their decisions make in terms of extra funding and workload. It's up to you to work with them and keep them informed.

On the other hand, do not refuse point blank to do work because you have no funding. Just make sure that you:

● clarify the cost and implications of the extra work
● discuss alternative solutions
● agree terms and conditions in writing with your line manager (together with their line manager if appropriate).

IF YOU ARE DOING EXTRA WORK WITHOUT FUNDING, TAKE ACTION

If you have taken on extra work with the promise of funding that somehow never arrived, you will more than likely be over-spent on your budget. Your priority now is to make sure that you are not labelled as the ward manager who is unable to manage their budget. Work out exactly how much the extra work is costing you in terms of staff time and supplies. Do this together with your finance advisor. Continually remind your manager(s) of the sum of money over and above your budget that you are spending on this extra work.

If you are working within your budget, then you have proved that you do not need extra staff and resources in order to have these extra beds. No manager will ask for extra money in the yearly business planning process for a team that is completing the required work within their given budget.

If you are expected to continue with the extra work without extra funding, you have two choices:

1. Get it in writing that your manager agrees you may go over budget by a set amount in order to deliver the extra work or staff the extra beds.
2. Work out with your team which aspects of work need to be sacrificed in order to keep within budget. Agree your actions in writing with your manager. If your manager does not agree, you must come up with alternative actions.

If you do not do either of the above, you are effectively sanctioning the compromising of health and safety standards on your ward. You are allowing your staff to cope with increased workloads and paving the way for mistakes to be made. You are taking the responsibility for the consequences of someone else's decision. Beware of being made a scapegoat.

KEEP THE COMMUNICATION CHANNELS OPEN

Do not wait until you are asked about what is going on in your ward; keep your manager informed. If your line manager's office is in a different building or even on a different site, do not use this as an excuse. Use email to keep your manager up-to-date with events. It's up to you to build up the relationship to ensure you have the right support and contacts for the good of your ward and your team. If your department is cut off from the rest of the directorate or overall organisation, you have only yourself to blame. You need to be proactive and do something about it. Blaming others for your predicament is a reactive approach and indicative of poor leadership.

Even if your line manager shows little interest in your ward or department, make sure you still keep regular contact and let them know what is happening. Leave out details that are not their concern, e.g. dealing with staff mistakes or problems with the 'off-duty'. Give them a general overview of the themes of complaints, incidents and staffing issues. Remember also to highlight any achievements.

WHY SOME MANAGERS 'MICROMANAGE'

When you go to your manager with any concerns, make sure you present solutions rather than dwell on the problem. If you always expect your manager to come up with the solutions and sort out your problems, you are at risk of being 'micromanaged'. This is a common situation which occurs when line managers begin to get too involved in the details of management at ward level. They will get personally involved in sorting out problems such as personnel problems, stafffing issues or even holding meetings with members of your team. This sort of behaviour can indicate that your manager does not have the confidence in your abilities to manage your unit.

If this is happening to you, try and focus on your own behaviour before changing theirs. Make more use of your mentor and/or clinical supervisor for support. Think through and find out what you could do to resolve your problem before seeing your manager. Phone your HR advisor or finance advisor and find out the information you need first. If, for example, a member of your staff comes to you complaining that they are being bullied, and you are not sure what steps to take, don't go immediately to your line manager. Call your HR advisor first for expert advice about the options you can take within the policy for bullying and harassment. Call your mentor and ask for their point of view. Ask your colleagues (other ward managers) if they have had similiar experiences that you could learn from. Once you have all the information, then go to your line manager and either:

- let them know what course of action you have decided to take, or
- present the options you have found for resolving the problem and ask for their opinion on the matter.

Show your manager that you have initiative. Don't burden them with even more problems on top of their own workload.

KEEP IN CONSTANT CONTACT

As you gain more experience over the years, you will need less support from your manager. On the other hand, don't fall into the trap of getting on with things so well that they don't bother with you and what is happening on your ward. Contact them regularly, at least each week, and give them a general update. This will ensure they are aware of the good practice on your ward and will remember to keep you involved in wider issues.

If you have any untoward incidents, let your manager know not only about the remedial action that has been taken but also what you are going to do to reduce the risk of it happening again. This prevents more senior managers telling you to change aspects of care on your ward as a result of receiving incident forms. It is wise to ensure that you and your team identify and implement the necessary changes first.

GIVE FEEDBACK

As with your team, it is necessary to give your line manager regular feedback on their performance. You want to be able to encourage all the positive aspects of their behaviour and make them aware of aspects which have a negative effect. They will not know unless you tell them. If your manager comes to see you regularly each week and you appreciate that, tell them so. If they interfere unnecessarily with the work of your team, they will not understand your frustration unless you tell them, and therefore will continue to interfere. They may think they are helping you when they are really hindering your work and will have no idea unless you maintain an open and honest dialogue.

In the same way, encourage lots of feedback from your manager so that you have some idea how you are progressing and what they are thinking. Some managers may not give feedback unless asked, so just keep on asking.

WRITE GOOD AND TIMELY REPORTS

Getting reports finished on time and done properly will help enormously in building a good relationship with your manager. Don't put all report writing tasks to the bottom of your in-tray. Start the process immediately. It prevents you spending precious time worrying about when you are going to get the time to do it. Once you have started and developed a basic outline, you will feel a lot better. You will also be clearer in your mind about what information is required and be able to delegate parts of the report where necessary.

When asked by your line manager to write a report, always confirm the objective of the report and who the reader(s) will be before you start work on it. Taking time to check this at the beginning can save you hours of wasted effort later on. It helps you to decide what information to include or leave out. It will also prevent your manager saying after all your hard work, 'this is not what I asked for'.

STAGE 1: WRITE A BASIC OUTLINE

Write a basic outline before you start researching or investigating the information that you will need. It will help direct your investigation. All reports should be based on the following headings, which can be individually adapted at a later stage:

● Introduction (based on the objective)
● Background (include the method of investigation/research)
● Results/implementations
● Conclusion
● Recommendations.

Start any report with these five basic headings to guide you. It prevents you from sitting down and staring at a piece of blank paper wondering where to begin.

STAGE 2: THE INTRODUCTION

The introduction is one of the most important sections of the report. The reader can form an opinion about the rest of the report based on the clarity and quality of the introduction. It's a good idea to use the objective you have agreed with your manager to form the basis of the introduction to your report.

STAGE 3: BACKGROUND DESCRIPTION

Describe the background to the report, i.e. make the context clear. Keep it in note form in the initial stages to stop you becoming too focused on this section. If your report is about how you have done something to come up with a solution, use this section to describe the process you used. It is often better to complete this section once you have finished the rest of the report.

STAGE 4: RESULTS/IMPLEMENTATION

This is the main part of the report. A good idea to get started is to list everything you want to include in the report then group them into key headings. You could write down each item on a 'post it' note then sort the 'post it' notes into general themes or key headings.

This gives you a good basic outline to the report. Once you have done this you can concentrate on researching or finding the information to put in under each heading, and delegating some parts to your team or others, if appropriate.

STAGE 5: CONCLUSION

Use this section to discuss the main findings or recommendations. It is a major part of the report. A busy manager should be able to see from the introduction and conclusion of your report what it is about, what has been found and what action (if any) they need to take.

STAGE 6: RECOMMENDATIONS

The recommendations should link directly with what has been stated in the conclusion. Don't introduce any new ideas in this section.

Further tips
When you come to the writing part, there are a few rules to remember:

1. Write in the first person, 'I'; not 'one' or 'the author'.
2. Don't use jargon such as 'obs' or 'resps'.
3. Use active, not passive phrases (e.g. 'they decided' rather than 'it was decided').
4. Avoid exclamation marks.
5. Try to avoid using superfluous phrases such as 'at this moment in time' instead of 'now', or 'in respect of' instead of 'about'.
6. Paragraphs should be wider than they are long.
7. Explain all abbreviations, keeping in mind that some people who read the report will not be health care professionals.
8. Ensure the report is page numbered.

As a general rule, any reports should be short and succinct, and include more facts than descriptions. Few managers will read long reports from cover to cover. Most will read the introduction, key headings, conclusion and recommendations, so concentrate on those aspects.

Always give reports in on time. Remember to under-promise and over-deliver. If you think it will take you two weeks, set a time limit of three to four weeks and aim to give it in at two weeks. Managers are always impressed by people who deliver work early or on time.

ACTIVELY MANAGE INCIDENTS, MISTAKES AND ACCIDENTS

Observe the trends from your incident forms and work closely with your team to reduce the risk of further incidents of the same nature happening again. Don't wait to be told what your main issues are from the organisation's risk management or clinical governance lead. Make your staff aware that sending off an incident form does not absolve them of the responsibility of ensuring that lessons are learned.

Remember that completing an incident form does not equate to an admission of liability. The culture of the health care is changing, and incident reporting is about supporting staff to learn from mistakes, not blaming them. Incident reports should concentrate on what happened and why, not who. The exceptions to this rule are:

- cases of gross negligence
- if someone has been malicious, deliberately negligent or carried out a criminal act
- where there have been similiar incidents and someone's actions have continued despite remedial actions being undertaken.

Copies of all incident forms are usually sent back to your manager, whose role is to make sure something is being done to reduce the risk of further incidents. Take the initiative and do this first with your team before waiting to be told what to do. It will make your life a lot easier in the long term.

SERIOUS UNTOWARD INCIDENTS

If the incident constitutes a serious untoward incident, your organisational policy will outline the steps you should follow regarding communications and dealing with the actual incident. You should not be grading incidents unless you have had the appropriate training. A serious incident still warrants the completion of an incident form but in addition you should gather any relevant information, photocopy any relevant clinical notes, keep faulty equipment and take statements from witnesses within 24 hours of the incident. This information will form the basis of further investigations.

An investigation team is usually nominated to undertake a further review in the case of serious untoward incidents. You may be nominated to assist with the investigation and writing of the report. It's advisable to use the root cause analysis (RCA) approach, for which you should have had training. If not, make sure you receive advice and support from someone who has. At the time of writing, The National Patient Safety Agency supply an RCA toolkit to all NHS staff free of charge (National Patient Safety Association 2005).

Root cause analysis

The root cause analysis approach focuses on identifying the sequence of events and allowing the root cause of the incident to emerge. A serious incident is often not just the result of human error but a chain of events that led to the human error. The investigation should result in recommendations for improving systems and processes to prevent the risk of human error occurring again.

When you have to write such a report, you may find it easier to use the following headings:

- Introduction (include terms of reference or objective of report)
- Executive summary (this is a summary of what is contained in the report)
- Sequence of events (description of what happened)
- Sources of information (methods used and witnesses interviewed)
- Findings (identification of reasons and underlying failures in the system which led to the incident)
- Conclusion (lessons to be learned)
- Recommendations
- Appendices.

The report should present the facts, not opinions, and demonstrate that the incident has been thoroughly and fairly investigated. Effectively managing adverse incidents, near misses or serious untoward incidents is a major part of clinical governance.

KNOW HOW TO CONDUCT A GOOD INVESTIGATION

You may be asked by your line manager to undertake a full investigation into matters involving issues such as:

- allegations of bullying or harassment
- poor performance or misconduct
- allegations of a criminal activity, negligence or deliberate harm.

Usually you would not investigate an incident on your own ward. It is good practice to appoint investigating officers who are not involved in the incident or line-manage the area in which it has taken place.

Before commencing any investigation, confirm the following with your manager:

1. Exactly what is to be investigated.
2. The time frame for completion. You will need to negotiate dedicated time in which to carry out the investigation. Do not attempt to do this in your own time, or in quiet times during your shift. You will require cover for your time out.
3. Who you can go to for support. You should have access to an experienced HR advisor throughout the process.

MAKE A PROVISIONAL PLAN OF ACTION

Agree a plan of action with your manager. This plan may change as new information comes to light but you should start off with a plan so you can estimate the time it will take.

Your first step in your plan is usually to arrange the interview dates. It takes considerable time to arrange venues, dates and times. Do not carry out the interviews until you have reviewed all the necessary documentary evidence, but try and do them as quickly as possible after the event in order to:

● ensure the event(s) is still fresh in everyone's mind
● stop rumours and gossip
● reduce unnecessary anxiety for all those involved
● reduce unnecessary waste of resources if anyone has been suspended.

When you arrange the interviews, you must ensure that each person is informed of their right to have a trade union representative or work colleague to accompany them. It is up to them to arrange this. You should also let them know of any support that your organisation offers such as trained counsellors for victims of alleged bullying. You should ensure that the alleged wrong-doer is informed of the investigation as soon as possible. It would be unfair for the witnesses or anyone else to hear of the investigation before them. You should also keep the ward/department manager informed as well as your own line manager.

REVIEW ALL THE DOCUMENTARY EVIDENCE

It's advisable to make photocopies of any documentary evidence to prevent tampering of records. Keep a record of all documents reviewed as part of the process. Relevant documents may include:

● 'off-duties'
● ward induction/development programmes
● patients' medical or nursing records
● local policies/guidelines
● any relevant professional or national guidelines.

Remember to follow the confidentiality guidelines if any patient information is involved in the investigation (see p. 131).

INTERVIEWS

Interviews usually start with the person who raised the issue. This is to establish the nature of the complaint or allegation and any further information which may be relevant. You will also need to interview the alleged wrong-doer(s) to give them the chance to put across their version of events. Any witnesses will need to be interviewed as well as the line manager. If you are investigating a matter of which you have no knowledge or experience you may also need to interview other professionals for their expert advice. Witnesses are usually entitled to time off in lieu or payment if interviewed outside of normal working hours. Check your organisational policy and inform their line managers of the time required if this is the case.

Before you start the interview you should prepare your questions to ensure you cover all the required areas. At the beginning of the interview, take time to:

1. Make the person feel comfortable with appropriate refreshments and seating.
2. Reiterate their right to be accompanied by a trade union representative or work colleague.
3. Explain that this is not disciplinary action and that your role is only to establish the facts.
4. Explain that they should not discuss the case with anyone else who is involved.

Keep a record of all the interviews. Give each person the opportunity to read through the notes of their interview and sign that they agree it is an accurate reflection of what was discussed. They may prefer to provide their own statements. Make sure they are aware that any statements may be used as evidence in the event of a subsequent disciplinary hearing.

Don't be concerned about calling people back to re-interview. You may find you have to do this as further information comes to light. Remember that all information obtained should remain confidential so do not share information about anyone else's interview with subsequent interviewees.

PREPARE A WRITTEN REPORT

The following headings can be used as a general guide, but check your organisation's policy for local guidance on what is expected within your report.

● Introduction – include terms of reference or objective
● Description of the issue and/or allegations and an outline of the investigative process including timetable of interviews
● Findings – list them clearly. You may wish to list them under headings of each complaint. Refer to witnesses either by their initials or as witness A, B or C, etc. throughout the report
● Conclusions – is the complaint or allegation substantiated?
● Recommendations
● Appendices.

The purpose of an investigation is to establish the facts. It does not equate to disciplinary action. It may or may not lead to a disciplinary hearing. If it does, the evidence provided in the investigative report will help inform the disciplinary panel.

ACTION POINTS

- If you haven't already had one within the past year, make an appointment with your manager for an appraisal and ensure your objectives are congruent with theirs.
- Arrange regular meetings with your manager throughout the rest of the year to review your set objectives and to keep them informed of progress on your ward.
- If your manager leaves you out of decision making or any changes, make a point of trying to improve your working relationship with them to reduce the risk of it happening again.
- If change takes place that is detrimental to patient care, gather the facts and approach the appropriate people with the support of your manager.
- Try not to present any problems to your manager; present solutions or options for action each time.
- Always calculate the monetary costs for any extra work, whether or not funding has been granted.
- Give regular feedback to your manager, particularly with a job done well. Invite lots of feedback from your manager to ensure you are continually improving your own performance.
- Use the main themes from incidents, mistakes and errors to make improvements on the ward, before being asked to by your line manager.
- Take on the delegation of an investigation as a challenge and opportune learning experience.
- Always start reports early and give them in early or on time.

References

Department of Trade and Industry 2004 Information and consultation of employees regulations. HMSO, London. Online. Available: http://www.dti.gov.uk/er/consultation/i_c_guidance_01.htm 2 Oct 2005

National Patient Safety Association 2005 RCA training and RCA toolkit. Online. Available: http://www.npsa.nhs.uk/health/resources/root_cause_analysis/conditions 2 Oct 2005

CHAPTER 13

MANAGE DIFFICULT PEOPLE AND DIFFICULT SITUATIONS

Manage a difficult manager 248

Managers who are prone to getting angry 248

Managers who don't manage 249

Managers who expect too much 249

Deal with that problematic colleague 250

Colleagues who tend to be continually negative 250

Colleagues who continually whinge about others 250

Colleagues who put themselves down all the time 250

Colleagues who are continually calling for advice and support 251

Manage any allegations of bullying or harassment 251

What is bullying or harassment? 251

What steps should you take? 252

What do you do if your initial approach does not work? 252

Manage staff complaints 253

What to do if staff raise concerns 253

What to do if you cannot resolve the complaint alone 254

Make sure staff are not being used or abused by others 254

The arrogant consultant 254

The pushy bed manager 255

Overloading link nurses 256

Don't tolerate any form of racism or other discrimination 256

Patients and relatives 256

Overseas nurses 257

Take action when staffing levels are dangerously low 258

What is dangerously low staffing? 258

Put everything in writing 259

Incident forms 259

Break up any cliques 259

New recruits 260

Take action 260

Don't be part of the clique 260

What if your own line manager is part of a clique? 261

Be specific about expanding nursing roles 261

Develop guidelines 262

Be proactive with enforced moves or mergers of services 262

The importance of being politically aware 263

Plan ahead 263

Developing a project plan 264

Involve the experts from the beginning 264

Managers have to deal with all sorts of different personalities ranging from the shy and passive to the explosive and aggressive types. Working in the health care environment can bring out the worst in people as the pressure increases with more work and less resources. It is important to understand the emotional vulnerability that underlies many difficult situations. A key managerial skill is to be able to recognise individual needs for recognition and self-esteem and to be confident in confronting challenging situations and people in a constructive and positive manner.

MANAGE A DIFFICULT MANAGER

People usually get promoted because they are good at their job. The problem with professionals being good at their job is that some are promoted to become managers and this is a totally different job to what they were doing before. They do not necessarily have the skills in managing people or resources. In some cases, people are promoted because they are no good clinically or because they have been in the organisation for a very long time.

That's not to say that all managers are no good because most are, even those who were not appropriate for the job originally. Many will thrive and become good managers. Unfortunately, there are a few who do not.

Some managers struggle in their role and may take out their frustrations on others or perhaps become very controlling and manipulative. Some adopt an aggressive manner and may shout or lose their temper on occasions, whilst others may shy away from difficult decisions and leave their team to their own devices.

MANAGERS WHO ARE PRONE TO GETTING ANGRY

If your manager has a tantrum and starts shouting at you, do not sit and take it and, whatever you do, do not scream back. Tell them that you are sorry about whatever it is, but would rather wait and discuss the matter when you have both had the chance to calm down. Say that you will leave if necessary. Only stay if they agree to talk to you in a civil manner. By saying that you both need a chance to calm down it does not look like you are blaming them. You need to be diplomatic. After all, this is your manager.

Unfortunately there are some managers who are continuously aggressive and intimidating. Tell them that their approach of shouting at you is not going to make you work any harder. It just serves to upset and intimidate you. If you have made a mistake, always admit to it. If you have not done something that was asked for, state clearly and succinctly the reasons why you have not achieved what's required. Don't make excuses; it will only serve to increase their anger.

If this is a situation that comes up time and time again, go and discuss it through with someone senior in your human resources (HR) department. All NHS organisations are required to have a policy for dealing with bullying and harassment. You should be well supported through the process.

MANAGERS WHO DON'T MANAGE

Some managers are reluctant to take on their managerial responsibilities. These tend to be people who are promoted because of their clinical experience. As mentioned previously, clinical skills are not the same as managerial skills. These types of managers may busy themselves with issues that require their clinical expertise and ignore their managerial role. It can be difficult to get them to make any decisions on important managerial matters.

It is difficult to deal with this sort of manager because they are normally well-liked and maintain a good rapport with everyone. They will spend a lot of time sympathising with you and your team over your issues, but don't actually do anything about them. People tend to label them as 'supportive' managers because they have spent time listening to their problems.

Often the only way to deal with this type of manager is to always present the full solution to your problem, or a number of alternative solutions from which the manager can choose. For each solution make sure:

● it has been fully researched and meets the appropriate guidelines or policy
● the appropriate people have been consulted
● the implications have been considered in depth.

Bear in mind that these managers tend to thrive on social acceptance amongst the clinical team so ensure you make it clear that your solutions have been generated by your team and reflect all their views too.

MANAGERS WHO EXPECT TOO MUCH

It is hard for managers whose working day used to revolve around patients' needs, to enter a world where it revolves around managing others from an office environment. Patients' needs were always the priority, but when the next role no longer entails looking after patients, some find it difficult to work out what the priorities are. Some will take on too much work in order to compensate for this and over the years may get into a pattern of being very busy but not actually achieving anything. They will take on extra projects or find it difficult to say no when bombarded with demands from their own senior managers.

This could result in you having some of their extra work being delegated down to you. If this is happening to you and it gets too much (and you are certain that you are managing your own time effectively) then you must say so. Work out what your priorities and time commitments are then go and discuss them with your manager (see Ch. 2). This can achieve two things:

1. They will hopefully stop delegating their extra work to you.
2. Having seen what you have done, they may be stimulated into defining and prioritising their own workload using the same formula.

DEAL WITH THAT PROBLEMATIC COLLEAGUE

The very nature of our work means we will always be working with people, sometimes some very difficult people. Unfortunately you can't choose your work colleagues, and in a clinically focused role, you cannot retreat to an office or work alone to avoid the problem.

So how do you handle a colleague who is proving rather difficult to work with? First, tell them. This sounds fairly obvious but you would be amazed at how many people put up with poor behaviour from colleagues. The individual then carries on blissfully unaware of the angst they are causing. The situation will get worse if you leave it and the longer you leave telling your colleague, the worse they will feel. Second, don't get personal, otherwise they will become defensive and you'll get nowhere. Focus on the issue, not the person.

COLLEAGUES WHO TEND TO BE CONTINUALLY NEGATIVE

Negative people are those who tend to be insecure and unsure of themselves. By saying negative things about others they are trying to cover up their own limitations. Make an effort to share your ideas with them. Get them on your side by offering to take on some work together. Boost their confidence by giving them positive feedback on things they do well.

COLLEAGUES WHO CONTINUALLY WHINGE ABOUT OTHERS

If you have a colleague who is always finding fault with people, ask them what they have done or plan to do about the problem:

'What have you done about her behaviour?'
'Have you told her?'
'Why are you telling me? Why don't you tell her?'

The more often you question what they have done about it, the less they will find fault.

COLLEAGUES WHO PUT THEMSELVES DOWN ALL THE TIME

Colleagues who turn the criticism on themselves, saying things like 'I'm not good enough' are usually lacking in confidence. It's easier to criticise themselves before anyone else does. With a colleague like this, you can help simply by telling them that they are doing a good job and to stop talking themselves down. Those who put themselves down in order to receive compliments and praise from others are equally annoying. You have to be blunt in this case and say something like 'look, you know how good you are at that sort of thing and you hardly need any more feedback from me to boost your confidence'.

COLLEAGUES WHO ARE CONTINUALLY CALLING FOR ADVICE AND SUPPORT

Some of your less experienced colleagues may have found you so helpful in the past that they continue to turn to you for every problem they encounter. If this happens, encourage them to seek a mentor/clinical supervisor for extra support. Tell them that relying on you alone for advice and guidance will restrict their learning; they have to seek support from others as well as you. Don't do things for them or you will encourage the behaviour. Whenever this person calls you, ask them what they think is the best action and enable them to come to their own conclusions and actions.

MANAGE ANY ALLEGATIONS OF BULLYING OR HARASSMENT

WHAT IS BULLYING OR HARASSMENT?

If members of your team do not treat their colleagues with dignity and respect it could be interpreted as bullying or harassment. Situations in which a member of your team feels threatened, insulted or intimidated in any way by another person's behaviour must be stopped immediately. If any of your staff come to you saying that someone else makes them feel this way, even if it was not intended, you need to take action. If you don't do anything:

1. The individual's confidence and self-esteem will plummet and therefore affect their standard of work.
2. Other staff will get involved and begin to take sides thus creating tension within the team.

You should take all complaints seriously, even if you personally believe that it is simply a case of firm management or a harmless joke. Bullying and harassment are defined as any sort of behaviour which makes an individual feel upset, threatened, humiliated or vulnerable and undermines their confidence. In other words, it is the *impact* of the behaviour, not the *intent* of the perpetrator which determines whether the person is being bullied or harassed.

Be aware that bullying can include:

- regular shouting or criticism in front of others
- refusing to speak to someone directly
- excessive supervision or checking up on a colleague's work
- constantly giving menial or trivial tasks
- deliberately excluding individuals from work-related social events
- unreasonably refusing requests for time off or training.

Harassment is any unwanted behaviour towards an individual regarding gender, race, disability, sexual orientation, religion, beliefs or any personal characteristic. This can include:

- intrusive questioning or gossiping about a person's private life, religion, activities, sexual orientation, etc.
- being condescending about the way a person dresses or speaks
- insensitive jokes or pranks
- unnecessary body contact.

WHAT STEPS SHOULD YOU TAKE?

When a member of staff complains to you that another person's behaviour is insulting or demeaning, your first step is to encourage them to tell the perpetrator, if they have not already done so. Sometimes people do not realise the effect they are having on others. Once informed, many will alter their behaviour.

The individual who came to you may be low in confidence and therefore may need your support to do this. It is far better to work through with the individual what approach to take and encourage them to do it for themselves. This will increase their self-esteem and enable them to deal with any future situations with more confidence. However, the situation may be such that you will need to act as mediator between the two parties. In this case, make sure you have both parties present, otherwise you will get caught between two different versions of events and not know who to believe.

WHAT DO YOU DO IF YOUR INITIAL APPROACH DOES NOT WORK?

If the perpetrator does not change their behaviour, the staff member may be encouraged to take a more formal approach by putting their concerns in writing. You should be liaising closely with your HR advisor throughout the process and ensuring that both parties involved in the allegation have access to support from their trade union representatives.

Once a formal allegation is made, a manager from outside your ward will usually be brought in to undertake a formal investigation. This means that those involved, other staff members and yourself will be interviewed and statements taken. A report will be written with recommendations to what action should be taken. The recommended actions could include a number of things such as:

- an apology
- transfer of either party to another ward or department
- counselling or time off
- identification of training needs
- a disciplinary hearing.

Every NHS organisation is required to have a specific policy and guidelines for cases of bullying and harassment. It is wise to make yourself familiar with this policy. Also ensure your staff are familiar with what your organisation defines as bullying and harassment. It will increase their awareness that bullying and harassment do not just concern people who shout and use violent threatening behaviour.

MANAGE STAFF COMPLAINTS

Hopefully you will have created a good healthy working atmosphere so that your staff will happily bring issues to your attention if they have any concerns about:

● their working conditions
● standards of patient care
● relationships with colleagues.

Your leadership style should also ensure that all staff are willing to work together to agree some sort of solution. This includes taking the time to listen to their concerns and being willing to help them work through the issue and ensure something is done to resolve the situation.

WHAT TO DO IF STAFF RAISE CONCERNS

Always keep a file note of any staff complaints. Note what was discussed and the actions you agreed on. Make a date to review these. Your notes will be invaluable should any member of staff decide to take the issue up formally.

If you are not particularly approachable or if staff are unhappy with your response, they can raise a formal grievance. A grievance is basically a written complaint from a member of staff. All NHS organisations are required to have a grievance procedure for you to follow, and it is usually very strict in terms of the timetable you have to keep to. If you receive a written complaint from a member of your staff about their working conditions, standards of care or relationships with colleagues, you should invite them to meet with you as soon as possible and inform them that they have a right to be accompanied by a friend, colleague or trade union representative. If the solution is outside your authority or if the grievance is against you personally, you should refer the matter to your line manager.

Most policies state that you must have a meeting with them within a certain number of days from receipt of the letter; always check your local policy. At this meeting you should:

1. Allow the staff member to explain their complaint and what they think the solution should be.
2. Discuss and agree a solution, or if you are not sure what to do about the complaint, you can then adjourn the meeting while you seek further advice.
3. Follow up the meeting with a letter confirming what was agreed. Your policy will state when this is to be done. It is usually within three to five days following the meeting.

WHAT TO DO IF YOU CANNOT RESOLVE THE COMPLAINT ALONE

If the complaint is not resolved, the individual can write to your line manager who, in turn, can either meet with them to discuss the issue or send a written response. Again, your policy will set a time limit for the response which is usually within three to five days from receipt of the letter.

If your line manager cannot resolve the issue, the individual can then take it to the next managerial level. Again, they will either meet with the individual or write a letter. If the individual is still not satisfied, they can raise an appeal at board level. At this stage, one of the board directors will arrange an appeal panel. They will consider all the evidence including statements from any witnesses or representatives. The appeal panel decision is final.

MAKE SURE STAFF ARE NOT BEING USED OR ABUSED BY OTHERS

You may be personally confident in dealing with difficult people when you are on duty but part of your role is to make sure that your staff are equipped with the skills to deal with difficult people and situations when you are not there.

THE ARROGANT CONSULTANT

Working partnerships between medical and nursing staff have not always been easy. The differences in pay, status, education and gender have often led to a clash in perspectives and tensions in the working environment. On the whole, things have changed for the better in recent times. Nursing is no longer a female-only profession and there are many more female doctors. In addition, nursing is now a university-based profession and the government has done much to improve the lot of nurses by supporting the expansion of nursing roles and responsibilities, e.g. nurse prescribing and nurse consultants.

The nursing profession nowadays is less hierarchical and more patient centred. However, the medical profession generally remains fairly rigid in its career structure, with the junior doctors doing all the running around and the consultants being the bosses who give the orders. There are some consultants who still feel they are the ultimate boss and everyone should do as they say and 'woe betide' those who dare to question their decisions. These types can be quite difficult to handle.

Sometimes the arrogance is a cover-up for the fact that they do have a highly stressful job and may well suffer from inner feelings of inadequacy. How many times have you given a consultant any positive feedback on their work, or seen others do so? It's quite an isolating role especially for those who have had no training and development in communication or leadership skills. How do they know what they need? They have only recently got used to the idea of having formal appraisals.

One way of dealing with an arrogant consultant is to build up a good working relationship with them right from the start. Give positive feedback regularly and any negative feedback will be taken more seriously. It you only give negative feedback they will assume that you are simply whinging all the time. You will be seen as the problem, not them.

Do not encourage your staff to confront them. Few people will acknowledge that they are arrogant and can be very patronising and hurtful particularly if some of your staff are shy or less confident in themselves. Instead, show your staff how to talk to all consultants with confidence and how to give regular feedback. Include your staff in all areas of decision making including ward rounds. Always encourage them to join in any discussions with your support rather than to be passive bystanders.

THE PUSHY BED MANAGER

Poor bed managers can never please anyone. A&E get fed up with them because patients are stacking up and the wards are fed up with them for constantly pestering about the 'bedstate'. They get hassled from all sides. It's no wonder that they may pressurise your staff to discharge too early or take patients when they are not ready.

When you are on duty, it shouldn't be a problem. But what do you do when your staff are coerced into making decisions when you are not there; decisions that may not be appropriate such as taking extra patients into an already overstretched team of staff? It is difficult to refuse, especially if a matron or general manager becomes involved. If you find this has happened when you return from days off, the first thing to do is to speak to the bed manager as soon as you can to ascertain the facts. It's not unusual for staff to exaggerate a little when in reality they did little to explain their position to the bed manager.

If you find out that members of your staff were forced into compromising patient care in order to meet targets, then explain to the bed manager that you are not happy and will not allow it to happen again in the future. Confirm the discussion plus your agreed actions briefly by email. Keep a file note of the conversation and if necessary send a copy of the email or file note to your line manager. This is usually enough to ensure it does not happen again. If it does happen again, do the same and copy senior managers into the email. The appropriate people must be made aware.

In the meantime, make sure that you set criteria with your team about bed decisions such as when to declare a bed is ready to take the next patient, i.e. the patient is no longer on the ward, or can wait in the dayroom only if they are fit and do not require any nursing care or attention whilst there. Make sure the bed manager, matron and general manager are fully aware of these guidelines. Your organisation may already have guidelines for this, so don't write new ones unless your ward or department is an exception.

OVERLOADING LINK NURSES

Always be aware about what your link nurses are being asked to do. Their role is to act as a link between the nurse specialist or practice development team and the ward team. These nurse specialists and practice development teams usually have a huge agenda and have targets to implement across the organisation. Often the only way they can communicate is through the link nurses. It is an effective system of disseminating information. Unfortunately, some will use the nurses to do their work for them. Your nurses may not realise that they are being used to fulfil the objectives of others.

Junior staff in particular may be eager to please and think nothing of doing the required work in their own time. Their dedication to improving patient care can be abused. Don't allow this to happen to your staff. Make sure you are fully aware of the demands placed upon them, and intervene if necessary. Give them permission to say no. They should be doing work which benefits the team and patient care on your ward, not the person who is leading the link nurses.

DON'T TOLERATE ANY FORM OF RACISM OR OTHER DISCRIMINATION

PATIENTS AND RELATIVES

If a patient or relative refuses care because they object to the nurse's appearance, skin colour, religion, etc. despite the fact that the person is a competent nurse, then it should not be tolerated. This sounds simple but there are still recent examples in which health care professionals were not supported by their managers when discriminated against by patients or relatives.

In 2004, a nurse was awarded £20 000 in compensation when a relative asked that she not look after her baby because she was black. The managers moved the baby to another ward (The Guardian 2004). They did not agree with the relative's comments but felt that their duty was towards the baby. In moving the patient, they simply condoned the relative's view.

If patients or relatives on your ward discriminate against your staff in any way, make sure you support them by telling the patient or relative that their comments are offensive. Remain polite and respectful. You will not be able to change the person's views, so it is not wise to attempt it. Just explain that their behaviour will not be tolerated. All members of your team should be assured that they will have your full support in any cases of this kind. Never dismiss any discriminatory comments as trivial and do not move the patient or nurse unless the nurse specifically requests not to look after them. If the patient or relative refuses care on discriminatory grounds, they should be made aware that they are effectively refusing services altogether.

If the patient or relative will not listen to you or the nurse involved, consult your organisation's formal policy. All NHS organisations are required to have a policy which outlines what steps you can take when discriminatory behaviour persists after you have told them that it is unacceptable. The next step usually involves giving a written warning setting out types of behaviour that will no longer be tolerated. You do have a right to withdraw care but consult with your HR department before you take any such action.

OVERSEAS NURSES

It is quite clear within our code of professional conduct that 'you are expected to work cooperatively within teams and to respect the skills, expertise and contributions of your colleagues. You must treat them fairly and without discrimination' (Nursing & Midwifery Council 2004; Standard 4.2).

Unfortunately, filling the gaps in the health service with internationally recruited nurses has revealed some alarming discriminatory practices within the UK. These include questioning of competence, giving special negative attention if mistakes are made and stereotyping (Allen & Larson 2003). This is more likely to be because the nurse is a foreigner or has a different cultural background rather than because of their colour or ethnicity.

Take action to ensure this does not happen within your team. Staff may resent the concept of recruiting from overseas. It does not help if they are seen as receiving better treatment than UK nurses, but that is no reason to treat the individual nurses any differently. Your role as a manager is to give overseas nurses the same treatment as any other new recruit. However, you should bear in mind that having come from another country, it will take them longer to settle in and adapt to UK working practice.

1. *Prepare your team for their arrival.* Get your staff to think how they would feel starting a new job in a different country. It usually takes at least three months to settle in. Allow them to make mistakes without judging them negatively. Make sure your team help them to learn from their experiences including their mistakes.
2. *Ensure all new recruits have a minimum two week induction programme* (even if your organisation has already provided a programme specifically for the whole group of overseas nurses).
3. *Ensure each new nurse has at least one mentor* and that those mentors have attended awareness sessions on equality and diversity. Some organisations set up specific sessions for staff to learn about the culture of the country where they have just recruited from.
4. *Make sure their personal development plan focuses on skills that they can transfer back home*, whilst ensuring they have the same career opportunities as the rest of your staff.

5. *Don't ever indulge in discussions* about 'the overseas nurses' where *they* are stereotyped as 'good workers, never complain, a bit slow, not very assertive, etc.'. Remember, no two individuals are the same, no matter what country they come from.

TAKE ACTION WHEN STAFFING LEVELS ARE DANGEROUSLY LOW

WHAT IS DANGEROUSLY LOW STAFFING?

Nursing 'off-duties', unlike many other professions, work to *minimum* safe staffing levels rather than *maximum* levels. Very few wards or departments are in a position where they can ever exceed their minimum staffing levels. This means that when someone goes off sick, you need bank or agency staff to cover. But there may be situations when:

● more than one member of staff phones in sick
● there are not enough bank or agency staff to cover
● staff go sick or are sent home during the course of a shift
● your workload suddenly and unexpectedly increases beyond your capacity to provide the required patient care.

Most staff are familiar with the following actions to take in such circumstances:

Step 1: Inform a senior manager to see if staff can be moved from elsewhere in the hospital.

Step 2: Phone around for staff to come in. Most wards and departments keep a list of staff home numbers which will be used in such emergencies. (Remember that this is confidential information and must be kept locked away.)

Step 3: Inform all relevant managers of the situation, including the bed manager to ensure that patients are admitted elsewhere, and cancel any further admissions where possible.

Once every avenue has been attempted, some nurses forget the most important last step; to *prioritise*. If your workload is far greater than your capacity to deliver, don't tell your staff to just do what they can. That is tantamount to muddling through and is dangerous. Important things may be missed.

Ensure your staff have the skills to sit down and work out with their team what care is essential and what is desirable for that shift. They should be able to decide within their team for example:

● which patients need a full blanket bath and which patients can just make do with a hands and face wash and those that can be left unwashed until that afternoon or even the next day
● which observations will get left undone
● which patients' wound dressings will not be taken down and redressed until the next shift, etc.

These must be conscious decisions and not left to chance. Don't expect your staff to do everything as if normally staffed saying that it's fine if things get missed or mistakes get made. Short staffing is not an excuse for mistakes.

Keep the patients and relatives informed; put up a notice saying something like, 'There are only three staff on today instead of the required five due to high sickness levels. Please bear with us. We have had to prioritise in order to maintain essential levels of care. The beds will not be made this morning and, if you need to see a nurse, could we please ask you to wait until this afternoon or tomorrow unless your request is urgent'.

A notice such as this will make sure that your patients and their relatives are still confident in your management skills despite the fact that you are obviously short staffed.

PUT EVERYTHING IN WRITING

Inform your line manager not only about the situation but also what you and your team have decided in terms of the care that is to be administered and which aspects of care will be left undone in order to maintain basic safe standards for all patients. Confirm the situation and the decisions that you made via an email to the appropriate manager. If the situation happens when you are not on duty, make sure your staff know to take such actions, keep written notes and inform the appropriate people of their decisions.

Try not to fill in the shift yourself each time unless absolutely necessary, and don't expect your staff to either. It undermines their professional status and your own by continually expecting to be used as 'just another pair of hands'. You and your staff are worth more than that. Your role is to look ahead and deal with the cause of the short staffing, not to continually 'plug the gaps'.

INCIDENT FORMS

You are usually required to fill in an incident form each time your staff are subject to dangerously low staffing conditions. It is good to ensure that the incident is being noted but incident reporting is not taking action; it is simply monitoring the situation. The forms will eventually reach your manager's office who will then hopefully consult and support you on what is to be done about it to prevent future occurrences.

BREAK UP ANY CLIQUES

Despite your best intentions, you may still find that cliques form within your team, particularly if you have staff who have been with you for many years. These long term staff can be invaluable in terms of stability and maintaining high standards. They tend to be loyal and can become almost like part of a family. However, it can have a detrimental effect, especially with newcomers to the team who find it difficult to fit in.

NEW RECRUITS

Cliques can result in the loss of self-confidence in a new member of staff. Their work may suffer and you could find you have a new staff nurse who is not quite living up to your initial expectations. Worse still, they may leave within a few months for another job but not tell you the real reason; in fact, they may not realise the reason themselves. If someone does not fit in to a new work environment, they tend to blame themselves for not having the right social skills. Few may admit that to their manager, so you will be left in the dark as to the real reason. Try and be alert to the signs.

TAKE ACTION

Powerful cliques like these need to be broken up. There are several ways you can do this. The first and most obvious is to arrange the 'off-duty' so that they do not always work together. When they are on duty together, encourage them to take different breaks as much as possible. Another option is to select one or two members of the clique and give them specific tasks or projects for which they must report to you. Give them lots of encouragement, praise and rewards for a job well done. This helps to divide them from the rest of the group.

A similar result may be gained if you ensure that each time you recruit a new member of staff, you assign one of the clique to be their mentor. Give the mentor lots of positive feedback around their work with the newcomer. This will help ensure new staff are not left out.

DON'T BE PART OF THE CLIQUE

You may find that when you become a ward manager it could well be on the same ward where you have been in a senior staff nurse or deputy ward manager role. You will be in the unenviable position of managing staff with whom you have been working alongside very well for a number of years. You may find that they are happy with the situation and continue to work well as a team. However, be wary of the perspective for new members coming into the team; you could unwittingly become part of a clique. This happens so easily.

So, if your first ward manager's post is on the same ward with the same team, it is advisable to take the following actions:

1. *Create a space between you and your previous colleagues.* This can be achieved by making sure that you give equal time to every single member of the team, including time spent with each one on tea and lunch breaks.

2. *Never talk about personnel issues with the long term staff*, even if you have known and worked alongside them for years. You are now their manager and it is not professional to do so. They will feel privileged compared to the others and the rest of the team will feel left out. It creates divisions within the team which you should avoid at all costs. Making sure you are not part of any clique is very important. You need to set the tone for how you expect your team to behave and model it.

WHAT IF YOUR OWN LINE MANAGER IS PART OF A CLIQUE?

You may find yourself in a situation where you are managing a team that has worked together for years and which includes your line manager. They may have even trained together. This is not an uncommon situation, but you must take control of it. Do not let your position be undermined by letting your staff bypass you and going to your line manager, who also happens to be an old friend, about issues pertaining to your ward.

If your line manager is taking time to listen to your staff concerns and starting to intervene without involving you, tell them how damaging the situation is. They may think that they are helping you out by listening to their friends/old colleagues and reporting back to you, but this can be more of a hindrance than a help. Once told, they will usually back off. The next line of action to take is to agree on a joint strategy with your line manager about what action you would prefer them to take when a member of your staff goes to them; i.e. refer them back to you and do not take the time to listen to their concerns until they have spoken with you first.

If your line manager allows the clique to continue and you find them liaising with your staff and not involving you, you could try explaining the situation to their line manager and asking for their intervention. Whatever you do, don't let the situation continue. It can gradually erode your confidence in your ward management skills and could be quite damaging for team morale.

BE SPECIFIC ABOUT EXPANDING NURSING ROLES

'Nursing is, apparently, what nurses do and nurses do whatever on earth needs doing' (Radcliffe 2005). This was written in response to the suggestion that foreign languages should be included in nurse training. Radcliffe concluded with the words, 'We don't always have to change nursing to fit the world's needs. Sometimes it's the things going on around it that need to change'. In other words, stop allowing nurses to continually take on extra roles just because someone else says it is needed. Extra roles should be taken on because it improves the patient care process and *causes no extra burden* for the staff. Expanded roles is an area where as a manager you have to be proactive. You can't afford to sit back and allow some staff to take on extra roles and other staff not to. It can cause great divides within your team. One example is intravenous cannulation. If you allow your nurses individually to decide whether or not to undertake training you may find that:

● those nurses who can cannulate will end up cannulating all the patients and not just their own
● doctors will resent the nurses who don't cannulate and will be less willing to undertake what they come to see as the nurses' role
● the nurses who don't cannulate will resent those who do, because they feel they are doing doctors' work and not their own
● patients will see nurses that do not cannulate as less experienced.

Before you allow any extra role to be taken on in your area, discuss it as a team first. Go through the advantages and disadvantages of the added responsibility. Decide together as a team whether to embrace the new role or reject it. It you decide to embrace it, then all members of the team must train and use the skills in practice.

DEVELOP GUIDELINES

Develop guidelines with the staff so that all agree the boundaries. For example, you may only wish to cannulate patients out of hours, because that is when the service is really needed and perhaps causes less disruption to the nurses' workload. The key to deciding whether to take on the role is to ask yourselves: Is the main reason for taking on this extra task to maximise the nurses' role or to minimise someone else's role?

Guidelines are less prescriptive than policies. Guidelines provide parameters within which your staff may practise safely. You should also clearly identify what the training needs are. Make sure you have the support of your organisation when taking on any expanded role. There may already be hospital-wide policies or guidelines on the subject. If you develop your own local ones, make sure they are validated by the standards committee so that you are protected through your organisation's vicarious liability. The law as it currently stands provides no barriers to the expanded role; it just requires nurses to be competent. The nurse only breaches their duty of care if the care falls short of what expert professionals would define as 'reasonable'.

As always, when you decide together with your team of staff to take on an extra role, you should also agree who will cover the work that you will not be able to do in order to take on the extra role.

BE PROACTIVE WITH ENFORCED MOVES OR MERGERS OF SERVICES

Health care managers are used to dealing with the frequent restructuring of services. On average organisations are now undertaking large-scale reorganisations at least once every three years (Whittington & Mayer 2002). It is widely recognised that in order to successfully reorganise, all staff should be given the opportunity to contribute and be involved in the changes. In other words, if your ward needs to be moved or merged with another, your managers should ensure that you and your staff are fully consulted and involved in making that decision including the consideration of all alternatives.

THE IMPORTANCE OF BEING POLITICALLY AWARE

Unfortunately you may find that you were not involved in making the decision. Some senior managers focus more on the outcome rather than the process of which communication and staff involvement is a great part. However, don't always blame the hospital board of directors or your managers if decisions are made without your involvement. You should also bear some of the blame. If you were making full use of your networking and political awareness skills, you would probably have ensured your full involvement. If you decide to concentrate on running your own ward without involving yourself in what else is going on within the organisation, you will be left out. So if you find yourself in such a situation, look at the skills and networks you need to develop to ensure it never happens again (see Ch. 9).

PLAN AHEAD

In the meantime, if you do suddenly find that your service is going to be restructured, you must plan ahead for this change. Even a relatively small change like moving your team to a different ward or site or merging with another team can result in long-lasting problems if not handled correctly. Staff morale can plummet, people will look elsewhere for jobs and the standard of care may well fall.

First, find out why the restructuring is required and explain the facts to your team. Take care not to procrastinate, backbite or talk negatively about the decision in front of your team. If you disagree with the enforced change, make your feelings known to your managers but only if you can offer a realistic alternative solution. If you cannot, you will have to accept the decision and then focus on your main objectives which are:

● supporting, involving and developing your team
● maintaining a good standard of patient care.

Develop a project plan with your team to manage the move or merger. Don't accept a plan developed by more senior managers. Only you and your staff will be able to identify and plan the finer details. Present the final project plan to your manager or, better still, involve your manager in the development of the plan.

DEVELOPING A PROJECT PLAN

So how do you develop a project plan? This is far easier than it sounds. The following steps will help you in the process:

Step 1: Find out what your deadline is for completing the move or merger.

Step 2: Inform your team as soon as possible. Take time to listen to their concerns and explain why the decision has been made. Make sure all valid concerns are relayed back to your manager in writing.

Step 3: Visit the area you are moving to or meet the manager of the team you will be merging with.

Step 4: Hold a team meeting for your staff in which you:

- brainstorm with all your team what issues need to be considered (e.g. equipment, extra skills that staff may need) and define the tasks that need to be undertaken
- break up the tasks into different phases, usually in terms of weeks (e.g. week 1, week 2, week 3, etc.)
- compile a simple Gantt chart (see Appendix 13.1)
- for each task, determine what needs to be done and by whom.

If you are merging with another team, hold the above meeting with both teams together.

Step 5: Set dates for regular review meetings with the team to review progress against the Gantt chart and identify any problems or issues that need further attention.

Always remember that you can never communicate enough in such situations. With a team covering 24 hours per day, seven days per week, you cannot communicate through team meetings alone. Use every other method open to you such as the ward communication book, handovers, staff noticeboard, etc.

INVOLVE THE EXPERTS FROM THE BEGINNING

Involve your finance manager in all stages of the plan to ensure that staff time and resources are appropriately costed and accounted for. Extra funding is usually allocated to assist with any move or merger: ensure that it is appropriately utilised.

Involve your HR manager, particularly if staff roles are changing. They will advise on the appropriate consultation and involvement of union representatives. Don't leave all this to your manager. You are the best person to lead the process. You understand the needs of your staff and patients better than anyone else. Your manager's role is to help, support and guide you through the process.

ACTION POINTS

- If you have difficulties with your manager, start thinking about the situation from their perspective and take positive steps to improve your working relationship.
- Read through your organisation's bullying and harassment policy and familiarise yourself with what is classed as 'unacceptable behaviour'.
- Take all staff complaints seriously to avoid the need for formal grievances to be made. If a formal grievance is made, read the policy and take action quickly to remain within the tight timescales of the policy.
- Concentrate on developing the skills of your staff to deal with arrogant or pushy senior health care professionals.
- Be aware and deal appropriately with any forms of discrimination particularly towards your staff from patients, relatives or other members of your team.
- Prepare your team carefully for new nurses recruited from overseas.
- Make sure your staff formally prioritise and make sure their decisions are relayed to the appropriate line manager in writing when staffing levels are dangerously low.
- Break up cliques using the 'off-duty' and using members of the clique to orientate new recruits. Devise a joint strategy with your own line manager to break up a clique if your line manager is involved.
- Decide jointly with your staff which expanded nursing roles you will all undertake ensuring the appropriate training and guidelines are available.
- Develop a project plan and Gantt chart with your team to help deal with any major changes, such as a ward move or merger.
- Don't ignore problematic colleagues. Take appropriate action now.

References

Allen H, Larson JA 2003 'We need respect': experiences of internationally recruited nurses in the UK. Report presented to the RCN, University of Surrey. Online. Available: http://www.rcn.org.uk/downloads/international/ irn-report-we-need-respect.pdf 2 Oct 2005

Nursing & Midwifery Council 2004 The NMC code of professional conduct: standards for conduct, performance and ethics. NMC, London. Online. Available: http://www.nmc-uk.org 2 Oct 2005

Radcliffe M 2005 Rear view (weekly column). Nursing Times 101(23):120

The Guardian 2004 Nurse wins £20 000 in race case. Press Association, Tuesday 18 May 2004. Online. Available: http:// www.guardian.co.uk/uk_news/story/0,,1219037,00.html

Whittington R, Mayer M 2002 Organising for success in the twenty-first century: a starting point for change. Chartered Institute of Personnel and Development, London

APPENDIX 13.1

EXAMPLE
OF SIMPLE GANTT CHART FOR WARD MOVE/MERGER

Actions	Week 1	Week 2	Week 3	Week 4	Week 5	Week 6	Week 7	Week 8
1. Equipment								
Compile equipment inventory	■	■						
Sort and label each piece							■	
2. Staffing								
Meet staff to clarify position		■						
Identify skills deficit			■					
Training and development								■
3. Review progress								
Meetings with whole team	■			■			■	
4. Documentation								
Gather all from both units	■							
Consult both teams		■	■					
Agree on best practice				■				
Communicate to all teams					■			
Sort out ordering process							■	
5. Guidelines and policies								
Identify all policies		■						
Set subgroups to merge				■				
6. Moving patients								
Agree plan with bed manager						■		
Stop admitting patients							■	
Transfer remaining patients								■

CHAPTER 14

MANAGE DIFFICULT STAFF

Staff who refuse to look professional or wear proper uniform 268

Is it an individual issue? 269

Is it a team issue? 269

Cultural, race and religious requirements 269

Staff who refuse to accept change 270

SWOT analysis 270

Staff who can't seem to prioritise their work 271

Getting staff to manage their time more effectively 271

Prevent burn-out 272

Maintaining good standards of care 273

Staff who are lazy 273

Dealing with those who lack motivation 274

Are they in the right job? 274

Staff who have alcohol problems 274

Staff who turn up for duty drunk 274

Staff who have a long-term drink problem 275

Members of staff who don't get on 276

Staff who are careless and sloppy 277

Use of competency packages 277

Use of positive feedback 278

Staff who manipulate situations for their own gain 278

Confront them directly 279

Don't be fooled by flattery 279

Laying the blame on you 279

Staff who moan and whinge 280

Challenge perceptions (including your own) 280

Don't allow a perpetual moaner to prevent progress 281

Holding a negative view of self 281

Staff who are continually late for duty 282

The problem with lateness 282

Getting to the root of the matter 282

Find a solution together 283

Prevention is better than cure 283

If you are having problems dealing with inappropriate behaviour from members of your team, you need to look firstly at your style of leadership. Have you established team objectives? Are you really listening to your team and providing them with regular feedback on their performance? Do you know them well and spend time enhancing their individual strengths within the team? If not, go back to Chapter 3 and review your own leadership style before you focus on dealing with the individual problem.

However, despite your excellent leadership skills, there may be the occasional instance when individuals in your team do behave in an unacceptable manner. These situations need to be dealt with swiftly. Be clear of your standards. Don't avoid the situation and don't let the individual(s) avoid you. The rest of the team will be watching you to see what you do. They will not respect a leader who ignores episodes of inappropriate behaviour.

STAFF WHO REFUSE TO LOOK PROFESSIONAL OR WEAR PROPER UNIFORM

If staff are deliberately flouting the uniform policy or dress code, it can be a sign of rebelliousness. Think first and foremost; is there any reason why your staff may wish to rebel against you? Disobedient behaviour is usually triggered when an individual feels that:

- they are not listened to
- their work is not fulfilling
- they have a controlling manager.

If you have shared objectives, listen and give regular feedback and know your staff well there should be little reason for individuals to want to rebel (see Ch. 3). But if you are having problems despite these measures, it is advisable to take action before the rest of the team follow suit and also start flouting the uniform policy. If you have any staff who refuse to dress or groom themselves appropriately for the job, they may be feeling unable to express themselves in any other way.

So what do you do? First, don't just tell them what the dress code is; you can be fairly certain they will know what the policy entails. The best way to approach them is to ask about their behaviour. But don't ask closed questions like:

'Do you object to wearing shoes rather than trainers?'
'Do you have a problem with removing your jewellery or tying your hair up?'

These questions can be interpreted as being confrontational. Instead, get the individual to cite the real reason by more open questioning. There will always be an underlying reason. Getting that reason to the surface depends on your questioning and listening abilities:

'Why are you wearing trainers/jewellery?'
'Why have you stopped tying your hair up?'

You may find you open a can of worms with answers such as:

'I don't feel we should be dictated to as to what we wear.'
'We are not at school any more, and I object to being treated like a child.'

These sorts of answers should be explored with further questioning. A simple 'why do you feel like that?' would suffice. They may wish to make a statement, so allow them to make it. Empathise with their predicament and support them to take action in another way.

Explain the rationale behind the policy, and the effects that their behaviour may be having on patients and others, such as:

● it may decrease people's confidence in their skills
● patients' health and safety may be compromised
● it is unfair to expose vulnerable people to an increased risk of infection
● the organisation will not be liable if a patient or member of staff is harmed in any way by the wearing of jewellery or trainers, etc. that are not recommended by the uniform policy.

IS IT AN INDIVIDUAL ISSUE?

If there is only one individual involved, make sure the discussion is held in private. People who want to make a statement may feel they have won if they feel that others have taken notice, or that they have got something in return for behaving this way.

Once you have listened to their issue, agree appropriate alternative action and ensure they agree to abide by the terms of the policy in future. Make sure they are aware that if they continually breach the uniform policy or dress code they are liable to disciplinary action. Remember to let them know that you will be making a file note of the discussion and agreed actions (see Ch. 4).

IS IT A TEAM ISSUE?

If you have recently taken over a new team as a ward manager, you may find yourself confronted with several members or even the whole team who are not adhering to the uniform policy. It can be a tricky situation if they have been doing this for years. It would be advisable in such a situation to raise the issue at a team meeting and have a general discussion about dress codes and uniform issues.

CULTURAL, RACE AND RELIGIOUS REQUIREMENTS

While all staff should adhere to the uniform policy, you must be sensitive to the needs of different cultures, races and religions. You should be able to accommodate these needs within the uniform policy. If there are particular difficulties, consult your human resources (HR) advisor. It would not be appropriate to discipline staff for noncompliance from having to adhere to a particular cultural, race or religious dress code.

STAFF WHO REFUSE TO ACCEPT CHANGE

Some staff are so set in their ways that they can be rather obstinate when you want to change something at work. Remember that most people don't like change and that we all (generally) would like to keep the status quo. In the majority of cases, staff who refuse to change are doing so because they have not been consulted or involved in identifying the need for the change. Keeping staff fully *informed* at each stage is insufficient. They must be fully *involved* at each stage of the process.

If, for example, you wish to implement team nursing where previously you have been using patient allocation you cannot expect your staff to simply conform even if you have explained your rationale and the advantages many times over. The key to implementing something like this effectively is to start right at the beginning by analysing the original problem with your team. In other words, get them together and look at what is wrong with the current system before you start suggesting the solution. Team nursing is a solution. Do the team have a problem with patient allocation? If so, what do they suggest should be done? Everyone will have different views; they must be listened to. You could use a theoretical model such as a 'SWOT analysis' to help you.

SWOT ANALYSIS

SWOT stands for 'strengths, weaknesses, opportunities and threats'.
Draw a matrix (Fig. 14.1) and get your team to identify:

● the strengths and weaknesses of your current system (internal)
● the opportunities and threats which may affect any future system (external).

Figure 14.1 SWOT analysis

Appendix 14.1 gives an example of a SWOT analysis. This tool helps teams to identify the weaknesses and threats of the current system. But don't leave it there, otherwise you will just be left with a long list of factors and no attempt to do anything about it.

Getting your team to 'own' the solution

Your next step is to identify with the team what can be done to overcome the weaknesses and threats and make the most of your strengths and forthcoming opportunities. Your team may identify team nursing or they may suggest an alternative solution. Only when you have all reached agreement about what needs to be done should you begin the process of planning and implementing the change. Doing it this way round will reduce the chances of staff refusing to change. If anyone does not want to change, they need to come up with a valid alternative solution. You will have given them ample opportunity to do this at your initial meeting.

Remember to make sure that all members of your team have the opportunity to take part. Keep notes of the meeting and make sure everyone gets to see them.

STAFF WHO CAN'T SEEM TO PRIORITISE THEIR WORK

Some staff will continually stay late in order to:

● complete their evaluations
● finish off a task that could easily be delegated to someone else
● see to other patients whom they have neglected by concentrating on giving a high standard of care to a select few patients.

People like this tend to be perfectionists. They may lose track of time and priorities by continually striving to maintain high standards of care. However, in this day and age with higher patient turnover, increasingly complex care requirements and continual staff shortages, maintaining exceptionally high standards of care all the time is not always realistic.

Sometimes staff have to be given permission to lower their standards in order to ensure that *all* patients receive adequate care rather than the ideal standard of exceptional care. If you allow them to continue striving to achieve these exceptionally high standards, it will result in either:

1. They become exhausted and end up going off sick or leaving, or
2. Some patients receive exceptionally high standards of care at the expense of others.

GETTING STAFF TO MANAGE THEIR TIME MORE EFFECTIVELY

Don't be tempted to send people on time management courses unless they are particularly aimed at clinical staff. These courses are usually geared towards office workers or people who have little experience of tending to the demands of sick people. Teaching people to manage their time at work becomes a lot more complex where unpredictable patient care is involved.

A more effective method of helping them would be to take some time to work alongside the individual, preferably for whole shifts at a time. That way you (or one of the more senior members of your team) can show them how to prioritise their work and break it up into sections with deadlines. Your seniority will also give them permission to lower their standards when necessary, such as in times of staff shortages. An example is helping a patient with partial paralysis from a recent stroke to get dressed. A high standard of care would be:

● to encourage the patient to do things for themselves throughout the process
● to spend time talking through the techniques they use, giving positive feedback and corrections where necessary
● to discuss any worries or concerns they may have
● to only physically intervene when absolutely necessary.

However, rehabilitation takes a lot of time and patience. If the nurse has six patients in a similar position, delivering an exceptionally high standard of care for every one of them may simply not be feasible within the time limits of their shift. They can either give all six an adequate standard of care, i.e. talk the patient through some of the process and physically help them through the rest, or purposefully delay some parts of their care until the later shift come on duty.

Many nurses have learned how to do this through experience, but some are reluctant to lower their standards and end up exhausted by not taking their breaks or staying on late to finish their work. People who work like this rarely complain. They simply get on with it thinking that they have to make sacrifices in order to deliver a high standard of care. Watch for people like this and take action before you end up with an exhausted and stressed member of staff. Often it is their home life and self-esteem that suffers long before the stress and exhaustion become an issue at work. By the time they reach the stage of taking time off sick, you will have a member of your team close to 'burnout'.

PREVENT BURN-OUT

By spending time working with the individual, you can show them how to work out which aspects of their work are the real priorities and which are their own personal priorities. You cannot just tell people how to plan and prioritise their care at the beginning of the shift; things always change. A patient's condition may unexpectedly deteriorate or there may be unexpected admissions or transfers. If you work the whole shift with the nurse, you can show them how to reprioritise as changes occur.

MAINTAINING GOOD STANDARDS OF CARE

While it is advisable to ensure staff do not exhaust themselves maintaining unrealistically high standards, don't become too complacent about lowering standards of care to fit in with increasing demand. It should not come to be seen as normal practice. If your workload is increasing, make sure you are doing something about getting more staff added to your establishment to deal with the extra work. If staffing shortages are becoming a regular occurrence, you should be working closely with your manager to find ways of reducing the workload temporarily until you can increase your staffing levels.

STAFF WHO ARE LAZY

People may slip into lazy habits when they see their work as boring or unrewarding. They become much slower at work, perpetuate gossip and spend time on less important tasks rather than the ones that really matter.

Lazy people, if left to their own devices, will try to get away with doing as little work as possible. This is usually because of one of three things:

1. They are lethargic due to physical or mental illness.
2. Their personal life takes all their energy.
3. They lack motivation.

Before you take action, try and identify which one of the three it is. If the laziness is intermittent, then it may be because they lack motivation. If it is a permanent feature, there may be an underlying cause, such as illness. If it is because of poor physical or mental health (e.g. stress, depression or a long-term back problem) consider referring them to their GP or the occupational health department for advice. Some time off sick may be all that they need to recuperate.

They may be having difficulty juggling their family commitments with work. If this is the case, find out what you can do to enable them to adapt their working hours around family life such as:

● more flexible shift patterns
● different start and finish times
● temporary reduction in hours.

You may feel that their family life is their own problem but such an attitude is unwise. Your role as manager is to enable your staff to provide their best efforts. Give less to your staff and your staff will give less to you. Whatever you do, you cannot ignore the issue otherwise they will continue to be paid the same as their colleagues for providing less work. It could lead to resentment from the rest of your team.

On the other hand, if a staff member is putting more energies into their personal life and thinks nothing of going out 'clubbing' between late and early shifts, they obviously do not value or appreciate their responsibilities as part of your team. This may well be a sign that they lack motivation at work.

DEALING WITH THOSE WHO LACK MOTIVATION

People who are lazy for reasons other than illness or overwhelming personal responsibilities have discovered a way of not doing something that they don't want to do. Spending time talking to someone or persistently 'telling them off' because of their perceived laziness will do no good at all. Their experience shows them that doing more is not in their best interests, so why should they change? The rewards for doing less work are probably far more preferable than the consequences of being reprimanded. Lazy people are clever people; you should try and channel this cleverness into areas that do interest them.

Find out how you can motivate them: it's all part and parcel of being a good leader – knowing what makes each individual in your team tick and taking time to work on those motivators (see p. 52). The unfortunate thing about managing people in health care is that you cannot provide monetary rewards, but there are other ways. Giving good feedback in front of others helps. Find out what part of their role they like and ensure they get to do this part only if they complete the 'boring' part. Reward-based systems have their place.

This is all about work/life balance. Whether the person is working too hard or playing too hard, the critical thing for you as their manager is to get them to re-evaluate and redress the imbalance.

ARE THEY IN THE RIGHT JOB?

If a member of your staff cannot summon up any enthusiasm at all for their job then it might be best to encourage them to consider whether this is the right job for them. If the work in your ward is not stimulating for them, despite your best efforts, then perhaps they are working in the wrong environment. Don't take this personally. Work with them to find out where their skills lie and what they really want to do, then help them towards that goal. Help to provide them with the appropriate training and development for their chosen role, and provide assistance with job applications, interviews and references on condition that they pull their weight at work in the meantime. At the very least, you are providing them with the required motivation to stop being lazy whilst they remain with you looking for another job.

STAFF WHO HAVE ALCOHOL PROBLEMS

STAFF WHO TURN UP FOR DUTY DRUNK

What do you do when a member of staff turns up for duty who is obviously under the influence of alcohol? The answer is simple: send them home again. This can only be done by someone who is the person's direct line manager. If you are not on duty, the nurse-in-charge should consult with your line manager or whoever is on call. That manager will then make the decision to send the staff member home.

There is usually no need to suspend the member of staff from duty or prevent their return the next day or when their next shift is due. Suspension of staff is usually only required if there is a risk of potential harm to patients or staff (or themselves). Check your policy, however, as some policies cite being under the influence of alcohol as grounds for automatic suspension.

The next step is to instigate a formal investigation into the incident. This is often done by an HR advisor, but could be anyone who is unrelated to the incident. They will interview all witnesses and formal statements will be taken. The staff member who was sent home will also be interviewed as part of the investigatory process. This gives them a chance to give their side of the story. Remember to ensure that any members of staff who are interviewed and required to give formal statements should be informed of their rights to have a trade union representative, colleague or friend present. Some investigators forget this very important part of the process.

The person appointed to carry out the investigation will gather all the evidence together in the form of a report and make recommendations. It all needs to be done as soon as possible after the event. The recommended action will depend on whether it is the individual's first offence and whether their actions were serious and detrimental to patient care.

If it is their first offence

If it is the person's first offence of this kind, you will probably be able to issue a verbal or written warning depending on the circumstances. When you ask them to attend a meeting to give a verbal or written warning, you must inform them that is what you are going to do and tell them of their rights to have representation at that meeting. They should also be given another chance to give their version of events.

If it is not the first offence or the offence is of a more serious nature

If this is not the first time that this has happened, or the person's actions were serious and detrimental to patient care, the investigation report may recommend a disciplinary hearing. Again, at this hearing you have the option to issue a formal verbal or written warning. If the circumstances surrounding the incident were very serious and compromised patient care, you could make a decision to dismiss at the disciplinary hearing.

STAFF WHO HAVE A LONG-TERM DRINK PROBLEM

Managing substandard work or misconduct due to prolonged alcoholism is an entirely different process. You usually have the option of using any one of the three following procedures, depending on the circumstances:

1. Disciplinary procedure.
2. Capability or competency procedure.
3. Sickness/absence procedure.

There may also be a drugs/alcohol policy that you would need to refer to. Always consult your HR advisor, who will guide you as to which policy is most appropriate.

You should offer reasonable support if any members of staff admit that they have a problem with alchohol or drugs and who are prepared to make a concerted effort to overcome this. Your role is to treat these staff with sympathy and in complete confidence. Make sure you involve the occupational health department at an early stage. Part of your support process should include the granting of leave to see their GP or attend counselling sessions. Such action will be considered in the event of disciplinary action but will not be seen as an alternative to disciplinary action if it is deemed necessary.

In any event, be aware that your prime concern is the protection of the patients. If any registered nurse fails in their duty of care towards their patients due to the influence of alcohol, you can dismiss them at a disciplinary hearing and you may also be obliged to recommend their removal from the register.

MEMBERS OF STAFF WHO DON'T GET ON

Allowing personal differences to get in the way of work is unprofessional and should not be tolerated. Since you are the one who is responsible for creating the right environment for good teamwork, you have a big role to play when members of your team don't get on. If left unattended to, the situation can end up affecting the whole team. You must step in at once or other members of the team will begin choosing sides. Those not caught up in the conflict will look to you to resolve it. They will see it as a failure on your part if you allow the situation to continue.

Five steps to resolving conflict within your team immediately are:

Step 1: Bring the two team members into your office to work together on some sort of solution. Give them each some time to explain their position. They need to know that you have given them the chance to air their grievances. Don't give them more than five to ten minutes each. You are their manager, not a counsellor. Don't let them interrupt each other, find fault or try to apportion blame.

Step 2: Once they have explained their sides, ask them each to say what they feel the other person should do differently. Make sure their solutions are clear and 'do-able'. Something like 'I want her to change her attitude' is too general and doesn't get you anywhere. Get them to be more specific; get them to say exactly what they want the other person to stop doing, such as 'I want her to stop pulling a face and walking off whenever I ask her to do something for me'. Then get them to say what they want the other person to do instead, such as 'I want her to tell me straight if she is unhappy with what I have asked her to do and why'.

Step 3: When these actions have been clarified, get each side to commit to doing at least one of the suggested solutions. Get them to agree to give each other feedback and show appreciation for the times when the other person has made the effort to change. This gets them to focus on the positive side of things.

Step 4: Let them know in no uncertain terms that it is down to them to make this work. If they do not make the effort and allow the situation to continue, inform them that you will have no choice but to take formal action.

Step 5: Make a brief file note of the discussion including an outline of the agreed actions. Let them read it through and sign if necessary.

Following this discussion, make it a priority to observe them closely over the next few weeks. Give them positive feedback when you notice a change in their behaviours. Hopefully the situation will resolve. However, if it does not improve within a few weeks (don't leave it any longer), bring them into your office again and outline the formal route that you will take should you see no improvement over the next couple of weeks. Again, make another file note.

Hopefully, the situation will be resolved following the second meeting. But if it is not, go straight to your HR advisor who will point you in the direction of the appropriate organisational policy and guide you through the formal process.

STAFF WHO ARE CARELESS AND SLOPPY

It can be really frustrating when dealing with members of staff who don't give enough attention to the important details when caring for patients. Their work can be hurried and sloppy but they are quite content and think that they are doing fine. Some people tend to make lots of mistakes but don't seem to see it as a problem. Important observations may not be done, discharge arrangements will be left for the next shift or patients requiring rehabilitation will be washed and dressed with no attention paid to assisting them to help themselves. They find paying attention to detail as tiresome and dull.

One of the problems with having someone like this in your team is that they cause resentment amongst the rest of the staff who consistently have to pick up the pieces. If you don't do anything about it, you are effectively sanctioning their behaviour. They will be perfectly happy to continue thinking that the rest of the team are at fault for making such a fuss.

USE OF COMPETENCY PACKAGES

Usually these types of people need to be told to slow down and take more responsibility for their patient care. You have to reiterate what the expected standards are. However, just telling them may not be sufficient. If the member of staff is junior and inexperienced, it may be a simple case of allocating a mentor to work through a competency package with them.

If the individual in question is more senior and experienced, why not get them to *develop* competencies or *review* the competency package that you already have in place. Make sure that the areas of care being overlooked are included in the package. For example, if your area cares for patients requiring rehabilitation, do the competencies specify how to assist the patients to help themselves rather than do everything for them? Does it assess the person's knowledge of when and why observations should be carried out? Does it set out each stage of the discharge process that should be covered and when?

Helping to write these standards down in the form of competencies usually helps to stimulate the member of staff about the quality of care they are expected to provide rather than what they have got away with over the years. You may prefer to do this as part of a team meeting or discussion to help raise standards generally across the team.

USE OF POSITIVE FEEDBACK

Reward the individual for when they have paid attention to detail by giving frequent positive feedback. When the work has not been done, get them to go back and correct or finish their work where possible. They need to learn that there are consequences for not producing an adequate standard of work.

Be prepared to stick at it. Staff who are careless and sloppy in their work will not change overnight. They have to unlearn their habits and acquire new ones, which takes time. If, after three to six months, you find that they have really not changed their ways, you should question their capability for undertaking the role. Most organisations have a policy which guides you through a specific process consisting of meetings and action plans to improve a person's capability (see Ch. 4). Ultimately you could make the decision to terminate their employment if the process is unsuccessful, but you must have explored all other avenues first and kept a full record of all your actions in the form of file notes.

STAFF WHO MANIPULATE SITUATIONS FOR THEIR OWN GAIN

Some staff are pretty astute when it comes to getting their own way. This behaviour often becomes apparent when it has something to do with requests and the 'off-duty'. There are some staff who, no matter what, will have their requests and they do not care what effect it has on other staff. You may be familiar with excuses such as:

'You told me if I put the request in first then I could have it'
'You promised me last year that I could have that weekend'
'I spoke to HR and they said that I could take four weeks' annual leave together and that you can't refuse to give it to me'.

Manipulators will often play off one person against the other. They will go to more senior people if they cannot get their own way. This is particularly rife if they are aware that you and your manager do not communicate well, or have any differences. Prevent this by ensuring that you never let staff know if there are problems between you or anyone else within your organisation. Manipulators are constantly on the lookout for these and will take advantage of any perceived breakdown in communications between you and your colleagues. Don't give them the opportunity.

CONFRONT THEM DIRECTLY

Often the only way to deal with these people is to confront them directly. Don't try and beat them at their own game, because that is what you will make it – a game. Tell them exactly what you think is going on; the chances are that they will be taken by surprise. Many people who do this do it as a way of life and are unaware that their behaviour might be determined as manipulation. Explain that if they had taken a more straightforward approach, and simply asked you rather than going to someone else, they could have got what they wanted without any hassle. However, as they have now gone to someone else to try and override your authority, you are seeing things in a different light and are reluctant to concede to their demands. Tell them in future they must be more direct in their approach.

Another way is to meet with the other person whom they used to try and manipulate you. Explain the situation to them and ask the manipulator to meet with you both and explain their actions, and perhaps even apologise. It could shame them into ensuring they don't do it again. Remember to praise them or give positive feedback in the future each time they do use a more direct approach for something they want.

DON'T BE FOOLED BY FLATTERY

Managing a ward or department can be very isolating and it is easy to be unduly influenced by a member of staff who tells you that you are wonderful, so knowledgeable, so capable or the best boss they have ever worked for. Be careful of the underlying agenda. Good factual feedback should be welcomed but a quick thank you is enough and don't let it sway your judgement or treatment of that person.

LAYING THE BLAME ON YOU

With the ever-increasing emphasis on accountability within health care, you may find that some staff are reluctant to take responsibility for their mistakes. You may hear phrases such as:

'Sister said I could do this'

'You told us that it didn't matter if we didn't do all the observations when it was busy'

'It wasn't my fault. If you hadn't agreed to admit those extra patients, this would never have happened'.

In situations such as these, don't be tempted to go into defensive mode with replies such as:

'I did not say that'

'When I said that I did not mean for you to go ahead and do this'

'It's not my fault either; don't blame me'.

Don't get into a discussion about who is to blame: concentrate on what is to be done about the situation. Get people to focus on generating solutions. Then once the problem has been dealt with, discuss and agree what steps to take to ensure there is no confusion or further misunderstanding in future similiar situations.

STAFF WHO MOAN AND WHINGE

There will always be people for whom nothing ever goes right. If life isn't perfect (which it never is) they feel hard done by. Life seems to be so much better for everyone else. Other people get their weekends off, get more pay, do less work, have better working conditions, etc. For some staff, anything that is less than perfect at work (and at home) is an excuse to whinge.

The thing about people who moan and whinge is that they never seem to do anything about the situation. If they did that, there would be nothing to moan about. They often perceive themselves as not being able to do anything and think that the solution always lies with others referred to as 'they' and 'them'. You can easily get used to this sort of behaviour and just accept that's how they are and get on with things. The problem with having people like this on your team is that their behaviour is infectious. Once someone starts moaning in the coffee room during break time, everyone will join in.

CHALLENGE PERCEPTIONS (INCLUDING YOUR OWN)

One way of dealing with such people is to review how you perceive them. Changes to systems often take place when someone is not happy with current circumstances. If nurtured, these people could become your agents for change.

Whenever you catch them moaning and whinging about something, your worst response would be to listen and sympathise. A better response would be to ask them to suggest a solution. This may catch them by surprise, as they would probably not be used to such a response. They may be more used to getting people to agree and moan with them. People who are challenged to do something about the situation tend to stop moaning at the very least because what you are really saying is 'if you're not prepared to do anything about it, then stop moaning'.

DON'T ALLOW A PERPETUAL MOANER TO PREVENT PROGRESS

If you have an idea that you want to raise with your staff, present it to each of them individually before raising it at a team meeting. Ask for their ideas and feedback. When you eventually raise the idea at a team meeting, you can ensure that most of the team will support your idea. If an individual realises that they are on their own with their usual negative opinions, they will rarely speak up. If they do, then ask them and the rest of the team what an alternative solution would be. Don't dwell on any negatives; focus on the positives. Always have an answer ready for the usual negative responses (Table 14.1).

HOLDING A NEGATIVE VIEW OF SELF

Some staff will consistently moan and whinge that they are not good enough:

  'Here's the work you asked me to do; it's not very good.'
  'I went to that meeting for you, but I was useless. I'm too shy to be any
    good at that sort of thing.'
  'I'm too fat/too thin/too old/not intelligent enough.'

All these sorts of comments do is demonstrate a lack of confidence. Sometimes it's done to protect them from negative feedback. If they've said it themselves then someone else is hardly likely to say it again. If you are continuously giving your team positive feedback (that is, every single day) then you will be very unlikely to hear these things. So if it is happening, question your style of leadership; are you giving enough feedback (see p. 51)?

Obviously you will get the odd one or two people who will put themselves down in order to get people to tell them how wonderful they are. Don't fall for that one. Tell them if you didn't think they were good enough they wouldn't be part of their team, and you don't want to hear them talking like that again, and leave it at that. Don't indulge them.

TABLE 14.1: Sample answers for negative responses within meetings

Negative response	Answer
'I don't see how it will work. They will never allow us to do that.'	Ask who it is when they refer to 'they' or 'them'. Ask why they think that, and then explain why there is clearly no question you will not be allowed to.
'It's all been tried before and it never makes any difference.'	'Well, I'm sorry it didn't work out for you before, but this time it is different because . . .'
'It's always back to us. Why should we have to do all the work?'	If you want to see things improve, then you have to make the effort. Moaning and whinging will achieve nothing, but taking action will.

STAFF WHO ARE CONTINUALLY LATE FOR DUTY

We've probably all done it; seethed in silence when a member of staff wanders into handover five or ten minutes late. Not only that, but some even have the nerve to grab a cup of coffee on their way.

THE PROBLEM WITH LATENESS

Lateness causes huge problems within teams, but some ward managers do little, if anything, to put a stop to it. Some don't even monitor lateness. In many other areas of work, people have less need to start on time because their jobs are outcome-focused. This means that as long as they get the job done, it doesn't really matter when or even where they work. But in nursing and any other jobs that involve shift work, getting to work on time has a greater importance. Arriving late results in:

- interruption and delaying of handover
- staff from the previous shift getting off late as they have to repeat everything for the latecomers
- the latecomer risking missing vital information about their patients and therefore compromising their ability to care for the patients when the previous shift goes home
- reduced morale and working relationships within the team becoming fragmented.

Ignore lateness at your peril. If allowed to continue, it may become accepted as normal practice. The staff will become divided into those that are conscientious and come in on time and those that simply don't bother. Consistent lateness is a reflection of poor attitudes about work.

GETTING TO THE ROOT OF THE MATTER

If you notice that a member of staff is regularly coming to work late, you should first try to uncover the underlying causes. If they are having genuine problems getting to work on time, such as their bus timetable being incompatible with shift start times, then it is better to compromise and formally agree to a later start time. That way, working practice can change in advance to accommodate this.

If you come to the conclusion that it is simply a poor attitude to work or because some staff are not committed, then you need to consider your leadership style again:

1. Are your team working towards shared goals?
2. Do you spend time really listening to what individuals have to say?
3. Do you give some positive feedback to each member of staff every time you work with them?
4. Do you know each individual in your team well?

If you hesitated or answered no to any of the above questions, then perhaps you need to ascertain what else you can do to provide a more motivating environment (see Ch. 3).

FIND A SOLUTION TOGETHER

If a member of staff continues to arrive late for duty despite you having ascertained that there are no extenuating personal circumstances and you know you have done everything outlined in Chapter 3 to maintain a motivating environment, the next step is to concentrate on finding a solution *with* them. Don't continually ask them why they are late each time. If you do, you will just receive a barrage of excuses. Turn the question round to make them suggest a solution: 'Despite our previous meeting, you still turn up late for most of your shifts. What can we do about it?'.

Don't allow the rest of your staff to accommodate lateness. They must not wait to give handover. Ensure they always start on time without them. Make sure they do not summarise what the latecomer has missed. They must be made to catch up themselves afterwards. They'll soon learn. If they don't, you have two options.

Option 1: Aim towards the disciplinary process

When dealing with persistent lateness, it is essential that you keep accurate records of all episodes, including lateness from lunch breaks. You must be able to demonstrate that you have met with the staff member to determine any possible solutions and agree actions. Make sure that during your meetings you have at some stage outlined when the lateness qualifies for disciplinary action. Always consult your HR advisor before making any decision to apply the disciplinary process. Before you take this route, you need to show that you have fully explored all possible solutions.

Option 2: Encourage them to look at other roles where they will be stimulated

Continual lateness, despite the actions outlined above, indicates that they are not committed to this job so perhaps it is not the right one for them. If you have a member of staff who is truly not happy in their work, they may simply be in the wrong specialty. Don't give up on them and wait for them to leave. Help them to identify what job would really stimulate them and assist them in developing the skills to be able to apply for a post in their chosen field. Whatever happens, you do not want staff leaving your ward and telling others how they hated working in your area. Helping them to attain their chosen job will see them leave on a more positive note.

PREVENTION IS BETTER THAN CURE

Make sure you have included in your induction package:

● what time shifts begin at and what time is considered late
● how to let staff know if they will be late
● when and how disciplinary action will be undertaken for lateness.

Many organisations now have some sort of code of conduct for their employees. This usually includes the above points, so inclusion of the document in the induction package may suffice.

Remember also that if you expect staff to be punctual in their arrival to work then you should also meet their expectations of getting off work on time. Don't expect staff to stay late (unless you are paying them extra). Giving time back is insufficient compensation for staff having to stay late regularly at work.

ACTION POINTS

- Ensure your staff adhere to the uniform policy. If any refuse, find out why, listen to their point of view and propose alternative solutions. Take the disciplinary route if appropriate.
- Involve all your staff in all changes by presenting them with the initial problem first and asking for proposed solutions. Do not present the solution first.
- Don't allow any staff to regularly stay behind to finish work or miss their breaks. Work with them if necessary to help develop their prioritising skills.
- If you feel a member of your staff is lazy, find out first if they have any illness, personal problems or simply lack motivation. Take action to increase their motivation either to work more efficiently or find another job.
- Be aware of the process to take should a member of staff turn up unfit for work through alcohol or drugs, so that the appropriate action is taken in any such event.
- Resolve any problems between members of your team by calling them to a meeting immediately and taking specific action. Do not allow any situation of conflict to be allowed to continue.
- Use competency packages to improve the skills of junior staff. Get any senior staff with poor standards to review the competency packages, thus improving their own skills in the process.
- Confront any staff who try to manipulate you.
- Encourage your staff to transform any negative statements into positive solutions.
- Take action immediately to put a stop to any staff who are persistently late for duty or back late from breaks. Show the rest of your team that you will not tolerate lateness.
- Ensure your ward induction package includes a section on how staff are expected to behave.

EXAMPLE OF A SWOT ANALYSIS OF CURRENT MODE OF NURSING CARE DELIVERY – PATIENT ALLOCATION

Strengths (*internal*)	Weaknesses (internal)
Nurses get variety of experience	Lack of continuity
Allocated nurse has full responsibility for patients	Lack of responsibility for long-term issues (e.g. discharge planning)
Patients get to see more nurses	Patients unable to build up relationship with same nurses
Each nurse brings different skills	Lack of information on ward rounds

Opportunities (*external*)	Threats (*external*)
Integrated care pathways being introduced – helps with continuity	Recruitment freeze, so less staff
Less writing, more time to care	Restrictive shift practices with EU directive
Proposed new ward layout in 6-bed bays	Proposed move and merger with neighbouring ward
	Flexible working policy affecting handover times
	Increased reliance on agency staff

CHAPTER 15

GET THE BEST ADVICE

Know where to go for legal advice **288**

Solicitors **288**

Trade union stewards **288**

Know where to go for professional advice **289**

The director of nursing **289**

The Nursing and Midwifery Council **289**

University lecturers **290**

Utilise the wide range of services from the chaplaincy department **290**

Bereavement **290**

Staff support **290**

Staff training and development **291**

Increase staff awareness **291**

Use but don't abuse the nurse specialists **291**

Different education and development responsibilities **292**

Be wary of de-skilling your staff **292**

Link nurse roles **293**

Help patients and relatives access the right advice **293**

Patient advice and liaison service **293**

Information leaflets **294**

Ward rounds and visits from other health professionals **294**

Keep up-to-date with risk management issues **295**

Performance indicators for risk management **295**

Hospital risk management committee **295**

Directorate risk management committee **295**

Consult policies, procedures and guidelines **296**

Why so many policies? **296**

Make sure they are accessible at all times **296**

Make sure your team know when elements have changed **297**

Evidence-based guidelines **297**

Maximise computer access **297**

The worldwide web **297**

Getting your staff to use computers **298**

European Computer Driving Licence **298**

Utilise the knowledge and skills of your nursing colleagues **299**

Channel the enthusiasm within your team **299**

Make finding information a staff development opportunity **299**

Draw on the experience of your peers **300**

Use email **300**

Utilise the practice development team **300**

When making decisions, try not to rely on just one source of advice. How do you know for sure that the person's advice is sound? How do you know they are giving you the best option? Try to seek advice from a variety of sources. That way you will be able to make a more informed decision based on as many facts and opinions as you can access. Include your team in this when you can. Enable them to have an input and influence over the decisions you have to make which affect them.

There are various departments within health care organisations to which you can go for advice. Some are underutilised by nurse managers. As a senior person within the organisation you have access to solicitors, senior professional advisors, educational advisors, counselling services, human resource advisors, computer experts and many more. You should never have to make decisions or struggle with any aspects of your work without being able to access the appropriate support.

KNOW WHERE TO GO FOR LEGAL ADVICE

SOLICITORS

NHS organisations appoint solicitors to act and advise on their behalf in respect of legal issues. If you require legal advice regarding a problem that has arisen or may arise at work, most NHS organisations have a procedure in place through which you can access these solicitors. This procedure is in place to ensure that they are not being asked the same questions from different areas within the organisation. The solicitors can usually be accessed through the person who deals with litigation and claims, known as the litigation and claims manager, legal services manager or clinical governance manager. The title differs within different organisations.

It is advisable to find out who the appropriate person is within your organisation and to keep a copy of their contact details available at all times for both you and your staff. Your director of nursing should be your first port of call for any professional issues. They have more experience and may be able to advise without calling on the solicitors.

If you have an emergency out of hours, contact the duty manager who will be able to access the solicitors. Some solicitors provide a 24-hour helpline for advice on clinical issues, but this number would usually be restricted for the use of a 'named' senior manager or on-call managers. Some NHS organisations hold contracts with solicitors that include free training for staff, which is well worth accessing, but often you will have to ask first. This service is not usually widely advertised.

TRADE UNION STEWARDS

Every NHS organisation has a trade union steward whose role is to protect members' rights and ensure they are treated fairly. Union stewards are specifically trained for the role. They will provide help and guidance with issues concerning employment rights, discrimination, health and safety legislation and concerns about poor practices. You can also get advice regarding legal or potential legal issues directly from your local regional office.

Both the Royal College of Nursing (RCN) and Unison provide their members with online advice services where you can get information on legal issues (Royal College of Nursing 2005a, Unison 2005).

KNOW WHERE TO GO FOR PROFESSIONAL ADVICE

THE DIRECTOR OF NURSING

One of the key responsibilities of your nursing director is to provide professional leadership to all nurses within the organisation. They will provide advice personally or they will direct you to the appropriate place to find the information you require. If you have a nonclinical line manager and need advice on a professional matter, there is no reason why you cannot contact your director or assistant director of nursing directly. Use the phone if it is an emergency; otherwise use email. Directors of nursing may be the most senior nurses within your organisation but they recognise that ward managers are a vital asset and will go out of their way to ensure you can access the appropriate professional advice and support.

Most nurse directors have at least one assistant director plus a small team of senior health care professionals to assist them in their corporate-wide role. The nursing director together with their team provide a support system for nurses and allied health care professionals and help them maintain high standards of care across the organisation.

THE NURSING AND MIDWIFERY COUNCIL

The main aim of the Nursing and Midwifery Council (NMC) is to ensure that registered nurses and midwives provide high standards of care, and to protect the public. This is achieved by:

- maintaining the professional register
- setting standards
- investigating and dealing with allegations of misconduct
- providing a professional advice service for nurses and midwives.

The advice service is free and confidential. It is provided by a team of professionals qualified in various specialties such as mental health nursing, paediatric nursing, adult nursing and learning disabilities. You can email or call one of the professional officers with your query or access information from their website: http://www.nmc-uk.org.

In addition you can access all current NMC publications such as 'Guidelines for records and record-keeping' or 'How to complain about a nurse or midwife'. These can all be downloaded free from their website.

UNIVERSITY LECTURERS

Your link lecturer is the obvious choice for advice regarding issues in your specialty, but there is no reason why you cannot access other university lecturers for expert advice. Most would be only too happy to provide information within their specialty. Email is usually the best approach to use as lecturers can be difficult to access by phone due to their Monday to Friday working pattern and tight teaching schedules.

Keep a copy of the annual course prospectus from your local university's department of nursing studies or health and social care. This will contain all the contact details of the lecturers in each specialty. You will find most lecturers helpful in professional matters and usually, if they do not know the answer, they will be able to refer you to someone who does.

UTILISE THE WIDE RANGE OF SERVICES FROM THE CHAPLAINCY DEPARTMENT

Chaplaincy services are under-used by some ward managers. They usually offer an excellent service which involves more than just providing spiritual care to patients of various faiths. They also provide a service for staff, including those who do not profess any particular faith. The chaplaincy services can be invaluable when your staff are going through a particularly hard time, such as dealing with difficult deaths or more deaths than usual. They can also be very supportive in times of staff shortages when staff are distressed at being unable to meet the usual high standards of care.

BEREAVEMENT

Part of the role of the chaplaincy department is to educate staff in dealing with bereavement (Department of Health 2003). They can also provide support to members of your team who suffer a personal bereavement. However, they will not come to you; you have to access these services in times of need. It can be difficult if you do not know them very well. It is better to prepare by building up a good relationship with your chaplaincy team before you get to the stage of requesting their services.

STAFF SUPPORT

It does not matter if you or your staff are not religious. Hospital chaplaincy services do not inflict their religious beliefs. Their role is to meet both religious and spiritual needs and they are not concerned about whether or not staff go to church.

It would be wise to include a meeting with a member of the chaplaincy service as part of your induction programme for new members of staff (if your trust-wide induction programme does not already include this).

STAFF TRAINING AND DEVELOPMENT

Chaplains working in health care receive specialist training, education and experience in working with people in challenging situations. They can contribute to your staff training programme in a number of subjects such as:

- listening skills
- dealing with difficult situations
- appreciation of religious and cultural diversity
- advanced directives or 'living wills'.

Their skills may also be helpful in the facilitation of clinical supervision groups for your staff.

Consider inviting one of the chaplaincy team to some of your ward meetings. Their skills may be particularly useful in debriefing sessions following distressing circumstances such as serious untoward incidents, accidents or mistakes.

INCREASE STAFF AWARENESS

Make sure your staff are fully aware of how to access the chaplaincy service and that they do not have to be religious in order to do so. Ensure they know they can call on the chaplaincy service for advice on a range of matters including advance directives (living wills), palliative care and even personal support for individual staff including bereavement or relationship issues. The chaplains are increasingly being used as someone to talk to who will listen and help individuals to reflect in absolute confidence. They also have the advantage in that they are not part of any internal hierarchy.

Obviously it will be far easier to call on their advice if you have built up a good working relationship with them in the first place. This is what networking is all about. It is a major part of your role as a manager. It's best not to leave it until your chaplaincy service contacts you or when you find yourself or your team in need their help and assistance.

USE BUT DON'T ABUSE THE NURSE SPECIALISTS

The role of the nurse specialist varies between organisations, but overall they tend to fall into two categories:

1. Organisation-wide nurse specialists.
2. Departmental nurse specialists.

The organisation-wide nurse specialists usually report directly to the nursing director and have responsibility across the organisation because their area of expertise involves a large majority, if not all, of the patients. The specialties include areas such as infection control and tissue viability. They are responsible for implementing and maintaining standards of care throughout the organisation.

The departmental nurse specialists are also responsible for standards of care within their specialty across the organisation. The difference is that their specialty involves a specific group of patients. These include areas such as diabetes, Parkinson's disease and dermatology. Their duties usually involve managing a caseload of patients often on an out-patient basis where they are responsible for activities such as running clinics, performing diagnostic tests and providing follow-up care and support.

DIFFERENT EDUCATION AND DEVELOPMENT RESPONSIBILITIES

The main priority for organisation-wide specialists is usually the education and development of staff. Their role is to reduce common problems such as infection and pressure sores through promotion of best practice.

The main priority for departmental nurse specialists is the provision of care for their caseload of patients. They also have a responsibility for the education and development of staff within the rest of the organisation but only as and when that can be fitted around their core responsibilities. It is not their main priority, but they will do their best to be available for specialist advice and support where possible.

BE WARY OF DE-SKILLING YOUR STAFF

It has become an issue in some areas where a nurse specialist may be called as soon as a patient within their specialty is admitted. The problem here is that nurse specialists are not employed to undertake the work that a general nurse should be quite capable of doing. If, for example, a patient is admitted to a general medical ward with angina, it should not be necessary to call in a cardiac nurse specialist to provide rehabilitation advice. That should remain within the remits of the general medical nurse.

The role of the nurse specialist is to provide appropriate education and advice to enable the general medical nurses to improve their own skills. If your staff fall into the habit of calling in a nurse specialist each time, they will lose their skills in that area. Your role as ward manager is to continuously improve the skills of your staff. Use the nurse specialists to help you in this role by asking them to provide education and development for your staff rather than the staff expecting them to take over.

Develop close links with all the organisation-wide nurse specialists plus those who are directly linked with your specialty. Usually the organisation-wide specialist nurses will be working towards specific targets and will be only too happy to come along at your request to assist in the education and development of staff. This also helps them in achieving their targets, as do link nurse roles.

LINK NURSE ROLES

Beware of having a link nurse role for each specialist subject. Ideally your staff should have no more than one link nurse role, otherwise they may not be able to make the most of the development opportunities for each subject area and the link nurse roles may become a chore.

There will always be more link nurse roles than there are available nurses within your team. The key is to prioritise. Usually the organisation-wide specialist areas would be your first priority. It is advisable to have a link nurse for infection control and tissue viability, for example. Other link nurse roles depend on the frequency of patients admitted with the specialist condition on your ward. You may find diabetes is the next key priority for a link nurse role on a medical ward where more than 50% patients admitted are diabetic.

If there are more link nurse roles than the number of staff in your team, get your team together and decide what your top priorities are. Make a conscious decision to leave out the rest. Inform your manager in writing (email will suffice) about the decision you have made with your team and why. You may have an outcry from nurse specialists who want a link nurse on your ward to maintain communications, but the welfare of your team comes before the needs of the nurse specialist. Work together with them to find some other less time-consuming way that you can maintain communications.

HELP PATIENTS AND RELATIVES ACCESS THE RIGHT ADVICE

PATIENT ADVICE AND LIAISON SERVICE

All patients and relatives have access to advice and support in making a formal complaint about their health services, but in England, the Department of Health has gone one step further through the development of patient advice and liaison services (PALS). Every NHS trust in England now has a PALS office employing several individuals to provide information and advice to patients and relatives about any concerns they may have whilst in hospital. (This service is currently unique to England: it is not available in Scotland, Wales and Northern Ireland.)

The main role of PALS officers is to resolve problems and concerns quickly by liaising with health care professionals and managers on the patient's behalf. They also offer services, such as providing information about the NHS and health care matters, and explanations about how to make a formal complaint and who to go to.

A great deal of money has gone into setting up these offices to provide patients in hospital with somewhere to go with their concerns; money that could have been spent on more staff. Why? Because patients have not been getting their issues and concerns resolved by clinical staff. It appears that health care professionals have not been listening to their patients and relatives nor providing advice and information sufficient for their needs.

Having to resort to setting up PALS offices in every NHS trust is a poor reflection on the service we provide, yet it is obviously needed. The problem is still there because some nurses and other health care professionals are actually referring their patients to PALS for advice and support. Think carefully about it; if patients and relatives from your ward are having to go to PALS for information or to resolve issues on their behalf, perhaps it's an indication that you and your team are not meeting their needs. If you find this is happening frequently it is worth using one of your team meetings to review all your dealings with PALS and identify areas where you need to improve. The PALS officers keep records of all visits to enable you to learn from the information.

INFORMATION LEAFLETS

It is imperative to ensure the supply of information sheets and leaflets are always plentiful, including those on how to make a complaint. However, given the huge array of literature which is now available, try to ensure that you and your staff select the appropriate ones for individual patients' and relatives' needs rather than expect them to help themselves. Patients who are given specific leaflets are more likely to read and take note than if they were just left to help themselves from the leaflet rack. It's also worth bearing in mind that they are more likely to read the information if their name is written on the front.

WARD ROUNDS AND VISITS FROM OTHER HEALTH PROFESSIONALS

Some patients and relatives become completely 'tongue-tied' when confronted with a group of doctors standing around the bedside. It's one of the main reasons why the patient's nurse should be part of the ward round. The nurse's role is to act as the patient's advocate, encouraging them to ask questions or asking on their behalf if necessary (see pp. 99–100).

Your staff should routinely advise patients and relatives to prepare for ward rounds and other visits by writing down their questions in advance. They should be reassured that this is normal and that the doctor (or other health care professional) would prefer that they did this so they can ensure they have met the patients' needs. Illness makes patients and relatives a lot more vulnerable than they would be normally. Don't expect them to be able to access all the right information by themselves. Sometimes patients and relatives need more than just pointing in the right direction.

KEEP UP-TO-DATE WITH RISK MANAGEMENT ISSUES

Risk management basically means taking measures to reduce the likelihood of any harm happening to your patients and staff. Managing health care delivery will always involve a degree of risk, but minimising those risks is a key part of your role.

PERFORMANCE INDICATORS FOR RISK MANAGEMENT

Your organisation will have a set of performance indicators to measure the effectiveness in the way they identify, reduce and manage risk. The main NHS performance indicators are set nationally and vary according to whether you are in England, Wales, Scotland or Northern Ireland. In England, the NHS Litigation Authority has specific risk management programmes against which your trust is assessed, such as the Clinical Negligence Scheme for Trusts (CNST).

It is important that you are aware of your organisation's targets for minimising risk and that your staff are trained in risk management. You should also access training for yourself in incident investigation and root cause analysis, if you have not already done so.

HOSPITAL RISK MANAGEMENT COMMITTEE

Many hospitals have some sort of risk management committee and employ a specific team of staff to ensure that you have access to the right advice and support. They also ensure the appropriate policies and procedures are in place to help you minimise risk. Find out who is responsible for clinical governance or risk management within your organisation and make sure they become part of your network. Perhaps even shadow them for a day. Not only will you benefit from their knowledge and find out what you should be doing, but you will get to know them well enough to be able to call on them for expert advice when required. You will also get to know their team and which individuals are the best to call for advice and support.

Aim also to include the following people in your network to be able to call on them for advice regarding risk management issues:

- the equipment manager
- the fire officer
- head of security
- manual handling advisor
- health and safety advisor.

DIRECTORATE RISK MANAGEMENT COMMITTEE

Your directorate will also have a specific group or committee which continually assess and manage risk. This could be part of your directorate clinical governance group or you may have a separate directorate risk management group. It would be advisable to make sure you are a member of this group.

Be careful if you decide to delegate the role of risk management to a member of your team. You still remain accountable to your organisation for ensuring that effective risk management measures are undertaken in your area. It is advisable that you retain the role of risk management lead for your area and ensure you get regular feedback from your link staff for issues such as manual handling and health and safety. You retain overall responsibility for all risk management issues so make sure you are kept well informed to be able to ensure your systems and processes are all in order.

CONSULT POLICIES, PROCEDURES AND GUIDELINES

WHY SO MANY POLICIES?

It seems that there are policies and procedures for everything we do these days. Some organisations even have a policy for the storage and filing of policies. But believe it or not, the more policies and procedures that your organisation has is an indication of how well you and your staff are looked after and valued. If you have relatively few compared to other organisations, it could mean that both you and your patients are at greater risk of harm.

Policies and procedures are very important in informing your day-to-day work. They indicate what the organisation expects with regards to staff behaviour and work standards. They guide you as to what is acceptable and what is not. Without this guidance, you would have no standard with which to measure others. If members of staff produce a lower standard of work, there would be little you could do about it without the appropriate policy or procedure in place. You and your staff would also have fewer rights.

MAKE SURE THEY ARE ACCESSIBLE AT ALL TIMES

Policies and procedures are useful documents and should be easily accessible for all staff to consult during the course of their shift. Make sure you keep files of all policies and procedures on your ward. Most will be accessible on your intranet system but it is still wise to keep hard copies in your office so that staff can consult them in times when they have no access to the computers.

Policies and procedures can often be a better source of advice than seeking someone else's opinion. They not only outline good practice but they also include the most current legislation. Try to read the appropriate policy regarding any staff management issues before consulting other individuals for advice. Policies and procedures give you a good idea about the correct line of action to follow in most situations.

MAKE SURE YOUR TEAM KNOW WHEN ELEMENTS HAVE CHANGED

Whenever you receive a new, revised or updated policy, find out exactly what has been changed in the policy. You can do this by calling the person responsible for the revised policy or procedure. Once you have done this, inform all your staff. If you just tell your staff that the policy has been replaced with a new one, it is highly unlikely that anyone will have the time or inclination to read it through. However, they will take note if you highlight what the changes are either in your ward communication book or via a team meeting. Asking staff to read through whole policies and procedures is unrealistic and you know it won't happen.

EVIDENCE-BASED GUIDELINES

Ensure that evidence-based guidelines and standards are also easily accessible for your team. All clinical guidelines you use on your ward should be based on the best possible evidence. Guidelines should not just be an outline of the current practice on your ward for new members. You must make sure they are up-to-date.

However, updating guidelines takes valuable time which you and your team often do not have. Try and use your specialist association for guidelines pertaining to your specialty and use national guidelines wherever possible. The Royal Marsden Manual of Clinical Procedures is an ideal example of evidence-based guidelines which are applicable for use in most wards (Dougherty & Lister 2004). Invest in having a book like this available on the ward for your staff. It will save you and your staff wasting time on having to develop your own and continually having to update them.

If you are really keen on developing your own, get the right help and support. Contact your organisation's practice development department. If they do not have the right expertise, they will still be able to help by finding the right person or the right information on your behalf. They will also be able to advise on how to formulate the guidelines and standards and how to get them validated by your organisation.

MAXIMISE COMPUTER ACCESS

THE WORLDWIDE WEB

Nothing beats the internet for providing instant access to information. It means that staff do not have to leave the ward area to find the information they need to enhance their practice.

It is a good idea to keep one computer on your ward available at all times for the sole purpose of enabling staff to be able to access the internet. Locating it at a work station outside the ward office may help to ensure that the internet is used for professional purposes only. There are many websites that you can access for up-to-date clinical information including those listed below:

1. The Cochrane Collaboration: http://www.cochrane.org. You can access the results of systematic reviews of evidence on health care interventions from this website.
2. Nursing, Midwifery and Allied Health Professions: http://www.nmap.ac.uk. Described as 'the UK's gateway to high quality internet resources in nursing, midwifery and allied health', this website is very simple to use. You can either browse through an A–Z index or search for a particular subject.
3. RCN online library and information service: http:// www.rcn.org.uk/library. As well as providing a literature search facility, this service also provides the opportunity to read full journal articles on your chosen subject, access to the Oxford Dictionary of Nursing and access to an A–Z of medicinal drugs (RCN membership is required to access this website).
4. Patient information websites are also very useful for general information especially when you have patients admitted with conditions you are not familiar with (see p. 95).
5. Many organisations enable you to access the university library databases such as Biomed, Cinahl and Medline as well as Ovid and Blackwell Synergy. These can also be useful for looking up information to assist your team in their day-to-day work.

GETTING YOUR STAFF TO USE COMPUTERS

Some nurses are still 'computer shy' and find it difficult to use computers. Don't force them into attending computer study days if they are not comfortable with using them. It is probably better to encourage members of your own team who are familiar with using computers to show those who aren't, on a day-to-day basis when dealing with real-life issues. In this way, they can learn at a pace more suitable to their needs. They may come across a patient with a condition that they have not nursed for some time. Having a colleague to help them access the information they need there and then would show them how useful and easy it is to incorporate in their everyday practice.

EUROPEAN COMPUTER DRIVING LICENCE

It would be a good idea to enable a number of your staff to undertake the European Computer Driving Licence (ECDL). This is an internationally recognised qualification which gives people the skills and confidence to use a computer. It is also the course commissioned and recommended by the NHS for all staff in England. The course consists of seven modules:

1. Basic concepts of IT.
2. Using the computer and managing files.
3. Word processing.

4. Spreadsheets.
5. Databases.
6. Presentations.
7. Information and communication.

It can be undertaken online or as a combination of taught lessons and online access. If you are not aware of how to access this course, contact your organisation's training and development manager or access the dedicated website (European Computer Driving Licence 2005). The course is offered to NHS staff throughout England, Wales, Scotland and Northern Ireland but is administered differently in each country.

UTILISE THE KNOWLEDGE AND SKILLS OF YOUR NURSING COLLEAGUES

CHANNEL THE ENTHUSIASM WITHIN YOUR TEAM

As pointed out in Chapter 3, a good leader knows the strengths and weaknesses of all their team members. Work on those strengths. It you have an issue where you need more knowledge in order to make an informed decision, delegating the task of fact-finding is often useful for the development of one of the individuals within your team. Don't delegate unless it serves a useful purpose for the person you are delegating to. Your junior sister/charge nurses need as much experience as they can get to prepare them for the next role. Make sure you learn together with each new experience.

MAKE FINDING INFORMATION A STAFF DEVELOPMENT OPPORTUNITY

If you come across a problem which you have never dealt with before, getting others to find out what the options are for dealing with the problem can be good experience for them as well as helping you. Don't always assume that if you don't know what to do, it's up to you to find out. You can still ask others to find out for you. Just point the individual in the right direction for finding out the information.

If, for example, you have a patient who divulges some confidential information to a member of your staff, who feels that others should know about it and comes to you for advice and support, your first instinct may be to contact your trade union, your organisation's solicitors and perhaps even the NMC advice line for further information on what to do. Delegating these actions to your junior sister/charge nurse as a learning oppportunity may be far more productive. They will feel they have accomplished something worthwhile and will be enthusiastic about the experience. If you delegate it because you do not have the time, it will quite rightly be regarded as a chore and there will be less learning from the experience.

Whenever you are confronted with staff who have a problem, be honest: 'I have no idea what to do in this situation. Who do you think might be able to help? Try calling them to see what they advise'.

DRAW ON THE EXPERIENCE OF YOUR PEERS

Meeting with other ward managers within your organisation on a regular basis is one way of learning from them, but it is also a good idea to set up some sort of network in between these meetings. This ensures that you have instant access to their knowledge and experience. Email is often the best way to do this. If you have not already done so, set up a group email address of all the ward managers within your organisation and encourage them to do the same. This can prove invaluable in cases where you need urgent information. Few ward managers with the appropriate knowledge would ignore the following email addressed to the group:

> 'A member of staff has come to me with an allegation of bullying from one of the agency nurses. I have not dealt with this situation before. If anyone else has experience of a similiar issue, I would be grateful to know how you handled it.'

Always remember to remain confidential and never divulge sensitive information which could result in the individuals involved being identified. You can contact each other by phone or face-to-face afterwards if details need to be discussed in depth.

USE EMAIL

All the ward managers within your organisation would benefit by maintaining close contact and learning from each other's experiences. In the past, it has been too difficult because of the nature of the role. Most would be reluctant to call colleagues and interrupt their work and you don't have time to keep leaving the ward to go around and talk to your colleagues. Email is the answer to all those problems. You do not have to leave the ward and you are not interrupting your colleagues in the course of their work. In addition, email takes up far less time and is a lot more succinct.

If you are not keeping a constant dialogue with your colleagues in this manner, you could be losing out on an extremely useful source of advice. There is nothing to stop you starting an email dialogue through the group address system. Contact your organisation's IT department for further ideas which could include having your own ward manager's webpage based on FAQs (frequently asked questions) or even a discussion forum. A little time invested at the beginning goes a long way in terms of help and support in the future.

UTILISE THE PRACTICE DEVELOPMENT TEAM

Most health care organisations have some sort of professional or practice development team. They are usually directly managed and report to the director or deputy director of nursing. Their role is to work with all members of the health care team but particularly with ward managers, to facilitate improvements in clinical practice and spread good practice across the organisation. They support and advise all health care professionals and provide education and development not accessed through the universities (although they often link closely with local academic institutions).

The work of the practice development teams usually involves the following:

- developing and implementing policies, procedures and best practice guidelines based on evidence
- provision of mandatory training, student and health care assistant support and further clinical training
- dissemination of examples of good practice across the organisation
- assistance for staff to learn and take action from their experiences and patient feedback (e.g. from the complaints process)
- improving staff access to the best evidence.

Try to involve the practice development team in any issue that involves changing or improving practice. If they are unable to give appropriate advice themselves, they will facilitate access to others who can. Some issues can be quite controversial such as nil-by-mouth policies or nurse prescribing. The practice development team will help and guide you throughout the process. Even if you do not feel confident in the skills of your practice development team, it is best to keep them informed of any changes and improvements in your area to avoid duplication of any work in other departments.

They can also be an invaluable source of information. The team usually includes at least the following members:

Practice placement facilitator and practice educators

These people are usually employed in part or fully by the local universities to ensure that student nurses have appropriate placements and support during those placements. If you have any problems with students or problems with too many or too few students, these people should be your first port of call.

NVQ coordinators

An NVQ coordinator is usually responsible for overseeing the training and development of health care assistants throughout the organisation. There is sometimes a coordinator who oversees cadet programmes for 16–18 year olds, some of whom plan to enter nursing at a later stage.

A clinical leadership facilitator

The NHS has recognised the importance of health professionals having good leadership skills and many hospitals now employ a facilitator to run management/ leadership programmes such as the RCN clinical leadership development programme (Royal College of Nursing 2005b). It would be wise to ensure you and your junior sisters/charge nurses undertake one of these programmes to aid their development for the next post.

A training and development coordinator

This person is usually responsible for coordinating the education contracts with the local academic institutions. Sometimes this role is incorporated into the assistant director of nursing role.

Nurses are also brought into the practice development team on secondments to facilitate the implemention of various national projects such as benchmarking (e.g. 'Essence of Care' in England or 'Fundamentals of Care' in Wales), IT projects (e.g. computerised rostering) or recruitment initiatives (e.g. the development of overseas nurses and nurses returning to practice).

Together the team form an invaluable source of advice and support. However, like you they have a set workload and will not have time to spend promoting their services. It's up to you to build up a good working relationship so you can call on them for advice in future situations.

ACTION POINTS

- Find out how to contact your organisation's solicitors both during and out of hours. Keep the details available in your ward office should the need arise.
- Find out who the main union stewards are in your organisation; get to know them and add them to your network.
- Locate a copy of the course directory from your local university on the ward, so that you can access lecturers/experts in various subjects if required.
- Get to know your chaplaincy lead, add them to your network and ensure that all new recruits meet with them during their induction programme.
- Review the link nurse roles to ensure that each member of your team has no more than one each. If necessary, prioritise with your team and set up different modes of communication to receive the necessary specialist information.
- Review your team's use of PALS and look for ways of improving the service you provide at ward level via appropriate information leaflets and staff education.
- Find out and familiarise yourself with *all* your organisation's performance indicators. Shadow or meet with the clinical governance manager or risk manager if necessary to find out what you need to know.
- Review all the policies and procedures on your ward, making sure they are up-to-date and easily accessible for all your staff.
- Pair up all staff who have poor computer skills with those staff who do have good computer skills. Encourage a certain number of your staff to undertake the European Computer Driving Licence course.
- Set up a group email address on your computer to include all other ward managers within your organisation for access to support and advice.
- Get to know your practice development team and include them within your professional network.

References

Department of Health 2003 NHS chaplaincy: meeting the religious and spiritual needs of patients and staff. Guidance for managers and those involved in the provision of chaplaincy-spiritual care. DH Publications, London. Online. Available: http://www.dh.gov.uk/assetRoot/04/06/20/28/04062028.pdf 8 Oct 2005

Dougherty L, Lister S 2004 The Royal Marsden Hospital manual of clinical procedures, 6th edn. Blackwell Publishing, Oxford

European Computer Driving Licence 2005 Basic IT skills. Online. Available: http://www.ecdl.nhs.uk 8 Oct 2005

Royal College of Nursing 2005a RCN online members only area. Online. Available: http://www.rcn.org.uk/members/direct 8 Oct 2005

Royal College of Nursing 2005b Clinical leadership – The programme so far. RCN, London. Online. Available: http://www.rcn.org.uk/resources/clinicalleadership/sofar.php 8 Oct 2005

Unison 2005 Unison membership benefits: legal services. Online. Available: http://www.unison.org.uk/benefits 8 Oct 2005

CHAPTER 16

QUESTION EXTERNAL DIRECTIVES

Is another link nurse role really needed?   306

Prioritise and reprioritise   307

Getting the most from the role   307

Monitor effectiveness of the role   307

Has the bed manager considered all other options?   308

Explain your situation clearly   308

Work together with the other ward managers   308

Don't use the dayroom   309

Was that audit really necessary?   309

Financial implications   310

What's in it for you?   310

Has your line manager questioned the decision? 310

Are performance targets worth lowering the quality of care for?   311

Putting patient care first 311

Challenging the system   312

Are senior managers aware of the implications of their decision?   312

Point out the implications of the decision   313

Are consultant/specialist decisions always right? 313

Teach your staff the art of diplomacy   314

What if the consultant/specialist is wrong but goes ahead anyway?   314

Whistleblowing   314

Ask your union steward for assistance   315

What help are unions?   315

Getting your voice heard 316

Don't hesitate in contacting the chief executive or other board directors if necessary   316

Statutory duty for maintaining quality   316

Inappropriate decisions need to be highlighted   317

Rely on your own common sense   317

Sometimes other health care professionals or managers make decisions which adversely affect patient care or staff. Sometimes you may feel that you are pressured into making decisions which you do not feel are appropriate. The message here is don't always accept that others' decisions are the right ones.

Don't hesitate to challenge people just because they are more senior or are more knowledgeable in certain subjects than you. Trust your instincts. You are an experienced professional, and sometimes have more insight than they do. Often it is not what you say but how you say it that makes sure you are heard. If you find that certain performance targets are reducing the standard of patient care or that undertaking audits is taking your staff away from patient care, you have a duty to speak up: 'You are accountable for your actions regardless of the advice or directions from another professional' (Nursing & Midwifery Council 2004; Standard 1.3).

IS ANOTHER LINK NURSE ROLE REALLY NEEDED?

Link nurses are a good way of maintaining links between the ward and various nurse specialists, educationalists or practice development nurses. The problem is that the number of nurse specialists and educationalists are increasing with the rise in national initiatives and targets. Some ward managers are now finding themselves in the position where the number of link nurse roles required is far greater than the number of staff they have on their team. Box 16.1 includes a small selection of the link nurse roles required from today's nurses.

BOX 16.1: A SMALL SELECTION OF THE LINK ROLES REQUIRED FROM TODAY'S WARD NURSES

Essence of care
Infection control
Nutrition
Palliative care
Risk management
Manual handling
Fire, health and safety
Diabetes
Tissue viability
Continence
Education
Child protection
Pain

PRIORITISE AND REPRIORITISE

Keep an up-to-date list of who is doing which link nurse role. Each time you are asked for another link nurse, don't automatically allocate the role to one of your staff. Get your team together first and reprioritise. Ask yourselves; is this new link role more important than the link roles you currently have. If it is, then identify which is the least important and drop it from your list. Find some other way of maintaining communication about the subject.

Try not to say to the nurse specialist that 'we are too busy and do not have the capacity to take on another role'. Be more specific. Show them the list of link roles you already have and explain why they are more important. Work out a compromise with them; it's in your best interests to maintain a good relationship with all nurse specialists.

Don't overburden your team with more than one link nurse role. Give each one the time and resources to gain full benefit from the work involved. The rest of your team and patients will also benefit.

GETTING THE MOST FROM THE ROLE

The role of the link nurse usually entails:

1. Attending and contributing to regular meetings and study sessions.
2. Making information available to the rest of the team.
3. Keeping all patient and staff information sources up-to-date.
4. Helping to set and implement standards in the subject.
5. Evaluating and monitoring practice on the ward.
6. Identifying educational needs of the team.
7. Contributing to induction packages and staff teaching programmes.
8. Assisting with monitoring standards and auditing where necessary.
9. Identifying own educational needs and maintaining a high standard of professional competence in the subject area.

It takes time to be able to carry out the above duties. Therefore, you should ascertain exactly how many hours per week or month will be required to undertake the role. Don't expect your staff to meet the demands of the link nurse role in their own time. It should be seen as a development opportunity, not a chore. Ensure the link roles are included in job descriptions and the budgeted staff establishment takes the role demands into account.

MONITOR EFFECTIVENESS OF THE ROLE

Monitor how these link roles are enhancing patient care on your ward. Are they making a difference, or are the link nurses being used as administrators to do work not directly involving or affecting patient care within your own ward? Do this by making sure that link nurses report back to the team and their mentors regularly regarding the additional work they are undertaking.

HAS THE BED MANAGER CONSIDERED ALL OTHER OPTIONS?

Work with your bed manager. You may dread them coming on to your ward or ringing you up every five minutes, but they have to know what is going on everywhere and place patients in beds as soon as possible. They are under constant pressure and sometimes do not realise the pressures you have, especially those who do not have a clinical background.

EXPLAIN YOUR SITUATION CLEARLY

Never accept administrative decisions that compromise patient care. Your patients' welfare should always come first. Obviously you cannot refuse admissions in emergency situations when it is clear that there is nothing else available, but you must not routinely accept additional patients knowing that the quality of care that they or your existing patients receive will be compromised.

If you have said to the bed manager that you do not have the staff required to care for the new patient appropriately at the moment but they still insist on sending the patient to you, you must explain clearly the implications of their decision, and put it in writing. It's usually preferable to do this by email sending a copy to your line manager and the appropriate duty manager.

WORK TOGETHER WITH THE OTHER WARD MANAGERS

Bed managers are used to the nurse-in-charge saying that they do not have enough staff. It seems to be a daily mantra. It can get to the situation where the bed manager has to decide for themselves which short-staffed ward is more worse off than the other. The decision is sometimes based on the persuasiveness of the nurse-in-charge. It would help a lot more if you use your leadership skills, i.e. influence and negotiate, to get all the wards to work together in these situations.

Use your close network with the other ward managers to create other solutions to the problem. You are the managers with the most clinical knowledge within the hospital and are probably in a better position to generate other options. The bed manager tends to work in isolation and does not have the knowledge and authority generated by a group of ward managers who communicate closely.

Working together as a group of ward managers alongside the bed manager will help reduce the problem of wards working against each other with regards to admissions. It may also help to stop some wards getting all the heavily dependent patients and makes sure that nurses get to nurse patients in their specialty rather than struggling to look after patients with illnesses they have little knowledge of who should be on another ward.

DON'T USE THE DAYROOM

Caring for patients in the dayroom is not usually costed within your staffing establishment and therefore should not be encouraged. The dayroom is not a waiting room. Hospital transport can be unreliable in terms of collection times, and sometimes patients are not fully fit and well at the time of discharge; they are usually still recuperating. You are still responsible for their welfare until they have left your ward.

You cannot leave patients waiting for transport in the dayroom unless you have the appropriate staffing levels to monitor them. Explain to the bed manager that you expect the bed to be available at a certain time, but will not accept a new patient until the previous patient has left.

If you are having your decision overturned by senior managers in your absence because of the pressure on waiting lists, make sure your staff book extra cover to look after the patients in the dayroom. Cost up the extra expense with your finance advisor and let your managers know in writing how much the decision is costing you. Unless you spell it out to managers and administrators, they may have no idea of the implications. Be specific: don't use vague terms, such as 'we are too busy' or 'we do not have enough staff' or 'it is affecting quality of care'. These phrases are heard every day and people become immune to such language. Use their language, e.g. 'we are requiring an extra £2000 per month to cover staffing costs with patients waiting in the dayroom, which amounts to an extra £24000 per year'.

WAS THAT AUDIT REALLY NECESSARY?

With the current national emphasis on targets everything has to be audited. Improvements in both quality and quantity of care cannot be demonstrated unless regular audits are undertaken. With the increase of computer databases, the days of recording numbers and actions on paper are becoming a thing of the past. However, auditing work is still taking up a lot of the time which could be spent on actually carrying out the work.

Some ward managers are still being inundated with various requests to monitor activities such as:

- documentation and record keeping
- numbers of pressure sores
- manpower forms
- numbers of requests for agency/bank nurses
- benchmarking assessments (e.g. Essence of Care).

FINANCIAL IMPLICATIONS

Audits take time. Has this time been costed within your staffing establishment? How many staff hours does it take every week/month to fill in the various forms? It's worth taking some time to work it out with your finance advisor to inform the various departments requesting the information.

Each time you are asked to undertake an audit or collect information, firstly ensure that it has been affirmed by your central audit department. All audits within the hospital need to be registered to ensure that someone else is not already collecting similiar information. Many also have to be passed through the ethics committee, particularly where patient information is involved.

WHAT'S IN IT FOR YOU?

If you are asked to undertake an audit on your ward, consider how the results are going to help you improve care. If you cannot see how they are going to help you, why do the audit? If the audit is for someone else's benefit then why are you doing all the work for them? What's in it for you? Don't undertake all audits without question. It is not your role to collect information for others. It is usually the role of your audit department. It is also the role of your audit department to assist you to collect information should you wish to carry out your own audit. They will be able to look up facts and figures to help you. They will also help you get your audit through the ethics committee if necessary.

Try to steer clear of undertaking your own patient satisfaction surveys. The NHS currently undertakes one each year, sending thousands of questionnaires to patients in each trust. Private health care companies also undertake their own. Find out the results of these surveys rather than duplicate with your own.

HAS YOUR LINE MANAGER QUESTIONED THE DECISION?

Don't always take 'no' for an answer from your line manager. If you have asked for something and your manager gives you a negative response, don't rant or rave, but on the other hand don't stand down and accept their answer either. How do you know how hard they have tried on your behalf or even if they have tried at all? Before you accept a negative response, find out the facts (Table 16.1).

If you are unsatisfied with the response, don't go to the next manager up, unless absolutely necessary. Undermining your own line manager can damage your future working relationship. Some line managers may not feel as passionately about the subject as you do and may not have tried very hard to get what you need. They may not fully understand what you want them to do or they may not know the right channels to go through.

Work with your manager to get the right results. Don't expect them to do things for you. When you receive a negative response and find they haven't tried hard enough, try again: 'perhaps we could try a different approach?' or 'perhaps if I

TABLE 16.1: How to find out the facts behind negative managerial responses

Negative response	Fact-finding response
'There's no money'	'Which budget have you tried to use?' 'Was it put forward as part of the business plan?' 'What happened to the money that was granted for the project?'
'I've asked and you're not allowed'	'Who did you ask?' 'What were the reasons?' 'How did you present the case to them?'
'No, it's not possible for you to have any more staff'	'What are the reasons?' 'Have you discussed all the options with . . . ?' 'Has it been included as part of next year's business plan?'

find out some further information, we could put it forward as a business case?'. Focus on using 'we' rather than 'you'; it's a less threatening approach and prevents unnecessary conflict.

ARE PERFORMANCE TARGETS WORTH LOWERING THE QUALITY OF CARE FOR?

Performance targets are devised for the sole purpose of enhancing the quality of care. Sometimes, in order to reach a performance target, some staff will accept the lowering of other aspects of care. It has not been unknown for patients to go without appropriate first line treatment in order to reach the 4-hour A&E waiting target for example. Had the government known that GPs would stop patients being able to book appointments in advance, they would probably not have enforced the original target of everyone seeing a GP within 48 hours. However, it was public demand that created the 48-hour target in the first place.

PUTTING PATIENT CARE FIRST

Targets have been devised from patient demand and the majority are reasonable targets. Unfortunately, some people can become so focused on targets that they will do anything to reach them, including the compromising of patient care. As a health care professional you are bound by the code of professional conduct which puts the patients' welfare first when facing any professional dilemmas. Unfortunately it can be difficult to challenge targets, when putting patients' welfare first is usually the original aim of the target.

CHALLENGING THE SYSTEM

Use your common sense. If you and your staff can see the quality of patient care is being drastically affected, question what is happening. Make sure everyone knows that clinical care is being compromised. Don't keep the knowledge within your directorate. If the target is affecting others too, get them all involved. Work together as a team to generate other ways of reaching the target that do not compromise patient care. If you cannot do this, challenge the target itself.

If you decide to challenge the target, make sure that you do this together with the appropriate senior managers. You must look after yourself and your team. It is not in your interests to be seen as 'difficult'. Your goal is to work with people and generate enthusiasm to support each other in challenging the target and suggesting alternative ways of improving care.

It is part of your professional code of conduct to put patients' welfare first. It is also part of the manager's code of conduct (Department of Health 2002).

ARE SENIOR MANAGERS AWARE OF THE IMPLICATIONS OF THEIR DECISION?

Senior managers provide an invaluable service within health care. Having their services within each organisation enables health care professionals to focus on their main area of expertise, i.e. health care. Human resources (HR) managers, for example, have expert knowledge on policies and procedures and are available for advice in all areas of people management. And if they are unable to help in certain areas, they will usually be able to find out the appropriate information for you.

However, there is one disadvantage in that the majority of staff within HR and senior management have no experience in the delivery of hands-on health care. Without this experience it is not easy to fully appreciate the pressures of dealing with unpredictable workloads, constant and varying demands from sick and vulnerable patients and the need to maintain clinical expertise in a continually advancing technical environment.

Administering and managing health care at the front line is a very different job to many other professions and, unless you have been in the role yourself, it is difficult to understand the complexities of the work. There are bound to be occasions where decisions are made which cause unintentional adverse effects in the delivery of health care. Some examples include:

1. The NHS trust chairman who decides to give all staff within the organisation a day off for Christmas shopping in order to thank them for all their hard work that year. This sort of decision can be an absolute nightmare for ward managers who are already struggling to cover their 'off-duties' and remain within budget.
2. A decision to instigate a recruitment freeze across the organisation. This is a common decision which in many departments can result in increasing

expenditure due to the need to book extra agency and bank staff. This is because they are required to cover both the original vacancies and the increasing sickness levels caused by the remaining staff trying to cover two or more jobs at a time.

3. All requisitions or 'off-duties' to be checked and signed by a senior manager. Again this only serves to cause delays for vital supplies which could put patient welfare at risk. It usually serves no purpose and senior managers may not be familiar with 'off-duties' or the supplies that have been requested.

4. Staff are not allowed to sleep at night on their breaks. Many staff who work nights are revitalised by having a short sleep on their break, particularly if working on a ward with heavily dependent patients. Some nonclinical managers may not appreciate that it could indeed be more dangerous if this was not allowed.

If decisions like this are being made and implemented without consultation in your organisation, don't accept it and moan and whinge amongst your peers. Ask yourself why you have not been involved in this decision. What can you do about it?

POINT OUT THE IMPLICATIONS OF THE DECISION

First, let the appropriate senior managers within the organisation know about the implications of their decision in writing. An email is more diplomatic than a formal letter. Make sure you offer alternative solutions after consultation with your team and peers.

Be positive; you do not want to be labelled as the difficult one. Point out that you understand the predicament but that you and your staff believe there are valid alternative solutions which will reduce the risk of the negative effects that you have outlined. Offer to discuss this further with them if they so wish. Do not be defensive; you are part of the organisation and part of 'the management'.

Second, consider why you were not involved in this decision and what you can do so that you are involved next time. Make yourself known and widen your networks. You and your peers want to be consulted next time decisions like this need to be made. Find a way of ensuring that you are.

ARE CONSULTANT/SPECIALIST DECISIONS ALWAYS RIGHT?

When an opinion has been requested by a specialist, always remember it is just that; an opinion. It does not mean that you have to do whatever is recommended. You and your staff know your patients better than most. Sometimes a specialist will come and give directions which are against your better judgement for that particular patient. A consultant may deem a patient fit for discharge whereas you know that the patient is not as independent as they seem. A nutritionist may recommend certain dietary restrictions for a patient that you are having problems getting any food down let alone put on a special diet.

Usually when you get to ward manager level, you have gained the skills and confidence to be able to question consultant or specialist opinions, but your staff may not have this confidence. On the other hand, they may become overconfident and literally say what they think of the specialist's opinion without thinking of the long-term consequences on team relations.

TEACH YOUR STAFF THE ART OF DIPLOMACY

Your job is to maintain good relationships with all members of the multidisciplinary team but also create an environment where your staff can challenge clinical decisions. The key is to ensure that they are diplomatic in their questioning, and discourage any moaning and whinging about the person's personality or behaviour afterwards. Be a role model and show your staff the most appropriate way to question decisions.

WHAT IF THE CONSULTANT/SPECIALIST IS WRONG BUT GOES AHEAD ANYWAY?

This rarely happens if you have spent time and effort in building up the relationship beforehand through the regular positive feedback approach (see p. 51). However, there may be occasions where a senior clinician is making decisions that are detrimental for your patient(s). If it is a one-off event, getting a second opinion is often all you need to do, e.g. 'I called the ICU anaesthetist because the patient deteriorated right after you left and I couldn't get hold of you'.

However, you cannot keep doing this if the senior clinician continues with the same decisions. Under the terms of your professional code of conduct, you are obliged to take your concerns to a more senior level. Your line manager should be your first port of call and if they are unable to solve the issue, then it is advisable to go to your director of nursing for professional advice and support. Your director of nursing should then take appropriate action.

WHISTLEBLOWING

After the Bristol inquiry, every NHS organisation is now obliged to listen to their employees' concerns over others' clinical practice. The Bristol inquiry recommendations also set out quite clearly that 'The reporting of sentinel events must be made as easy as possible, using all available means of communication (including a confidential telephone reporting line)' (Kennedy 2001; Recommendation 113). Most NHS organisations now have an appropriate policy in place that ensures your concerns will be heard.

However, while we should try to be positive about the subject of accountability, it is worth considering first what could be the consequences before you or any of your staff decide to raise your concerns. It may be appropriate to abide by your code of conduct and take action that is best for your patients but if you do decide to whistleblow it is advisable to consider the worst case scenario. There is still a chance (albeit a small one since the implementation of clinical governance) that you can become subject to defensive or ignorant behaviour from senior managers, so make sure that you prepare very carefully.

Keep copies of all documents including emails. Any conversations not recorded on paper can easily be denied. Use email rather than letters; letters may go unheeded. People can always deny they received a letter or say they forwarded it on but it got lost. See your trade union steward for advice or contact the Nursing and Midwifery Council (NMC). For more independent advice you can contact 'Public Concern at Work'. This is a charity set up in 1993 which is an independent authority on public interest whistleblowing. It offers free advice to people concerned about danger or malpractice at work and who are unsure about whether or how to raise the matter (Public Concern at Work 2005).

ASK YOUR UNION STEWARD FOR ASSISTANCE

WHAT HELP ARE UNIONS?

Unions were set up to protect living standards and improve working conditions. As an individual you do not always have the power to be able to negotiate with your board of directors or to make your voice heard. Union stewards have a strong voice and meet regularly (usually every month) with board members to represent the views of the workforce.

Stewards from different unions meet together regularly as a formal group called the Joint Staff Side Committee (JSSC). This group liaises directly with the board of directors via another formal group called the Joint Consultative and Negotiating Committee (JCNC). The JCNC usually has at least one of the board directors attending each time. This is how local policies governing many aspects of your working conditions are agreed. Most JCNC meetings have to consist of 50% managers and 50% union stewards.

The role of the JCNC is to provide a forum for discussing or negotiating matters that affect employees, including issues stemming from:

● organisation change (e.g. ward closures, poor consultation)
● health and safety (e.g. unsafe working conditions)
● employee welfare (e.g. provision of catering facilities, withdrawal of changing facilities).

The committee also provides a mechanism for formal consultation regarding proposed future changes and serves to formally agree any changes and approve changes to terms and conditions for staff.

GETTING YOUR VOICE HEARD

Only recognised union stewards can attend the JCNC so if you wish to raise any issue which involves or affects your staff and others within your organisation, you need to discuss it with your union steward first. They can raise the issue on your behalf.

You may wish, for example, to raise concerns about the decision to reduce the canteen facilities for your night staff or a directive not to wear uniform outside the premises. These issues are wider than your remit as a ward manager and, as they affect other staff, they are probably better raised at the JCNC. There are certain situations where the union stewards' voices can be far louder and more effective than yours.

DON'T HESITATE IN CONTACTING THE CHIEF EXECUTIVE OR OTHER BOARD DIRECTORS IF NECESSARY

The chief executive is responsible for ensuring that finance and quality are properly controlled. They are Accountable Officers which means they are held responsible for ensuring that the organisation meets all it's statutory and legal requirements.

STATUTORY DUTY FOR MAINTAINING QUALITY

Following the 1999 NHS Act, all chief executives within the NHS now have a statutory duty to put and keep in place arrangements for monitoring and improving the quality of care provided to individuals. This means that your chief executive wants to make sure that all systems are in place within their organisation to maintain standards. If any part of the system is failing in any way they do not want to be the last to know.

Don't always assume that the chief executive must know or that someone must have told them. This is not always the case. In 2001, someone took photographs of deceased patients on the floor of the chapel of rest at Bedford Hospital and published them in the media. An investigation found that the bodies were put there temporarily due to a minor fault with the mortuary doors which was reported on the Monday, but by Thursday nothing had been done (NHS Executive Eastern 2001). The chief executive was obliged to resign as a result. It is not their personal job to sort out these issues but to make sure there are systems in the organisation to ensure these issues do not occur.

Guidance had already been issued earlier by the Department of Health to NHS trusts regarding standards of dignity and respect for deceased patients. They had not been implemented at Bedford Hospital. These roles are delegated by the chief executive who would not personally implement guidelines or mend mortuary doors. However, even though they do not do the job personally they are still accountable for the actions of others.

Chief executives are always keen to keep informed about what is going on (or not going on) in the clinical area. The other board directors also like to keep informed, particularly your director of nursing.

INAPPROPRIATE DECISIONS NEED TO BE HIGHLIGHTED

If the board has made a decision which adversely affects staff or patient care, do not hesitate to tell them directly. It may be unintentional. Don't moan and whinge about the effects; they may have no idea. Tell them. A short email saying 'I'm not sure whether anyone has realised but the new car park has no disabled access which means that patients have not been able to attend their clinic appointments over the past three weeks. My apologies if this has already been raised but could you let everyone know what the plan is as it is causing considerable angst for our patients'.

It is unlikely that anyone would complain at receiving such an email, but only send it if you have already tried the appropriate channels such as the facilities manager first. The board director should be your very last option and definitely not the first port of call.

RELY ON YOUR OWN COMMON SENSE

No matter what the problem is, the number one principle of managing a ward should be to employ your common sense. There are many rules and regulations in health care to help you in making decisions. They were not made to be broken but there are times when the rulebook should not be taken literally. You can use your common sense and strive to uphold the intent of the rule rather than the actual rule itself.

Nothing beats the common sense approach learned through years of experience. It is common sense to:

- consult others before you make any decisions
- establish shared annual objectives with your team
- give consistent feedback to enable your team to grow
- take time to listen to your staff's concerns
- get to know all your staff well and treat them all equally
- take care of yourself and your health.

None of this is rocket science and you do not need to know all the management theories and models in order to manage a ward. In fact, most management theories and models have been included in this book. The jargon has just been removed. You remove jargon yourself every day by continually explaining concepts to your staff and your patients in a language that they understand. It is common sense, for example, to tell a patient they have had a heart attack rather than a myocardial infarction.

Absence
  allowance, 108–109
  procedure, 276
  unplanned, 113–115
    maternity leave, 115
    other leave, 115
    sickness levels, 114
Abuse
  of specialists, 291–293
  of staff, 254–256
    bed managers, 255–256
    consultants, 254–255
    link nurses, 256
Accidents, 241–243
Accountability, 315
  care plans and, 87
  professional, 3–4
Accountable Officers, 316
'Acting up', 12, 196
Action
  agreed, 136–137
  learning, 194–196
  plans, 80, 141
    investigation, 243–244
    team, 49
Administrative duties, 16–17
Adoption leave, 115
Advanced directives ('living wills'), 291
Advertisements and applications, 150–151
  application packages, 151
  writing, 150–151
Advice, 6–7, 287–303
  chaplaincy department, 290–291
  colleagues, 299–300
  computer access, 297–299
  legal, 288–289
  nurse specialists, 291–293
  for patients and relatives, 293–294
  policies, procedures and guidelines,
      296–297
  practice development team, 300–302
  professional, 289–290
  risk management, 295–296
  support and, 251
Agency, nurses, 109–110, 121, 149, 159, 236,
    309
Agenda and timetable, 134–135
Alcohol problems, 274–275
  drunk on duty, 274–275
  long-term, 275–276

Allen, H., 257
Allen, I., 19
Allocated patients, 56
'An organisation with a memory' (DoH),
    202
Annual leave, 32, 108–109, 112–113
  spreading, 113
  taking, 113
Antenatal classes, 115
'Any other business' (AOB), 37
Apology, 136, 140
Appearance, personal, 210–211, 268–270
  cultural, race, religious needs, 269–270
  grooming, 211
  individual issues, 269
  standards, 210–211
  team issues, 269
  uniform policy, 210
Applications *see* Advertisements and
    applications
Appointments, 37
Appraisals, 53–54, 67–69
  as formal confirmation, 68
  forms and, 69
  reasons for, 67–68
  successful, 68–69
  unpopularity of, 68
Articles, 35
Assessment and care plans, 86–87
  accountability, 87
  as communication tools, 87
  evaluations and, 57, 218–219
  models, 86
  standardised, 86–87
  as teaching tools, 87
Attitudes
  negative, 250
  positive, 213–214
    optimism, 213–214
    solutions, 214
Audits, 96–97, 309–310
  benchmarking, 97
  financial implications, 310
  improving care, 310
  standards, 96
  tools of, 96–97
Awareness, 291

Balance, work, 16–17
  caseload reduction, 16–17

Bank staff, 109–110, 121, 149, 159, 309
Bed managers, 255–256, 308–309
  dayroom, 309
  decisions, 234
  other wards and, 308–309
  patient care and, 308
Bedford Hospital, 316
Beds, extra, 236
Bedside handovers, 89–91
Behaviour
  leadership, 220–221
  unacceptable, 69–71
    meeting guidelines, 70
    stopping, 71
Benchmarking see Audits
Bereavement, 290
Berne, E., 216–217
Biomed (library database), 298
Blackwell Synergy, 298
Blame, 279–280
BMI Healthcare, 170
Board directors, 171–172, 175, 316–317
  chairman, 171
  chief executive, 172,
    statutory duties, 316–317
  decisions, inappropriate, 317
  executive, 172
  meetings, 173
  as mentors, 181
  networks and, 172–173
  nonexecutive, 171
Breaches of conduct, 72–73
Breaks, 31
Bristol Royal Infirmary Inquiry, 202, 314
British National Formulary (BNF), 84
Budgets, 22, 105–123
  absence, unplanned, 113–115
  amount, 106–107
    monitoring or managing, 106
    'off-duty' and, 107
    staffing establishment, 106–107
  annual leave and, 112–113
  business planning, 118–119
  finance advisor meetings, 121–122
  funding, identified, 119–121
    written, 120–121
  monthly checks, 110–111
    columns, 111
    team involvement, 111
  NON PAY, 107, 110–111, 116–118

  PAY, 107–111, 116–117
  pay priorities, 107–110
  study leave, 115–116
Bulletins, 35
Bullying, 233
  harassment and, 59, 251–253
    action, 252
    definition of, 251–252
    initial approach, 252–253
BUPA, 170
Burnout, 204–205, 272
Business cards, 176
Business planning, 118–119
  business cases, 119, 120, 122
  contents of, 118–119

Caldicott Committee (1997), 132
  principles, 131, 132
Capability procedure, 276
Cardiopulmonary resuscitation (CPR), 77,
    158
Care plans see Assessment and care plans
Care standards, 273, 308, 310, 311–312
Carelessness, 277–278
  competency packages, 277–278
  positive feedback, 278
Carers' leave, 113, 115
Caseload reduction, 16–17
Centre for Policy Studies, 13
Chairperson role, 38–39, 155, 171
Challenge, 195–196
  perceptions, 280
  the system, 312
Change
  difficult staff and, 270–271
    SWOT analysis, 270–271
  to policies, procedures and guidelines, 297
Chaplaincy department, 290–291
  bereavement, 290
  staff awareness, 291
  support, 290–291
  training and development, 291
Charities, 116
Chief executives, 172, 316–317
Chief Nursing Officers (CNOs), 36, 169–170
Cinahl (library database), 298
Clayden, J., 204
Clinical Government Support Team, 97
Clinical Negligence Scheme for Trusts
    (CNST), 295

Clinical skills, 84–85
  learning from experience, 84–85
  teaching and learning, 85
  textbooks and journals, 85
Clinical supervision, 6–7, 59–60, 85
  courses, 60
  group, 60
  reasons for, 59
  staff access to, 59–60
Clinical work, 16–17
  expertise, 36
  induction period, 158
  interference, 230–231
  standards, 22–23
Cliques, 259–261
  action, 260
  line managers and, 261
  recruits, 260
  rejecting, 260–261
Cochrane Collaboration, 298
Code of Confidentiality (NHS), 131
Code of Professional Conduct, 3–4, 87–88,
    283, 312, 314–315
Coffee, 203
Colleagues
  advice, 299–300
    email, 300
    peer experience, 300
    staff development, 299–300
    team enthusiasm, 299
  difficult, 250–251
    advice and support, 251
    negative attitudes, 250
    self critical, 250
    whingeing, 250
Combination handovers, 90
Comment cards, 144
Common sense, 317–318
Communication, 23, 47
  books, 67
  clear, 214–216
  constant contact, 239
  feedback, 239
  with managers, 238–239
  'micromanaging', 238–239
  team, 101
  tools, 87
Compassionate leave, 115
Competency
  packages, 277–278

  procedure, 276
Complaints, 80, 125–146
  content of, 126–128
    verbal, 127
    written, 127, 129
  file notes, 253
  final response letters, 137–142
  follow up action, 142–144
    comment cards/information boards,
      144
    team involvement, 144
  investigation
    accurate notes, 134
    before, 128–129
      contact complainant, 128
      draft response, 128–129, 130
    halting, 132–134
      disciplinary action, 132–133
      legal action, 133–134
    progress sheet, 146
    sensitive, 129–132
      appointing investigator, 129–130
      collating information, 131
      confidentiality, 131
      staff information, 131–132
  meetings, 134–137
    six steps of, 135–137
  moaning and, 223–224
  staff, 253–254
    action, 253
    appeal panel, 254
    resolution, 254
    support, 133
Complaints procedure (NHS), 126
Computer access, 297–299
  European Computer Driving Licence
    (ECDL), 298–299
  staff and, 298
  worldwide web, 297–298
Conduct
  breaches of, 72–73
  code of, 3–4, 87–88, 283, 312, 314–315
Conferences, 180
Confidence, personal, 201
Confidences, 199–200, 261
  criticism, 200
  grapevine, 200
  line manager, 200
  networking, 200
  team, 199

Confidentiality, 300
  complaints and, 131
  handovers and, 91
  patient, 57–58
Conflict, 58–59, 216–217
  bullying or harassment, 59
  disagreements, 58–59
  disciplinary action, 58
  resolving, 276
Confrontation, 279
Consultants/specialists, 254–255, 313–315
  diplomacy and, 314
  mistakes, 314
  whistleblowing, 314–315
Consultation, 231–233
  staff, 48–49
Contact, constant, 239
Control, 216–218
  conflict, 216–217
  empathy, 217–218
  temper, 177, 216, 248
Coping, 234–235
Cost pressures, 118
Covering letters, 184
CPR (cardiopulmonary resuscitation), 77, 158
Criminal Records Bureau clearance, 156
Criticism, 176–177, 200
  self, 250, 281
Culture
  changes, 202
  diversity, 291
  needs, 269–270
Cunningham, G., 5
Curriculum vitae (CV), 183–184

Data Protection Act (1998), 57, 66, 131
Dayrooms, 309
Decision-making, 79, 231
  ward rounds and, 101
Decisions
  audit, 310–311
    implications of, 312–313
  board directors, 316–317
  consultant/specialist, 313–315
  documenting, 98–99
  HCAs and, 88
  informed, 6–7
    clinical supervisors and, 6–7
    Finance department and, 7

    HR department and, 6–7
    line managers and, 6
    mentors and, 6
    ward managers and, 7
  managers' autonomous, 231–233
    action, 232
    bullying, 233
    organisation-wide, 232
    prevention, 232
Definitions and priorities, 26–28
Dehydration, 202–203
Delay, 42
Delegation, 39–41
  approach to, 41
  care, 91
  deputies and, 41, 196–198
  of emails, 32
  to health care assistants (HCAs), 40
  promotion and, 40–41
  task, 91–92
Department of Health, 95, 117, 150, 168–169, 202
  advice and, 290, 293
  complaints and, 131, 142
  external directives and, 312, 316
  managing staff and, 68, 80
  and Social Services in Northern Ireland, 95
  Social Services and Public Safety (DHSSPS) (Northern Ireland), 170
  website, 36
Department of Trade and Industry, 232
Deputies, 41, 163, 196–198
Development
  coordinator, 302
  staff, 299–300
  see also Training
Diary control, 30–32
  annual leave, 32
  breaks, 31
  time limits, 31
  'to-do' lists, 30–31
  using pencil, 31
Difficult people and situations, 247–266, 291
  abuse of staff, 254–256
  bullying or harassment, 251–253
  cliques, 259–261
  colleagues, 250–251
  discrimination, 256–258

Difficult people and situations (*contd*)
  expanding roles, 261–262
  managers, 248–249
  moves or mergers, 262–264
  staff complaints, 253–254
  staff shortage, 258–259
Difficult staff, 267–285
  alcohol problems, 274–275
  appearance, 268–270
  careless, 277–278
  change and, 270–271
  late, 282–284
  lazy, 273–274
  manipulating, 278–280
  moaning, 280–281
  priorities and, 271–273
  relationships and, 276–277
Diplomacy, 176–178, 314
  criticism, 176–177
  disagreements, 178
  opinions, 176
  service users, 178
  taking sides, 177
  temper control, 177
  thinking as manager, 177–178
Directives *see* External directives
Director of nursing, 178–179, 288–289, 314
  mentoring, 179
  professional development team, 179
  shadowing, 179
Directorate meetings, 174
Directors *see* Board directors
Disability Discrimination Act, 152
Disagreements, 58–59, 178
Disciplinary action, 132–133, 269
  conflict and, 58
  hearings, 275–276
  procedure, 276
Discipline, 72–73
  breaches of conduct, 72–73
  warnings, 275
Discrimination, 160–162, 256–258
  enrolled nurses, 161
  overseas nurses, 161–162, 257–258
  part time nurses, 160–161
  patients and relatives, 256–257
Doctors, 17–18
Documents
  evidence in, 244
  for meetings, 135

Dougherty, L., 297
Dress *see* Appearance, personal
Drinks *see* Alcohol problems; Eating and
    drinking
Drugs budget, 117
Duty to report, 11

Eating and drinking, 202–204
  fizzy drinks, 203–204
  night shifts, 204
  regular, 204
  tea/coffee, 203
  water, 203
Education, 21
  development and, 292
Emails, 32–33, 219–220, 300
  delegation of, 32
  filing, 29, 33
  time management and, 33
Emergencies, 15–16, 235, 288
  contact, 34
Empathy, 136, 217–218
Empowering staff, 88–89
Enrolled nurses, 161
Environment, positive working, 29–30,
    45–61
  budget, 117–118
  clinical supervision, 59–60
  conflict, 58–59
  feedback, 51–52
  interview, 154–155
  knowing staff, 52–54
  listening, 49–51
  plans for, 46–48
  staff responsibilities, 55–56
  talking of others, 54–55
  team objectives, 48–49
  visitor system, 56–58
Essence of Care benchmarking
  assessments, 309
  project, 15
  standards, 96
  tool, 97
European Computer Driving Licence
    (ECDL), 298–299
Evaluations, 57, 218–219
Evidence, documentary, 244
Executive directors, 172
Exit interviews, 148
Expanding roles, 261–262

Expectations, 228–230, 249
Experiences
  learning from, 65, 77–78, 84–85
    complaints, 134
    peer, 300
  sharing, 225
Expertise, abuse of, 36
Experts, 264
  see also Consultants/specialists
Explanation
  and apology, 136
  of facts, 140–141
External directives, 305–318
  audits, 309–311
  bed managers, 308–309
  common sense, 317–318
  consultant/specialist decisions, 313–315
  implications of, 312–313
  link nurses, 306–308
  performance targets, 311–312
  union stewards and, 315–317

Feedback
  360 degree reviews and, 9
  positive, 278
  role model, 221–222
  sincere, 51–52
    as learning opportunity, 51–52
    receiving, 52
    thanking staff, 51
  to managers, 239
File notes, 66–67, 255, 277
  complaints, 253
  written, 259
Final response letters, 137–142, 143
  apology, 140
  facts explanation, 140–141
  finishing, 141–142
  layout, 142
  plan of action, 141
  staff confirmation, 142
  starting, 139
Finance department, 7
Flattery, 279
Flexibility, 109–110
Forms, appraisal, 69
Foundation trusts, 168
Freedom of Information Act, 66
Frost, R.O., 201

Fundamentals of Care performance
    standards, 96
Funding
  extra work, 235–237
  see also Budgets

'Games people play' (Berne), 216
Gantt charts, 264, 266
Goals, 47, 80, 87
  see also Objectives
Gossip, 54–55
  moaning and, 223–224
  reasons for, 223–224
Grapevine, 200
Grievance procedures, 253
Grooming, personal, 211
Group
  address system, 300
  'Group facilitator', 38
  supervision, 60
Guardian, The, 256
Guidelines, 296–297

Handovers, 89–91
  bedside, 89–90
    confidentiality, 91
  combination, 90
  office, 89
Handwriting, 218
Harassment see Bullying
Health boards (in Scotland), 169
Health care assistants (HCAs), 49, 91–92,
    119
  decisions and, 88
  delegation and, 40
  empowering, 88–89
  recruitment and, 149, 158, 163–164
Health care professionals, 17–18, 294
Health, personal see Eating and drinking
Health and Personal Social Services
    (Northern Ireland), 36
Health and Safety Executive, 78, 90, 99, 188,
    190
Health and safety training, 158
Health and social services (HSS), 170
  trusts, 170
Healthcare Commission, 168
Healthcare Inspectorate Wales (HIW),
    169

Help requests, 42
High Dependency Unit (HDU), 121, 234
Holland, K., 86
Home calls, 2–3
Horbury, C., 92
Hospital management, 18
Human Resources advisors, 6–7, 64–65
  experience, 65
  informal involvement, 65
  meetings, 64–65
  team knowledge, 65
Hurst, K., 106

Impressions, first, 211–213
  new staff, 212
  spotlighting, 212–213
  visitors and, 212
Improving Health in Wales, 169
Incidents
  mistakes and accidents, 241–243
  record forms, 259
Incompetence, 71, 249
  procedure, 71–72
Induction, 76, 157–158
  before, 157
  mentors, 158
  programme, 77, 257
    checklist, 158
    clinical work, 158
    mandatory training, 158
    welcome, 158
  supernumerary period, 157–158
Information
  boards, 144
  collation, 131
  Commissioner, 66
  dissemination, 34, 36–37
  leaflets, 294
'Information and Consultation of
    Employees Regulations' (2004),
    232
Informing and involving
  complaints and, 80
  decision-making and, 79
  meetings and, 78–79
  planning and recruitment, 79
  study leave, 79
Informing patients, 93–96
  information boards, 94

leaflets, 94–95
  suggestions, 94
Internet, 36, 297–298
Interruptions, 33–34
  informing staff, 34
  'open door' policies, 34
  ward rounds, 33
Interviews, 151–153
  follow up, 155–157
    promising candidates, 156
    taking risks, 157
    unsuccessful candidates, 156
  getting best, 153–155
    chairperson, 155
    environment, 154–155
    interviewers, 154–155
    practical skills, 154
    questions, 153–154
  investigation, 244–245
  preparation, 152
    team, 153
  shortlisting, 151–152
  skills, 164
Investigations, 243–245
  documentary evidence, 244
  interviews, 244–245
  plan of action, 243–244
  written reports, 245
  see also Complaints
Investing for Health (Northern Ireland NHS
    plan), 170

Jargon, 139
Job
  descriptions, 149–150
  enthusiasm, 274
Joint Consultative and Negotiating
    Committee (JCNC), 315–316
Joint Staff Side Committee (JSSC), 315
Journals, 35, 85

Kawamura, K., 201
Kennedy, I., 101, 314
Kennedy, J., 90
Kings Fund, 6, 13
Kitson, A., 5
Knock on effects, 233–235
Knowledge and skills framework (KSF), 9,
    68, 76, 199

Knowledge sources, 8–9
Kouzes, J., 5, 220

Language choice, 222–223
Lardner, R., 90
Larson, J.A., 257
Lateness, 282–284
    prevention, 283–284
    problem with, 282
    root of matter, 282
    solution, 283
Laziness, 273–274
    job enthusiasm, 274
    motivation and, 274
Leadership, 4–6
    behaviours, 220–221
    clinical, 301
    management and, 4–5
    skills, 5–6, 21
    strong, 13–14
    transformational, 5
Leaflets, 94–95, 294
League of Friends, 116
Learning
    action, 194–196
    experience, 65, 77–78, 84–85
        complaints, 134
    mandatory, 77
    opportunities, 51–52, 101
    sharing, 225
    teaching and, 85
Leave
    adoption, 115
    annual leave, 32
    compassionate, 115
    maternity, 113, 115, 149
    other, 115
    sick, 73–76, 114
    study, 79, 115–116
Lecturers, link, 78
Legal matters
    accountability, 4
    action, 133–134
    advice, 288–289
        solicitors, 288
        trade unions, 288–289
    responsibilities, 9–11
        duty to report and, 11
        expanded roles, 11
        role tensions, 9–10

staff shortages, 10–11
        vicarious liability, 11
    statutory duties, 316–317
Legislation
    Data Protection Act (1998), 57, 66, 131
    Disability Discrimination Act, 152
    National Health Service (NHS) Act
        (1999), 316
Letters
    complaint, 127, 129
    covering, 184
    holding, 132
    news, 35, 180
    response, 128–129
        see also Final response letters
Line managers
    advice, 6
    audits and, 310–311
    cliques and, 261
    confidences, 200
    role, 11–13
        'acting up', 12
        shadowing, 12
        working relationships, 12–13
    talking about, 54
    see also Managers
Link nurses, 77–78, 236, 256, 306–308
    roles, 293
        effectiveness, 307–308
        getting most from, 307
        priorities, 307
Link universities, 116
Listening, 49–51, 135
    skills, 291
    understanding and, 50–51
Lister, S., 297
Lists, 28–29, 30–31
Litigation Authority (NHS), 295
'Living wills', 291
Local health boards (LHBs), 169
'Local resolution' of complaints, 126
Loyalty, 230

Managers, 227–246
    communication and, 238–239
    decisions, autonomous, 231–233
    difficult, 248–249
        angry, 248
        expectations, 249
        incompetent, 249

Managers (*contd*)
   expectations, 228–230
   extra work, 235–237
      without funding, 235–237
   incidents, mistakes and accidents, 241–243
   investigations, 243–245
   knock-on effects, 233–235
   reports to, 239–241
   senior, 175
   working with, 230–231
      clinical interference, 230–231
      decision making, 231
      loyalty, 230
      meetings, 230
      workload, 233
   see also Bed managers; Line managers
'Managing not to Manage' (Sergeant), 13
Managing staff, 21–22, 63–82
   appraisals, 67–69
   discipline, 72–73
   HR advisors, 64–65
   informing and involving, 78–80
   poor performance, 71–72
   self-rostering, 80–81
   sick leave, 73–76
   training and support, 76–78
   unacceptable behaviour, 69–71
   written records, 66–67
Mandatory training, 116, 158
Manipulation, 278–280
   blame, 279–280
   confrontation, 279
   flattery, 279
Manual handling, 77, 158
Maternity leave, 113, 115, 149
Mayer, M., 262
Medical secretaries, 174
Medical supplies, 117
Medline (library database), 298
Meetings, 36–38, 44
   abuse of expertise, 36
   'any other business' (AOB), 37
   attendance, 158
   chairing, 38, 155, 171
   choosing, 173–174
      board, 173
      directorate, 174
      impromptu, 174
      sisters', 173
      staff attendance at, 174

   disseminating information, 36–37, 78–79
   finance advisors, 121–122
   getting best from, 37–38
   guidelines, 70
   HR advisor, 64–65
   investigation, 134–137
      complainant, 134–135
         learning experience, 134
         preparation, 134–135
      key steps
         agreeing action, 136–137
         closing, 137
         empathy, 136
         explanation and apology, 136
         follow up, 137
         listening, 135
      managers', 230
      notes, 39, 67, 135
      waiting for, 37
Mehrabian, A., 210
Mentees, 181–182
Mentors, 179, 257, 260
   advice, 6
   induction, 158
   mentees and, 181–182
   personal needs and, 192–193
      approach, 193–194
      avoiding, 194
   role of, 181
Mergers *see* Moves or mergers
'Micromanaging', 238–239
Minute-taker at meetings, 39
Mistakes, 201–202, 233, 237, 259, 314
   confidence, 201
   dealing with, 202
   perfectionism, 201
Mistakes and accidents, 241–243
Moaning and whinging, 223–224, 250,
         280–281, 313–314, 317
   challenging perceptions, 280
   progress prevention, 281
   self criticism and, 281
Modernisation Agency, 96–97
Motivation, 274
Moves or mergers, 262–264
   experts, 264
   Gantt chart for, 266
   planning ahead, 263
   political awareness, 263
   project plans, 264

Name badges, 211–212
National Assembly for Wales, 169
National Health Service (NHS), 6, 9, 35, 95, 310
  advice, 298–299, 301
  budgets and, 117–118
  in England, 168–169
  Executive Eastern, 316
  NHS Act (1999), 316
  'NHS Plan', 168
  in Northern Ireland, 170
  organisations, 248, 252–253, 257, 288, 314
  political awareness and, 171, 181
  in Scotland, 95, 169
  staff and, 68, 76, 242
  trusts, 168–169, 171, 293, 316
  in Wales, 95, 169
  website, 36
National Leadership and Innovation Agency for Health (NLIAH), 6
National Patient Safety Agency, 242
National service frameworks (NSFs), 168–169
Needs *see* Personal needs
Networks, 172–173, 174–176
  building, 175–176, 200, 291
  informal, 200
  opportunities, 175
  senior managers and directors, 175
  ward managers, 175
Newsletters, 35, 180
Night shifts, 204
NON PAY, 107, 116–118
  budget, 110–111
  medical supplies, 117
  pharmacy/drugs, 117
  stationery, 117
  ward environment, 117–118
Non-clinical managers, 15
Nonexecutive directors, 171
Northern Ireland Office (NIO), 170
Notes
  accurate, 134
  file, 66–67, 253, 255, 277
  meeting, 39, 67, 135
  written, 259
Nuffield Hospitals, 170
Nurses
  agency, 109–110, 121, 149, 159, 236, 309
  bank, 109–110, 121, 149, 159, 309
  enrolled, 161

  overseas, 161–162, 257–258
  part time, 149, 160–161
  returning, 159–160
  specialist, 291–293
  staff, 162–163
  student, 159
  see also Link nurses
Nursing, director of, 178–179, 288–289, 292
Nursing, Midwifery and Allied Health Professions, 298
Nursing and Midwifery Council (NMC), 3–4, 87–88, 159, 192
  advice and, 289–290, 299
  external directives and, 306, 315
  standards, 257
NVQs (National Vocational Qualifications), 88, 91, 119, 163
  coordinators, 301

Objectives, 8–9, 268
  feedback and, 9
  goals, 47, 80, 87
  knowledge sources and, 8–9
  regular review of, 8
  team, 48–49
Occupational health (OH) department, 74–75
'Off-duty', 81, 107–109, 112–115
Office organisation, 28–30
  good environment, 29–30
  handovers, 89
  lists, 28–29
'Open door' policies, 34
Opinions, 176
Optimism, 213–214
'Our National Health' (Scottish NHS plan), 169
Overseas nurses, 161–162, 257–258
Ovid, 298
Oxford Dictionary of Nursing, 298

Paperwork, 42–43
Part time nurses, 149, 160–161
Paternity leave, 115
Patient advice and liaison service (PALS), 14, 293–294
Patient-centred care, 83–103, 117, 308
  assessment and care plans, 86–87
  audit and benchmarking, 96–97
  clinical skills, 84–85
  handovers, 89–91

Patient-centred care (*contd*)
  health care assistants (HCAs), 88–89
  informing patients, 93–96
  performance targets and, 311
  primary nursing, 92–93
  standards and short-staff, 98–99
  task-orientated care, 91–92
  ward rounds, 99–101
Patients
  advocates, 13–14, 99, 294
    strong leadership for, 13–14
    vulnerability and, 13
  allocation of, 56, 92
  confidentiality, 57–58
  information websites, 298
  involvement, 100–101
  relatives and, 18, 256–257, 293–294
    health professionals' visits, 294
    information leaflets, 294
    patient advice and liaison service
      (PALS), 293–294
    ward rounds, 294
PAY and NON PAY, 116–118
Pay, prioritising, 107–110
  flexibility, 109–110
  'off-duty', 107–109
  sharing staff, 109
Peer support, 194–196, 300
  action learning, 194–195
  challenge and, 195–196
Perceptions, 280
Perfectionism, 201, 271
Performance
  assessment framework, 169
  indicators (NHS), 295
  poor, 71–72
    incompetence, 71
      procedure, 71–72
  targets, 311–312
    challenging, 312
    patient care and, 311
Person specifications, 150
Personal development
  plan, 257
  through delegation, 39
Personal needs, 182–183, 187–207
  burnout, 204–205
  confiding in staff, 199–200
  deputies, 196–198
  eating and drinking, 202–204
  mentors, 192–193

  mistakes, 201–202
  peer support, 194–196
  staff stress, 190–192
  stress, 188–190
  union representatives, 198–199
Pharmacy/drugs budget, 117
Piper Alpha disaster, 90
Plans, 46–48
  of action, 141
    investigation, 243–244
  business, 118–119
  communication, 47
  forward, 263
  knowing team, 47–48
  own needs, 182–184
    covering letters, 184
    curriculum vitae (CV), 183
      tailoring, 184
      writing, 183–184
    special interests, 182–183
  priorities and, 28
  project, 264
  recruitment, 79
  team objectives, 47
  see also Succession plans
Policies, procedures and guidelines, 296–297
  accessibility, 296
  changes to, 297
  evidence-based, 297
  reasons for, 296
Political awareness, 167–186, 263
  boards of directors, 171–172
  diplomacy, 176–178
  director of nursing, 178–179
  meetings, 173–174
  mentors and mentees, 181–182
  national issues, 168–170
  networking, 174–176
  own needs, 182–184
  recognition, 180
Posner, B., 5, 220
Practice
  development team, 300–302
  placement, 301
Pre-registration house officers (PRHOs), 17,
  212
Pressure
  of work, 14–16
    emergencies and, 15–16
    non-clinical managers and, 15
  see also Stress

Primary care trusts (PCTs), 168, 225
Primary liability, 11
Primary nursing, 92–93
  best methods, 93
  patient allocation and, 92
  in practice, 93
  team nursing and, 92–93
Priorities
  board of directors', 171–172
  definitions and, 26–28
  difficult staff, 271–273
    burnout, 272
    care standards, 273
    time management, 271–272
  link nurses, 293, 307
  staff shortage, 98–99
  workload, 258
  see also Pay, prioritising
Private health care, 170
Proactive, being, 41–43
  delay and, 42
  help requests, 42
  paperwork, 42–43
  under-promise, over-deliver, 41–42
Procedures and guidelines, 296–297
Professional advice, 289–290
  director of nursing, 289
  Nursing and Midwifery Council (NMC),
    289–290, 299
  university lecturers, 290
  visits, 294
Professional issues, 225
  code of conduct, 3–4, 87–88, 283, 312,
    314–315
  development team, 179
Progress prevention, 281
Projects, 236, 264
Promotion, 161, 248
  delegation and, 40–41
Pronunciation, 214–215
Prouse, M., 90
'Public Concern at Work' (charity), 315
Punctuality, 282–284

Quality Improvement Scotland (NHS), 169
Questions, 153–154

Racial needs, 269–270
Racism see Discrimination
Radcliffe, M., 261

Reading, unnecessary, 34–36
  internet, 36
  journals, 35
  newsletters, 35
Recognition, work, 180
  conferences and study days, 180
  newsletters, 180
  ward comparisons, 180
Records, written, 66–67, 120–121, 259
  communication books, 67
  file notes, 66–67, 253, 255, 277
  meeting notes, 39, 67, 135
Recruitment programme, 79, 147–165
  advertisements and applications, 150–151
  discrimination, 160–162
  induction, 157–158
  interviews, 151–153
    follow up, 155–157
    getting best, 153–155
  new recruits, 260
  other avenues, 158–160
    bank and agency staff, 159
    lead liaison, 160
    returning nurses, 159–160
    student nurses, 159
  reviewing post, 148–150
  succession plan, 162–163
  team involvement, 163–164
Redesigning jobs/roles, 149–150, 163
Refresher training, 159
Registered nurses, 163
Regulation and Improvement Authority, 170
Regulations and guidelines (NHS), 170
Rehabilitation, 272
Relationships, 276–277
Relatives, 18, 256–257
  advice for, 293–294
Religion
  beliefs, 290
  diversity, 291
  needs, 269–270
Report, duty to, 11
Reports
  to managers, 239–241, 245
    stages of, 240–241
Responses
  complaint, 127
  managerial, 311
  negative, 281
  see also Final response letters

Responsibilities
  staff, 55–56
    allocated patients and, 56
  see also Role and responsibilities
Restructuring *see* Moves or mergers
Revans, R., 195
Reviews
  360 degree, 9
  documentary evidence, 244
  of objectives, 8
  vacant posts, 148–150
    job description, 149
      person specification, 150
    reasons for leaving, 148–149
Reward-based systems, 274
Risk management, 295–296
  directorate committee, 295–296
  hospital committee, 295
  performance indicators, 295
Risks
  minimising, 3
  staff stress, 192
  staffing, 157
Robbins, A., 201
Role
  expanding nursing, 261–262
    guidelines, 262
  link nurse, 293, 306–308
Role models, 209–226
  appearance, 210–211
  first impressions, 211–213
  gossip, 223–224
  handwriting, 218–220
  language choice, 222–223
  others' perceptions, 220–222
    feedback, 221–222
    strengths and weaknesses, 220
    work satisfaction, 220–221
  positive attitudes, 213–214
  relaxed control, 216–218
  speaking clearly, 214–216
  stagnation, 224–226
Role and responsibilities, 1–23
  24-hour, 2–4
  impact on others, 17–19
  informed decisions, 6–7
  leadership, 4–6
  legal matters, 9–11
  line managers and, 11–13
  link nurse, 293

nurse specialists, 291–293
objectives, 8–9
patients' advocate and, 13–14
pressure, 14–16
work balance, 16–17
Root cause analysis (RCA), 242–243
  toolkit, 242
Roper, N., 86
'Roper's' model, 86
Rostering *see* 'Off-duty' and Self-rostering
Royal College of Nursing (RCN), 5–6, 13,
    198, 225, 289, 301
  website, 298
Royal Marsden Manual of Clinical
    Procedures, 297

Satisfaction, work, 220–221
Scotland's Health on the Web, 169
Scottish Executive, 169
  Health Department, 169
Select Committee on Health, 160
Self criticism, 250, 281
Self management, 23
Self-disclosure, 217
Self-rostering, 80–81, 159
  advantages, 81
  'off-duties', 81
  in small teams, 80
Sergeant, H., 13
Service developments, 118
Service and Financial Framework (SAFF),
    118
Service level agreements (SLAs), 168
Service users, 178
Shadowing, 12, 179, 226
Shortages, staff, 10–11, 98–99, 258–259,
    273, 292
  coping, 98
  incident forms, 259
  low staffing, 258–259
  priorities and decisions, 98–99
  written notes, 259
Shortlisting, 151–152
Sick leave, 73–76, 113, 114
  long-term, 75, 149
  short-term, 74–75
  unauthorised absence, 76
Sickness/absence, 108–109
  procedure, 276
Sisters, 163, 173

Skills
    clinical, 84–85
    de-skilling staff, 292–293
    interviewing, 164
    leadership, 5–6, 21
    practical, 154
SMART (Specific, Measurable, Achievable,
        Realistic, Timetable), 49
Solicitors, 288, 299
Solutions, 214, 280–281, 283
Special interests, 182–183
Specialists
    nurse, 291–293
        de-skilling staff, 292–293
        education and development, 292
        link nurse roles, 293, 306–308
    see also Consultants/specialists
Speech, clear, 214–216
    pronunciation, 214–215
    telephone manner, 215–216
Speed-reading, 35
Spotlighting others, 212–213
Staff
    abuse of, 254–256
    awareness, 291
    clinical supervision of, 59–60
    complaints, 131–132, 142, 253–254
    computer access and, 298
    confiding in, 199–200
    consultation, 48–49
    development, 299–300
    empowering, 88–89
    informing, 34
    knowing, 52–54
        appraisals, 53–54
        equal time, 53
        strengths and weaknesses, 53
    management, 21–22
    meeting attendance, 174
    new, 164, 212, 260
    nurses, 162–163
    responsibilities, 55–56
    sharing, 109
    shortages, 10–11, 98–99, 258–259, 273,
        292
    stress, 190–192
    support, 290–291
    talking about, 54–55
        being positive, 55
        managers, 54

    see also Difficult staff; Managing staff;
        Teams; Training
Staffing
    establishment, 106–108, 121, 162
    minimum, 108
    see also 'Off-duty'
Stagnation, 224–226
    learning and experiences, 225
    professional issues, 225
    shadowing, 226
    wider organisation, 225
Standards
    of appearance, 210–211
    of care, 273, 308, 310, 311–312
    clinical, 22–23
    falling, 96
    Nursing and Midwifery Council (NMC),
        257
    short-staff and, 98–99
Staphylococcus aureus (MRSA), 8, 121
Star rating assessment, 169
Stationery, 117
Statutory duties, 316–317
Strategic health authorities (SHAs), 168
Strengths and weaknesses, 53, 220, 285
Stress, 19, 188–190
    breaks, 189
    positive and negative, 191
    reducing pressure, 190
    role tensions, 9–10
    staff, 190–192
        dealing with, 191–192
        signs of, 191
Student nurses, 18
Study leave, 79, 108–109, 115–116, 180
    funding sources, 116
    mandatory training, 116
Succession plans, 162–163
    charge nurse level, 163
    health care assistants (HCAs), 163
    staff nurse level, 162–163
    staffing establishment, 162
Suggestions, 94
Supernumerary periods, 157–158
Supervision see Clinical supervision
Support, 251
    staff, 290–291
    to practitioners, 133
    see also Peer support; Training
SWOT analysis, 270, 270–271, 285

Task-orientated care, 91–92
  care delegation, 91
  task allocation, 92
  task delegation, 91–92
Tea Council, 203
Teaching
  and learning, 85
  tools, 87
Teams
  appearance, 269
  budget involvement, 111
  communication, 101
  complaints involvement, 144
  confidences, 199
  enthusiasm, 299
  informing and involving, 78–80
  knowledge of, 47–48, 65
  objectives, 47, 48–49
    action plans, 49
    consultation, 48–49
  preparation for interviews, 153
  professional development, 179
  recruitment involvement, 163–164
    interviewing skills, 164
    new staff in, 164
  self-rostering in, 80
  team nursing, 92–93
  see also Managing staff; Staff
Teasdale, K., 13
Telephone manner, 215–216
Temper control, 177, 216, 248
Tensions, role, 9–10
Textbooks and journals, 85
Time limits, 31
Time management
  emails and, 33
  staff and, 53
    difficult, 271–272
Timetables, 134–135
Trade unions, 299
  representatives, 198–199, 232, 275
    stewards, 198, 288–289, 315–316
      help, 315
      raising issues, 316
Training, 274
  cardiopulmonary resuscitation (CPR), 77,
    158
  clinical supervision, 60
  coordinator, 302
  deputies, 196–198

'acting up', 196
  delegation and, 196, 197–198
  strengths of, 197
  support of, 197
  as threat, 197
development and, 291
in-house, 77
mandatory, 116, 158
manual handling, 77, 158
refresher, 159
and support, 76–78
  experience and, 77–78
  induction, 76
  link lecturers and, 78
  mandatory learning, 77
  ward-based teaching, 76–77
Trust boards, 172–173
Trustees of London Clinic v Michael Alan
    Edgar, 4

Under-promise, over-deliver, 41–42, 132,
    137, 155
Understanding, listening and, 50–51
Uniform policy, 210, 268–270
Unions see Trade unions
Unison, 198, 289
University
  lecturers, 290
  link, 116

Vacant posts, 148–149
Visitor system, 56–58, 212
  first impressions, 57
  patient confidentiality, 57–58
  welcome, 56–57
Voicemail, 34
Vulnerability, patients', 13

Waiting lists, 309
Ward
  -based teaching, 76–77
  comparisons, 180
  environment, 117–118
    fund, 79
  managers, 175
    advice, 7
  rounds, 33, 99–101, 294
    clarifying issues, 100
    decision-making, 101
    as learning opportunity, 101

Ward (*contd*)
 patient involvement, 100
  team communication, 101
 welcome, 56–57
Warnings, 275
Water, 203
Weaknesses, strengths and, 53, 220
Websites, 36, 95, 298
Welcome
 information boards, 94
 ward, 56–57
Welsh Assembly Government, 96, 169
Whistleblowing, 314–315
Whittington, R., 262
'Whole time equivalent' (WTE), 110,
  115–116
Williams, S., 98
'Wills, living', 291
Work
 environment *see* Environment, positive
   working
 extra, 235–237
  beds, 236
  emergencies, 235
  managers and, 237
  nonemergencies, 235

 project work, 236
 relationships, 12–13
 satisfaction, 220–221
Workload, 25–44, 233
 being proactive, 41–43
 defining, 26–28
  planning and prioritising, 28
 delegation, 39–41
 diary control, 30–32
 emails, 32–33
 interruptions, 33–34
 meetings, 36–38
  chairing, 38–39
  terms of reference for, 44
 office organising, 28–30
 priorities, 258
 reading, 34–36
Worldwide web, 36, 95, 297–298
Wright, M., 92
Writing, 218–220
 care plans and evaluations,
  218–219
 emails, 219–220
 handwriting, 218
 reports to managers, 239–241, 245
 see also File notes